English-Portuguese Medical Dictionary and Phrasebook

Portuguese-English

first edition 2013

ISBN is 1490507795
EAN-13 is 978-1490507798

by A.H. Zemback

© All rights reserved

Special thanks to Larissa Venhaus, Isabela Matta,
Sister M. Kateri and Sister Maria
for their assistance with editing.

Contents

Phrasebook and History & Physical template..................4
English-Portuguese medical dictionary..........................21
Portuguese-English translation....................................163
Postscript..305

	English	Portuguese
Introduction	How are you?	Como está?
	Good morning, good afternoon, good evening.	Bom dia, boa tarde, boa noite.
	My name is ...	Me chamo...
	I am a nurse.	Sou enfermeiro (enfermeira).
Demographics	What is your name? Can you write it in English?	Qual é o seu nome? Como se chama? Pode escrevê-lo em Inglês?
	Pleased to meet you.	Prazer em conhecê-lo.
	Do you speak English?	O senhor fala inglês?
	Speak more slowly, please.	Pode falar mais devagar?
	Say that one more time, please.	Pode repetir, por favor?
	Come with me, please.	Queira vir comigo.
	Take a seat over there, please.	Tome uma cadeira se faz favor.
	What province do you live in ?	Em qual província você mora?
	What is your address?	Qual o seu endereço?
	What is your telephone number?	Qual o seu número de telefone?
	Can you give us the name and telephone number or address of someone to be contacted?	Você pode me dar o nome, número de telefone e/ou endereço de uma pessoa para contato de emergência?
	Are you married?	Você é casada (o)?
	What is your age?	Qual é idade tem?
Chief complaint	What is your health concern? (What can we do for you today?)	Qual é o problema que te traz aqui hoje (O que podemos fazer por você hoje?)
	When did you become ill?	Quando ficou doente? Quando adoeceu?
	Have you had an accident?	Teve um acidente?
	Do you feel pain... At night? Before meals? After eating?	Você sente dor? A noite? Antes de comer? Depois de comer?
	When did it start? (show on the calendar and clock)	Quando começou? (pode me mostrar aqui no calendário ou relógio?)
	What is your level of pain? 1 (no pain) 2 3 4 5 6 7 8 9 10 (severe pain)	Qual é o seu nível do dor? 1 (não tem dores) 2 3 4 5 6 7 8 9 10 (dor severo)
	The pain, is it constant or does it come and go?	A dor é constante? Ou vai e vem?
	Sharp or dull?	A dor é aguda ou não?
	Where does it hurt?	Onde doi?
	Use one finger to point exactly where the pain is.	Mostre-me com o dedo o sitio exacto onde lhe doi.
	Is there anything that makes it better or worse?	Há alguma coisa que torne a dor pior ou mais suportável?
	Have you been seriously ill before?	Já teve problemas de saúde sérios antes?
	What were you treated for?	Qual tipo de tratamento?

	English	Portuguese
Common complaints	My lower back hurts.	Tenho dor nas costas(na parte lombar).
	My neck is stiff.	Meu pescoço.
	I have a sore throat.	Tenho dor de garganta.
	It hurts when I swallow.	Sinto dor quando engulo.
	I have an earache.	Tenho dor de ouvido.
	I have a toothache.	Tenho dor de dentes.
	I have shoulder pain.	Tenho dor nos ombros.
	I have elbow pain.	Tenho dor nos cotovelos.
	I have wrist pain.	Tenho dor nos punhos.
	I have knee pain.	Tenho dor no joelho.
	I have ankle pain.	Tenho dor no tornozelo.
	I am dizzy.	Sinto-me aturdido.
	I am very nervous.	Estou muito nervosa (o).
	I can't sleep.	Não consigo dormir.
	I am always tired.	Estou sempre cansada (o).
	I have chest pain.	Tenho dor no peito.
	My heart beats very fast.	Meu coração bate muito rápido!
	I have a headache.	Tenho dor de cabeça.
	I have trouble breathing.	Estou tendo dificuldade de respirar.
	I am coughing a lot.	Tusso muito.
	It hurts when I take a deep breath.	Doe quando eu respiro profundo.
	I am pregnant.	Estou grávida.
	I have a stomach ache.	Tendo dor no estômago.
	I am nauseated.	Estou com náusea.
	I want to vomit.	Sinto-me vou vomitar.
	I have indigestion.	Tenho indigestão.
	I have no appetite.	Não tenho vontade de comer.
	I have diarrhea	Tenho diarréia.
	I have constipation.	Estou constipada.
	I feel sick.	Sinto-me muito doente.
	I sprained my ankle.	Eu torci meu tornozelo.
	I think I broke my arm (leg).	Acho que quebrei meu braço (perna).
Past medical history	Do you have a past history of the following:	Já teve:
	anemia	anemia?
	asthma	asma?
	cancer	câncer?
	cirrhosis	cirrose?
	diabetes	diabetes?
	epilepsy	epilespsia?
	hypertension	pressão alta (hipertensão)?
	thyroid disease	doença tiróide
	heart problems (heart attack)	ataque cardíaco?

	English	Portuguese
	hepatitis	hepatite?
	tuberculosis	tuberculose?
	HIV/AIDS	HIV/AIDS
	What date did you start taking HIV medicine?	Quando começou a tomar os remédios para HIV?
	What was the date of your last CD4?	Qual foi a data da última vez que fez o CD4?
	What was the result of your last CD4?	Qual foi o último resultado do seu CD4?
	Have you had pneumonia or meningitis?	Você já teve pneumonia ou menigiti?
Past surgical history	Have you ever had an operation?	Já fez alguma operação?
	What type of surgery was done?	Que tipo de cirurgia?
	What year was the surgery done?	Qual o ano que fez tal cirurgia?
Medications	Are you taking any medication now?	Está a tomar agora algum medicamento?
	What is the name of the medication?	Qual o nome do medicamento?
	Can you show me the medication bottle?	Você pode me mostrar o rótulo do remédio?
	Do you take illegal drugs?	Você usa drogas?
	Are you taking bactrim?	Esta tomando "bactrim"?
Allergies	Have you had reactions to medications?	Tem alergia a algum medicamento?
	Which medicines?	Qual medicamentos?
Family history	Is your mother living?	Sua mãe ainda esta viva?
	Is your father living?	Seu pai ainda esta vivo?
	Do your brothers/sisters have health problems?	Seus irmãos/irmas tem problema de saúde?
Social history	Do you drink alcohol?	Você toma bebidas alcoólica?
	How many drinks per day?	Quantas bebidas por dia?
	Do you drink alcohol every day?	Você bebe bebidas alcoólicas todos os dias?
	Do you smoke?	Fuma?
	How many cigarettes per day?	Quantos cigarros por dia?
	What is your job?	Qual a sua profissão/trabalho?
Review of systems	Do you have a skin rash?	Você tem alguma urticária o condição dermatologica?
Skin	Do you have any blisters or sores?	Tem alguma bulha ou feridas?
	Have you had lice?	Tem tido piolhos?
	Have you been bitten by ticks?	Tem sido mordido por carraças?
	Have you seen rats, sand flies, mosquitos or bugs in your quarters?	Tem visto ratos, mosquitos, percevejos no seu quarto?
	Were you bitten by a dog or another animal?	Foi mordido por algum cão ou outro animal?

	English	Portuguese
Lymphatic	Do you have lymph node enlargement?	Notou se seus nódulos linfáticos estao grandes?
Bone	Do you have bone pain?	Você sente dor nós ossos?
	Do you have joint pain?	Você tem dor nas juntas?
	Do you have joint swelling?	Você tem enxamento nas juntas?
	Do you have pain in the back or neck?	Você tem dor nas costas ou no pescoço?
Blood	Do you have bleeding problems?	Você tem problemas com sangramento?
Endocrine	Do you urinate frequently?	Você tem que urinar frequentemente?
	Are you frequently thirsty?	Você sente sede frequentemente?
	Have you lost weight?	Perdeu peso?
Head	Have you suffered from a head trauma in the past?	Você já sofreu traumatismo crâniano no passado?
	Do you have dizziness?	Você sente tonta?
	Have you blacked-out?	Você já desmaiou?
Eyes	Can you see well?	Você pode ver bem?
	Do you have double vision?	Você tem dupla visão?
	Do you have vision loss?	Você tem perda de visão?
	Do you have blurred vision?	Sua visão esta turva?
	Do you have pain in bright light?	Você sente dor quando esta exposta a luz?
Ears	Can you hear well?	Você pode ouvir bem?
	Do you have an earache?	Você tem dor de ouvido?
	Do you have drainage from the ears?	Você tem drenagem saído de seus ouvidos?
	Have you had gradual hearing loss in only one ear?	Você teve perda de audição gradual em um ouvido somente?
Nose	Do you have nosebleeds?	Você tem sangramento no nariz?
Mouth	Do you have a toothache?	Dor de dente?
	Do you have a broken tooth?	Dentes quebrados?
	Does hot or cold make it worse?	Quente ou frio faz a dor nós dentes piorar?
	Do you have lumps or swelling in your mouth?	Você tem bolhas ou enxamento na sua boca?
Throat	Do you have hoarseness? (Have you had a change in your voice?)	Você esta perdendo a voz? Ou notou que sua voz mudou?
	Do you have a sore throat?	Você tem dor garganta?
Neck	Do you have neck stiffness?	Seu pescoço esta duro? Consegue movelo?
Breast	Have you noticed breast lumps?	Você já notou algum caroço no seio(s)?
	Do you have nipple discharge?	Tem algum corrimento saído dos seios?
	Do you have swelling around or below your nipples?	Enxasso nos seios?
Respiratory	Are you short of breath?	Tem falta de ar?

7

	English	Portuguese
	Do you sit up at night to breathe?	Você tem que sentar a noite para respirar?
	Do you have pain when you take a deep breath?	Tem dores quando respira fundo?
	Do you have wheezing?	Você tem respirar ruidosamente?
	Do you have a cough?	Tem tosse?
	How long have you had the cough?	A quanto tempo tem essa tosse?
	Do you cough anything up?	Tem expectoração?
	What color is your sputum... white? yellow-green? bloody? brown?	De que cor... branca? amarelo-esverdeada? vermelha? castanha?
Cardiovascular	Do you have chest pain?	Você tem dor no peito?
	Do you have palpitations?	Você tem /sente papitaçoes?
	Do you have leg edema?	Você tem problema com enxasso nas pernas?
	Do you have weakness?	Você tem fraqueza nas pernas?
Gastrointestinal	Do you have abdominal pain? (Do you have pain in your belly?)	Você sente dor no seu abdómen/ barriga?
	...after you eat?	...depois que come?
	When did this problem start?	Quando começou o problema?
	Has it been weeks, months, years?	Faz semanas, meses, anos?
	Are you in pain now?	Sente-se mal agora?
	Touch the spot where you have pain with one finger.	Mostre-me com o dedo o sitio exacto onde lhe doi.
	Does it hurt all the time?	Doi-lhe sempre?
	Does the pain come and go?	A dor é intermitente?
	Is the pain better than yesterday?	A dor esta melhor hoje do que ontem?
	Do you have ...fever?	Está febre?
	...chills?	Está calafrio?
	Do you sweat much?	Transpira muito?
	How is your appetite?	Como esta o seu apetite?
	Have you vomited?	Vomitou?
	What did the vomit look like?	Descreva o vómito?
	Have you vomited blood?	Vomitou sangue?
	Do you have nausea?	Tem náusea?
	Do you have regular bowel movements?	Vai à retrete regularmente?
	Are you constipated?	Tem prisão de ventre?
	Do you have diarrhea?	Tem diarréia?
	How many times today?	Quantas vezes ao dia?
	What do the stools look like?	Descreva as fezes?
	Have you passed black stools?	As suas fezes são escuras?
	Do you pass blood in your stools?	Há sangue nas suas fezes?

	English	Portuguese
	Have you recently traveled outside the country?	Você recentemente viajou para fora do país?
	What color was the stool?	Que cor eram as fezes?
	Do you have anal itching?	Você tem coceira no ânus?
	Do you have pain with swallowing?	Tem dores quando se engole?
	Do you have difficulty swallowing?	Tem dificuldade em engolir?
	Do you often suffer from a bloated feeling?	Você frequentemente se sente cheia?
	Do fatty foods agree with you?	Comidas com muita gordura te afetam?
	Have you had a gastroscopy in the past? (A camera that passes through your mouth to see your stomach)	Você já teve um procedimento pelo qual uma câmera e inserida pela sua boca para acessar seu estômago?
Genitourinary	Do you have burning on urination?	Você sente queimação quando urina?
	Have you had penile discharge?	Você tem corrimento no pênis?
	Do you have a sore (chancre) on the penis?	Você tem alguma bolha ou urticária no pênis?
	Is your urine cloudy?	A urina esta escura ou não-clara?
	Do you have sharp pains in your back or groin?	Você tem dor aguda na suas costas ou pélvica?
	Do you have an aching pain under your scrotum?	Sente dor atrás do escroto?
	Do you have difficulty starting to urinate?	Você tem dificuldade para urinar?
	How often do you void at night?	Quantas vezes urina durante a noite?
	Do you have the urge to void after just urinating and are you urinating only small amounts?	Você sente que tem que urinar mesmo tendo acabado de urinar?
	Is the urine stream slow?	A urina sai de forma lenta?
	Do you leak urine when you cough or sneeze?	Você urina quando tosse ou espirra?
	Do you have blood in the urine?	Você percebeu sangue na urina?
	Have you ever passed a kidney stone?	Você já passou alguma pedra de rim?
Women's health	Are you pregnant?	Você esta grávida?
	How many months pregnant are you?	Quantos meses de gravidez?
	Could you possibly be pregnant?	É possível que esteja grávida?
	Can we do a pregnancy test?	Podemos realizar um teste de gravidez?
	Are your periods regular?	Seus ciclos de menstruação são regulares?
	Are your periods painful?	Você sente muita dor quando menstrua?

	English	Portuguese
	Is the flow heavy or light?	Quando menstrua, o sangramento e muito ou pouco?
	When did your last period start?	Quando começou o seu último período menstrual?
	How many days do your periods last?	Quanto tempo dura sua menstruação geralmente?
	Do you bleed between periods?	Você tem sangramento entre ciclos de menstruação?
	Do you take birth control pills?	Você toma pílula para evitar gravidez?
	Do you have pain during intercourse?	Você sente dor quando faz sexo?
	Do you have vaginal itching?	Sua vagina coça?
	Do you vaginal pain?	Você sente dor na vagina?
	Do you have unusual discharge from the vagina?	Você tem corrimento na vagina?
	...a lot or a little?	...muito ou pouco?
	How many times have you been pregnant?	Que número de gravidez e essa pra você?
	How many children do you have?	Quanto filhos você tem?
	Were your deliveries normal?	Quantos partos normais/vaginais?
	Have you had any miscarriages?	Já teve perda de gravidez?
	Did you have problems in your previous pregnancies?	Você teve problemas com sua (s) gravidez anteriores?
	Did you have any severe bleeding after any of your deliveries?	Você já sofreu de hemorragia pós-parto?
	Do you know your blood type?	Você sabe qual o tipo do seu sangue?
	During your pregnancy did have you had any of the following: bleeding or swelling of the ankles?	Durante sua gravidez você teve: sangramento ou enxasso dos tornozelos/pés?
	If you are in labor, please answer the following questions:	Se esta em trabalho de parto, por favor me responda as seguintes perguntas:
	When did your contractions start?	Quando suas contraçoes começaram?
	Are they (contractions) regular or irregular?	As contraçoes são regulares ou irregulares?
	How many minutes between contractions?	Quantos minutos entra cada contração?
	Did your water break?	Sua bolsa de água rompeu?
Peripartum/ neonatal	How old is the baby?	Qual a idade do bebé?
	What was the baby's birth weight?	Qual o peso de nascimento do bebé?
	How are you feeding the baby, with breast or bottle?	Esta planejando amamentar o bebé ou dar mamadeira?
	Is the baby nursing well?	O bebé esta amamentando bem?

	English	Portuguese
	Has the baby had any convulsions?	O bebé teve convulsão?
	Apgar at 1 minute.	Nota apgar de 1 minutos?
	Apgar at 5 minutes.	Nota apgar de 5 minutos?
	Moro reflex.	Reflexo moro.
	Fontanelle.	Moleira.
Amniotic fluid	What color was the amniotic fluid? Clear, cloudy, green (meconium)?	Que cor era o fluido amniótico? Era claro, verde?
Pediatrics	How old is the child?	Qual a idade da sua criança?
	Does the child cry often?	A criança chora frequentemente?
	Is the child gaining weight?	A criança esta ganhando peso?
	Does the child have a good appetite?	Como esta o apetite da criança?
	What kinds of pain does the child complain of?	Que tipo de dor a criança esta reclamando?
	Is he (she) drinking ok?	Ele esta bebendo bem?
	Is he (she) eating ok?	Ele esta comendo bem?
	Have you seen worms in the vomit or the stool?	Você via algum verme no vómito ou nas fezes?
Neurologic	Do you have: facial weakness?	Você sente: fraqueza facial?
	facial numbness?	entorpecimento facial?
	leg weakness?	fraqueza perna?
	leg numbness?	entorpecimento perna?
	arm weakness?	fraqueza braço?
	arm numbness?	entorpecimento braço?
	Were you unconscious?	Perdeu os sentidos?
	Have you had any convulsions?	Teve convulsões?
	Do you have tremors? (Do your hands shake or other parts of your body?)	Você tem tremores? (Nas mãos ou outra parte do corpo?)
	Have you had recent vision loss in one eye?	Você teve perda de visão em um olho recentemente?
	Have you had problems with your balance?	Tem problemas com balanço?
	Do you walk without problems?	Você anda sem problemas?
	Do you have pain in your back that travels to your buttock and down the back of your leg?	Você tem dor nas suas costas que vai da bunda até a sua perna?
Psychiatric	Do you have anxiety?	Você tem problemas com ansiedade?
	Do you have depression?	Você tem depressão?
	Do you feel nervous or tense?	Você se sente nervoso ou tenso?
	How are your spirits?	Como vai o moral?
	Do you hear voices?	Você escuta vozes?
	Do you sleep well?	Dorme bem?
Extremities	Is the ankle pain so severe you cannot walk on it?	A dor no tornozelo e tanta que você não consegue andar?

	English	Portuguese
	Do your have a grinding pain in your knee? Do you have the knee lock up occasionally?	Você sente uma dor nos joelhos (como artrose)? Ou os seus joelhos trancam de vez em quando?
	Do you have pain in your calf when walking that is better with rest?	Sente dor na panturrilha quando anda que melhora quando esta sentado ou deitado (descansando)?
	Do you feel pain when you move your shoulder?	Sente dor quando move os ombros?
	Do you have pain or numbness in your hand, wrist or fingers, especially when flexing your wrist?	Você sente dor ou dormência nas suas mãos, punhos ou dedos? Especialmente quando flexiona os punhos?
	Do you have pain when gripping a doorknob and does the pain go from the outside of the elbow to your wrist?	Sente dor quando segura a maçaneta da porta? Ou a dor vai da parte de fora do cotovelo até seu punho?
Physical exam General	appearance, height	aparecimento, altura
	pulse bp resp temp weight (in pounds/ kilograms)	pulso pressão sangüínea freqüência respiratória temperatura peso (libra/ quilograma)
	skin	pele
HEENT	visual acuity	acuidade visual
	conjunctivae, sclerae	conjuntiva, esclera
	pupils	pupila
	optic disc	disco óptico
	ear canal, tympanic membrane	ducto auditivo, membrana timpânica
	nasal mucosa	mucosa olfatória
	sinuses	seio
	teeth	dentes
	mouth, gums, teeth, uvula "Open your mouth, please."	boca, goma, dentes, úvula "Abra a boca."
	"Stick out your tongue, please."	"Mostre-me a língua, por favor."
	"Say ahh."	Abra a boca e diga "ahhhhh".
Pulmonary	auscultation "Breathe deeply with your mouth open."	auscultação "Inspire e expire profundamente, com a boca aberta."
	percussion	percussão
Back	"Lie down on your back, please."	"Volte-se, se faz favor de costas. "
	"Lie on your left side."	"Volte-se, se faz favor sobre o lado esquerdo. "
	"Lie on your right side."	"Volte-se, se faz favor sobre o lado direito. "
	tenderness "Does it hurt here?"	sensibilidade "Doe aqui?"
	cva tenderness	sensibilidade ângulo costovertebral

	English	Portuguese
Cardiovascular	heart rate, rhythm "Breathe normally."	freqüência cardíaca "Respira normalmente."
	heart murmur?	sopro cardíaco?
	carotid "Hold your breath."	carotídeo "Pare de respirar um momento."
	jugular venous pressure	pressão venosa jugular
Breasts	nipple discharge?	descarga mamilo?
	tenderness "Does it hurt here?"	sensibilidade "Doe aqui?"
	breast exam	exame peito
Vascular	carotid, radial, aortic pulsation	pulsação carotídeo, radial, aórtico
	femoral, dorsalis pedis, posterior tibial	femoral, dorsal do pé, tibial posterior
	leg edema	edema perna
Abdomen	"Lie down, please."	"Deite-se, por favor?"
	"Show me where it hurts, please."	"Me mostre onde doe, por favor?"
	"Does it hurt here?"	"Doe aqui?"
	umbilicus	umbigo
	hernia, inguinal	hérnia inguinal
	palpation	palpação
	auscultation	auscultação
	fluid wave, superficial abdominal veins?	onda líquida, veia abdominal superficial
Maternal/gyn	uterine height (cm)	altura uterino
	Fetal heart sounds	tons cardíacos fetal
	urinalysis	urinálise
	presentation	apresentação
	head presentation	apresentação cefálica
	breech presentation	apresentação de nádegas
	transverse presentation	apresentação transversa
	speculum exam	exame espéculo
	vaginal exam	exame vaginal
	gestational age	idade gestacional
	amniotic fluid	fluido amniótico
Genitourinary; male	circumcision?	circuncisão
	genital herpes?	herpes genital?
	testicular exam	exame testicular
Rectal exam	hemorrhoids, nodules, prostate?	hemorróidas, nódulo, próstata
	"I want to check your rectum (for hemorrhoids), bend over please."	"Preciso de checar seu ânus para ver suas hemorróidas, por favor?"
	guaiac; positive or negative	guáiaco, positivo ou negativo
Neurologic	N1 olfactory: coffee, peppermint? "Close your eyes and tell me what you smell."	N1 nervo ofatório: café, hortelã? "Feche os olhos e me diz que cheiro você respira."

	English	Portuguese
Cranial nerves	N2 optic: snellen, confrontation "Follow my finger with your eyes, without moving your head."	N2 nervo óptico: teste de Snellen, confrantação. "Siga meu dedo com seus olhos sem mover a cabeça."
	N3,4, 6, oculomotor, trochlear, abducens: EOM's "Follow my finger"	N3,4,6 nervo oculomotor, troclear, abducente: movimentos oculares cardinais: "Siga meu dedo."
	N5 trigeminal	N5 nervo trigêmeo
	"Clench your jaw."	"Feche sua mandíbula."
	"Move your jaw back and forth."	"Mova sua mandíbula pra frente e pra trás."
	forehead (ophthalmic), cheek(maxillary), chin (mandibular) "Do you feel this?"	fronte (oftámico), bochecha (maxilar), mento (mandibular) "Sente quando eu toco aqui?"
	N7 facial: "Raise your eye brows." ("Do like this.")	N7 nervo facial: "Levante suas sobrancelhas."
	"Close your eyes tightly, smile big."	"Feche seus olhos bem fechados e sorria bem grande."
	N8 acoustic: whisper, Rinne "Can you hear me talking? Try to repeat what I say."	N8 nervo acústico: cochicho, teste de Rinne "Ouve-me. Procure repetir o que eu digo."
	"Can you hear this?"	"Você escuta isso?"
	"Tell me when you can't feel vibration"	"Diga-me quando não sente mais a vibração."
	N9 glossopharyngeal: swallow, (hoarseness), "Swallow now."	N9 nervo glossofaríngo: engolir, (rouquidão) "Engole agora."
	N10 vagus: swallow, soft palate, gag reflex	N10 nervo vago: engolir, palato mole, reflexo de ânisia
	"Stick out your tongue, please."	"Coloque sua língua para fora, por favor."
	N11 spinal accessory nerve: "Turn your head to the right, now to the left. Shrug your shoulders."	N11 nervo espinhal acessório "Vire sua cabeça para a direita, agora para a esquerda. Levante e abaixe seus ombros."
	N12 hypoglossal: tongue midline	N12 nervo hipoglosso: língua inha do meio
Glasgow coma score	opens eyes to: spontaneous (4),to speech (3), to pain (2), none (1)	Abertura ocular: olhos se abrem espontaneamente (4), olhos se abrem ao comando verbal (3), olhos se abrem por estímulo doloroso (2), olhos não se abrem (1)
	best motor "Hold up 2 fingers." obeys commands (6), localizes (5), withdraws (4), abnormal flexion (3), abnormal extension (2), none (1)	Melhor resposta motora: "Me mostre dois dedos." obedece ordens verbais (6), localiza estímulo dolorso (5), retirada inespecífica à dor (4), padrão flexor à dor (decorticação) (3), padrão extensor à dor (2), sem resposta motora (1)

	English	Portuguese
	best verbal: clear (5), confused (4), inappropriate (3), garbled (2), none (1)	Melhor resposta verbal: orientado (5), confuso (4), palavras inapropriadas (3), sons ininteligíveis (2), ausente (1)
Motor	Motor function	função motora
	biceps brachii, elbow flexion	bíceps do braço; flexiona o antebraço
	"Pull your arm up."	"levante seu braço."
	wrist extensors	extensão do punho
	"Bend your wrist up."	"Dobre seu punho."
	triceps brachii, elbow extension	tríceps do braço, estende o braço
	"Straighten your arm out."	"Estique seu braço."
	finger flexors; distal phalanx middle finger	flexão de falange distal do dedo médio
	"Bend the tip of this finger."	"Dobre a ponta deste dedo, por favor."
	finger abduction, little finger	abdução do quinto dedo
	"Hold the small finger tightly" (don't let me squeeze your fingers together.)	"Com seus dedos separados; não deixe que aperte seus dedos juntos."
	iliopsoas, hip flexors	iliopsoas, flexão quadril
	"Move your knee to your chest."	"Traga seu joelho ao seu peito."
	quadriceps, knee extensors	quadríceps, extensor do joelho
	"Straighten your leg out."	"Estique suas pernas."
	tibialis anterior, ankle dorsiflexors	tibial anterior, dorsoflexão do tornozelo
	"Pull your foot up." (point your foot up)	"Aponte seu pé para cima."
	extensor hallucis longus, long toe extension	extensor longo do hálux, extensão do primeiro dedo do pé
	"Raise your toe up."	"Levante seu dedo do pé."
	gastrocnemius, ankle plantar flexors	gastrocnêmio, flexão plantar do tornozelo
	"Push your foot down."	"Empurre o seu pé para baixo."
Sensory	Sensation "Say 'yes' if you can feel this"	"Diga "sim" se você pode sentir isto."
	"Can you tell if it is sharp or dull?"	"Sente se isto é rombo ou pontiagudo?"
	C-4 (top of acromioclavicular joint)	C-4 (sobre articulação acromioclavicular)
	C-5 (lateral side of antecubital fossa)	C-5 (aspecto lateral do fossa cubital)
	C-6 (thumb)	C-6 (polegar)
	C-7 (middle finger)	C-7 (dedo médio)
	C-8 (little finger)	C-8 (quinto dedo)
	T-4 (nipple line)	T-4 (linha do mamilo)
	T-10 (umbilicus)	T-10 (umbilicus)
	L-2 (mid-anterior thigh)	L-2 (coxa mid-anterior)

	English	Portuguese
	L-3 (medial femoral condyle)	L-3 (côndilo medial do fêmur)
	L-4 (medial malleolus)	L-4 (maléolo medial)
	L-5 (dorsum of the foot, at third MTP joint)	L-5 (pé dorsal, terceiro articulação metatarsofalangiana)
	S-1 (Lateral heel)	S-1 (calcanhar, aspecto lateral)
	S-2 (popliteal fossa of the knee, in the midline)	S-2 (fossa poplítea, linha do meio)
	S-3 (ischial tuberosity)	S-3 (tuberosidade isquiática)
	S4-5 (perianal area)	S4-5 (área perianal)
reflex	Reflexes	Reflexos
	triceps right and left	tríceps, direito e esquerdo
	biceps, right and left	bicipital, direito e esquerdo
	brachioradial, right and left	braquiorradial, direito e esquerdo
	patella, right and left	patelar, direito e esquerdo
	ankle, right and left	tornozelo, direito e esquerdo
	Babinski, right and left (great toe extension= positive)	Babinski, direito e esquerdo
Screening	Tandem walk	ambulação uma atrás outro
	"Walk like this, one foot in front of other." (Or, say walk like this and demonstrate.)	"Ande assim: colocando um pé na frente do outro."
	heel walk, toe walk	ande calcanhar, ande dedos
	"Walk on your heels."	"Ande no seu calcanhar."
	"Walk on your toes."	"Ande na ponta dos seus dedos."
	Romberg "Stand up, hold your arms out, close your eyes."	sinal de Romberg "Levante-se, coloque seus braços esticados na sua frente e feche seus olhos."
Coordination	rapid alternating movement (2nd finger, thumb) "Do this, fast".	"Faca isso bem rápido."
	heel-shin "Move your right heel from your left knee to the ankle with your eyes shut."	calcanhar-canela: "Mova seu calcanhar direito do seu joelho esquerdo para o calcanhar com seus olhos fechados."
	finger nose finger "Touch my finger with your finger then touch your nose."	"Toque no meu dedo com o seu dedo e depois toque na ponta do seu nariz."
Discriminative	stereognosis (key, pencil, cup) "Close your eyes; what is this in your hand?"	estereognose (chave, lápis, xícara) "Feche os seus olhos e me diz o que esta nas suas mãos."
	graphesthesia (draw #3 in hand) "Close your eyes, what is the number written in your hand?"	grafestesia: "Feche os olhos, diga-me o número que esta sendo escrito em suas mãos."
	point localization: "Close your eyes, tell me what part of your body is being touched."	localização ponto: "Feche os olhos, diga-me qual a parte do seu corpo esta sendo tocada."
	two point discrimination "Do you feel one or two points of contact?"	Você sente um ou dois pontos de contato?"
Memory	SLUMS Examination	O teste SLUMS

	English	Portuguese
	Saint Louis University Mental Status Examination	Saint Louis University Mental Status Examination
SLUMS	What day of the week is it? (1)	Que dia da semana é hoje? (1)
SLUMS	What is the year? (1)	Em que ano estamos? (1)
SLUMS	What state are we in? (1)	Em que distrito estamos situados? (1)
SLUMS	Please remember these five objects. I will ask you what they are later. Apple Pen Tie House Car	Lembre-se por favor das 5 palavras seguintes. Mais tarde vou pedir-lhe para as recordar. Maçã Lápis Saia Casa Táxi
SLUMS	You have $100 and you go to the store and buy a dozen apples for $3 and a tricycle for $20. How much did you spend? (1) How much do you have left? (2)	Se for a um supermercado com 100€ para aí comprar um dúzia de maçãs por 3€ e um ferro de engomar por 20 €, pergunto: (1) Quanto gastou?, (2) Quanto lhe sobrou?
SLUMS	Please name as many animals as you can in one minute. (0) 0-4 animals, (1) 5-9 animals, (2) 10-14 animals, (3) 15+ animals	Diga por favor o maior número de animais que souber durante um minuto. (0) 0 a 4 animais, (1) 5 a 9 animais, (2) 10 a 14 animais, (3) 15 ou + animais
SLUMS	What were the five objects I asked you to remember? Apple Pen Tie House Car. One point for each correct answer.	Quais são as 5 palavras que eu lhe pedi há pouco para recordar? (1 ponto por cada recordação correcta)
SLUMS	I am going to give you a series of numbers and I would like you to give them to me backwards. For example, if I say 42, you say 24. (0) 87, (1) 649, (2) 8537	Vou dizer uma série de números e depois gostaria que os repetisse do fim para o princípio. Por exemplo se eu disser 4-2, gostaria que dissesse 2-4. Compreendeu? (0)87; (1) 6 4 9; (1) 8 5 3 7
SLUMS	This is a clock face. Please put in the hour markers and the time at ten minutes to eleven o'clock. (2) Hour markers correct? (2) Time correct?	Este círculo é um mostrador de relógio. Escrava as marcas da hora e indique o tempo seguinte: 11 horas menos 10 minutos. (2) Marcas da hora correctas, (2) Tempo correcto
SLUMS	Place an X in the triangle. □△◊, (1) Which of the figures is the largest? (1)	Coloque um X no triângulo (1). Qual destas figuras é major? (1)

	English	Portuguese
SLUMS	I am going to read you a story. Please listen carefully because afterwards, I'm going to ask you some questions about it. Jill was a very successful stockbroker. She made a lot of money on the stock market. She then met Jack, a devastatingly handsome man. She married him and had three children. They lived in Chicago. She then stopped work and stayed at home to bring up her children. When they were teenagers, she went back to work. She and Jack lived happily ever after.	Eu vou contar-lhe uma história. Preste muita atenção, porque no fim eu vou fazer-lhe algumas perguntas sobre a história que ouviu. A Elsa era uma economista de grande sucesso. Ela ganhou imenso dinheiro negociando na Bolsa. A certa altura conheceu o Daniel, um homem muito elegante. Casou-se com ele e teve 3 filhos. Eles viveram na cidade de Vila Nova de Gaia. Ela deixou de trabalhar e ficou em casa voltou a trabalhar. Ela e o Daniel viveram felizes para sempre.
SLUMS	What was the female's name? (2)	(2) Qual era o nome da mulher?
SLUMS	What work did she do? (2)	(2) Que profissão tinha?
SLUMS	When did she go back to work? (2)	(2) Quando regressou ao trabalho?
SLUMS	What state did she live in? (2)	(2) A que distrito pertencia?
SLUMS	Add total score, with high school education: 27-30 normal, 21-26 mild cognitive disorder, 1-20 dementia. Without high school education: 25-30 normal, 20-24 mild cognitive disorder, 1-19 dementia.	
Counseling	Do you understand?	Você me entende?
Laboratory/ imaging	I need to send you for an x ray.	Preciso de o encaminhar para a radiografia.
	I need to take a sample of your blood.	Preciso de lhe tirar sangue para análise.
	I need a sputum sample.	Eu preciso de uma amostra de saliva.
	Please pass water in this container.	Por favor, urine para este recipiente.
	We need to do an EKG (electrocardiogram).	Tenho que fazer um eletrocardiograma.
Pulmonary	I have the result of your sputum.	Tenho os resultados do teste de saliva.
	You have...	Você tem...
	tuberculosis	tuberculose
	pneumonia	pneumonia
	Your lungs are...	Seus pulmões são/estao...
	one is affected, the other is healthy.	um esta afetado, o outra esta normal/saudável.
	You must stop smoking.	Você precisa de parar de fumar.
	You are suffering from...	Você esta sofrendo de...
	Your illness can be healed.	Sua doença e curável.

	English	Portuguese
Gastroenterology	There is an ulcer in your stomach.	Tem uma úlcera no seu estômago.
	You need to quit drinking beer completely.	Você tem que para de beber cerveja completamente. (Tem que para de beber bebidas alcoólicas.)
Surgery	You need to have an operation today.	Você precisa de uma cirurgia hoje.
	We need to sew up (suture) this wound.	Tenho que dar pontos nessa ferida.
	When did you last eat and drink?	Qual foi a última vez que comeu ou bebeu algo?
	You need to stay in the hospital.	Precisa de ficar no hospital.
Pharmacy	I will give you a prescription.	Vou te passar um remédio.
	You can get the medication at any pharmacy.	Pode levar o pedido a qualquer farmácia.
	You take this medicine two (one, three, four) times per day.	Tome esse remédio (uma, duas, três, quatro) vezes ao dia.
	Do not stop this medication!	Não para de tomar esse remédio!
	Take this medication only if you want to.	Tome esse medicamento somente se quiser.
	Take this medication before meals.	Tome esse medicamento antes das refeições.
	Take this medication at bedtime.	Tome esse medicamento na hora de dormir.
	Take this medication after meals.	Tome esse medicamento depois das refeições.
Maternity/Ob	Congratulations! You are pregnant.	Felicidade! Você esta grávida!
	The delivery date will probably be...	A data prevista para o nascimento provavelmente sera...
	The nurse is on her way.	A enfermeira esta a caminho.
	She will help with the delivery.	Ela vai ajudar com seu parto.
Procedures	I need to pass this tube.	Preciso de fazer passar este tubo.
	I need to treat you with medication in an IV.	Tenho que tratar com medicamento no soro intravenoso.
	I need to give you an injection.	Preciso de lhe dar uma injecção. Agora vou dar-lhe uma injecção.
Orthopedics	You have a broken leg.	Fracturou uma perna.
	You have a broken arm.	Fracturou um braço.
	You have tendinitis.	Você tem tenditini.
	You have fluid in your joint.	Você tem fluido na sua junta.
	We have to put a cast on your arm/leg.	Precisa de levar gesso no(a) perna/braço.
General	What you have is not serious.	O que você tem não e sério.
	Your condition is grave.	Sua condição e grave.
	Please come back if you have more problems.	Volte se tiver mais problemas.

English	Portuguese
Please return within a couple weeks.	Por favor, retorne aqui em duas semanas.

English	Portuguese
abasia *Inability to walk due to impaired coordination.*	abasia
abdomen *The portion of the body bordered by the diaphragm and the pelvis.*	abdómen (P), abdômen (B)
abdomen, lower	barriga
abdominal girth *Waist circumference.*	medida de cintura
abdominal reflexes *Elicited by stroking the abdomen lightly from mid-axillary line to umbilicus. A normal response is contraction of the umbilicus toward the stimulated side.*	reflexos abdominais
abdominocentesis *Puncturing of the abdominal wall for drainage purposes.*	abdominocentese
abducens nerve *A motor nerve (6th cranial nerve) that controls the lateral rectus muscle of the eye.)*	nervo motor ocular externo (P) nervo abducente (B)
abducent *Abducting or to separate.*	abducente
abductor pollicis brevis *Abducts the thumb.*	músculo abdutor curto do polegar
abductor pollicis longus *Abducts and flexes the thumb.*	músculo abdutor longo do polegar
aberrant *Different than normal.*	aberrante
ablation *Surgical removal or amputation.*	ablação
abnormal	anómalo (P) anormal (B)
ABO system *The system using human blood antigens to determine blood type.*	sistema do grupo sanguíneo ABO
abortion *Premature expulsion of the fetus from the uterus.*	aborto
above	acima de
abrupt *Suddenly or hastily.*	abrupto
abruptio placentae *The premature detachment of a normally implanted placenta resulting in maternal decompensation.*	descolamento prematuro da placenta
abscess *A localized collection of pus.*	abcesso (P), abscesso (B)
absence of	ausência de
absolute	absoluto
absorption (intestinal absorption)	absorção (absorção intestinal)
abuse (sexual abuse)	abuso
acalculia *The inability to perform mathematical calculations.*	acalculia
acanthoma *An adult cornifying squamous carcinoma.*	acantoma
acanthosis *Hypertrophy of the prickle cell layer of the skin.*	acantose
acanthosis nigricans *A skin disorder characterized by dark, thick, velvety skin in the body folds and creases.*	acantose nigricans
acapnia *A condition of lower than normal carbon dioxide level in the blood.*	acapnia
acariasis *Mite infestation.*	infestações por ácaros
acaricide *A treatment for mite infestation.*	acaricida
acarus *A mite.*	ácarus
acatalasia *A condition characterized by the congenital absence of the enzyme catalase.*	acatalasia
acathisia *The inability to sit quietly or to have motor restlessness.*	akathisia
accelerate *(To accelerate the healing process).*	acelerar
access *Means of entry.*	acesso
accessory *Complimentary or concomitant.*	acessório
accessory nerve (XI) *Supplies motor innervation to the sternocleidomastoid and trapezius.*	nervo acessório, nervo espinhal

English	Portuguese
accident	acidente
acclimatization *The process of becoming adapted to a new environment.*	aclimatação
accommodation *A term used to describe the ability of the eye to adjust to various distances.*	acomodção
accomplish, to *Achieve.*	alcançar
according to	conforme
accretion *The expected growth of tissue from the intake of nutrients.*	acreção
acephalous *A absence of a head.*	acéfalo
acetabular *Referring to the acetabulum.*	acetábulo, relativo ao
acetabulum *The cup-shaped cavity with which the head of the femur articulates.*	acetábulo
acetaminophen *Mild analgesic drug used for pain relief.*	acetaminofen
acetonemia *The presence of acetone in the blood.*	acetonemia
acetonuria *The presence of acetone in the urine.*	acetonúria
acetylcholine *A reversible acetic acid ester of choline.*	acetilcolina
acetylsalicylic acid *The chemical name for common aspirin.*	ácido acetilsalicílico
achalasia *Inability to relax the smooth muscle fibers of the gastrointestinal tract. In the case of esophageal achalasia one has dilatation and hypertrophy of the esophagus.*	acalasia
achieve, to *To complete something one was striving for.*	realizar
Achilles tendon reflex *The normal response to tapping the achilles tendon with a reflex hammer is the plantar flexion of the foot.*	reflexo do tendão de Aquiles; reflexo aquiliano
achilliodynia *Pain around the calcaneal tendon.*	aquiliodinia
achillobursitis *Inflammation around the calcaneal tendon.*	aquilobursite
achlorhydria *The absence of hydrochloric acid in gastric secretions.*	acloridria
acholia *The lack of bile.*	acolia
achondroplasia *A congenital inadequacy of enchondral bone formation resulting in a type of dwarfism.*	acondroplasia
achromatic spindle *The threads between the poles of the spindle in karyokinesis.*	fuso acromático
achromatopsia *Inability to differentiate yellow, blue, red or their intermediates.*	acromatopsia
achylia *The absence of chyle.*	aquilia
acid phosphatase *A phosphate derived chemical that is optimally active in an acidic environment.*	fosfatase ácida
acid *Substance with a pH less than 7.*	ácido
acid-base balance *The equilibrium of the electrolytes in the body.*	balanço ácido-básico
acidemia *A lower than normal pH in the blood.*	acidemia
acidity *Referring to an acid state.*	acidez
acinous gland *The exocrine part of the pancreas.*	glândula acinosa
acinus *A very small grape shaped portion of an acinous gland.*	ácino
acne *Inflamed or infected sebaceous glands.*	acne
acne rosacea *A chronic disease characterized by the presence of flushing of the skin of the nose, forehead and cheeks.*	rosácea
acne vulgaris *Chronic acne occurring on the face, chest and back of youth.*	acne vulgar
acorea *The absence of the pupil of the eye.*	acoria
acoustic crest *A prominence on ampulla of the semicircular ducts.*	crista acústica

English	Portuguese
acoustic neuroma *A nonmalignant tumor that can cause deafness, tinnitus and vertigo.*	neuroma acústico
acoustic *Referring to the auditory system.*	acústico
Acquired Immunodeficiency Syndrome (AIDS) *Presence of an AIDS defining illness or having a CD4 of less than 200/mm3.*	síndrome da imunodeficiência adquirida (SIDA)
acrocephaly *A condition characterized by a pointed head.*	acrocefalia
acrocyanosis, Raynaud's disease *A benign condition in which the feet and hands are cyanotic, cold and sweating.*	acrocianose
acrodermatitis *Inflammation of the skin of the hands and/or feet.*	acrodermatite
acrodynia *An infantile condition exhibited by swollen bluish-red extremities and later polyarthritis..*	acrodinia
acromegaly *Hyperplasia of the nose, jaw, fingers and toes.*	acromegalia
acromioclavicular joint *Referring to the junction of the acromion and clavicle.*	articulação acromioclavicular
acromion *The flattened process extending laterally from the spine of the scapula which forms the most prominent point of the shoulder.*	acrômio
acrophobia *The morbid fear of heights.*	acrofobia
acrotic *Referring to great weakness or absence of a pulse.*	acrótico
actin *A protein in the muscle that, along with myosin, facilitates muscle contraction and relaxation.*	actina
actinic dermatosis *A skin disease caused by exposure to radiation from the sun, ultraviolet waves or gamma radiation.*	dermatose actinico
actinomycosis *A chronic bacterial infection that effects the face and neck and is caused by Actinomyces israelii. In rare cases it can cause a pulmonary infection.*	actinomicose
actinon *A radioactive element, radon-219; short lived isotope of radon.*	radônio-219
action potential *The alteration in electrical potential associated with the movement along a nerve cell.*	potential de ação
activity	atividade
actomyosin *Myosin and actin complex present in muscles.*	actomiosina
acuity *1. Relating to accuracy of hearing, as in hearing acuity. 2. Severity of illness as in, "What is the patient's acuity?"*	acuidade
acupuncture *Traditionally an aspect of Chinese medicine involving insertion of needles into the skin.*	acupunctura
acute *Abrupt onset.*	agudo
adactylia *A congenital condition exhibited by the absence of toes and fingers.*	adactilia
Adam's apple *A prominence on the anterior neck caused by the thyroid cartilage of the larynx.*	Pomo-de-Adão
Adams-Stokes Syndrome *Characterized by bradycardia, syncope and convulsions.*	síndrome de Adam-Stokes; doença de Adam-Stokes
add, to *To count.*	adicionar
addiction *An abnormal dependency.*	adicção
Addison's disease *A disease of the adrenal gland exhibited by anemia, hypotension and a bronze tone to the skin.*	doença de Addison
adduction *To bring toward the midline.*	adução
adductor *A muscle that brings a part to the midline.*	adutor
adenectomy *The removal of a gland.*	adenectomia
adenitis *The inflammation of a gland.*	adenite
adenocanthoma *Malignant tumor comprised of glandular tissue.*	adenocantoma
adenocarcinoma *Cancer from glandular tissue.*	adenocarcinoma

English	Portuguese
adenofibroma *Connective tissue with glands that form a tumor.*	adenofibroma
adenohypophysis *The anterior portion of the pituitary gland.*	adeno-hipófise
adenoid *Referring to a gland.*	adenóide
adenoidectomy *Removal of the adenoids.*	adenoidectomia
adenoiditis *Inflammation of the adenoids.*	adenoidite
adenoids *Pharyngeal tonsils.*	adenóides
adenolymphoma *A salivary gland tumor, also called Warthin's tumor.*	adenolinfoma
adenomyoma *A tumor characterized by the overgrowth of endometrial and uterine muscle tissue.*	adenomioma
adenomyosis *A condition characterized by the overgrowth of endometrial and uterine muscle tissue.*	adenomiose
adenopathy *Generally referring to a condition of the lymphatic glands.*	adenopatia
adenosine triphosphate (ATP) *A chemical that represents the energy reserve of the muscle.*	trifosfato de adenosina
adenosine diphosphate *A product of hydrolysis of ATP.*	difosfato de adenosina
adenosine monophosphate *A nucleotide, it is produced when ATP is converted to ADP.*	monofosfato de adenosina
adenovirus *A type of a virus that can cause upper respiratory tract infections.*	adenovírus
adequate *Sufficient.*	adequado
adherence *To stick to something figuratively or literally.*	aderência
adhesion *The abnormal adherence of tissue exposed to inflammation or after surgery.*	adesão
adhesive capsulitis *Also known as frozen shoulder.*	capsulite adesiva
adhesive tape *Tape used to secure dressings or intravenous lines to the body.*	fita adesiva
adiadochokinesia *The inability to perform rapid alternating movements.*	adiadococinesia
Adie's pupil *Characterized by a weak light reaction and a strong but slow near response.*	pupila de Adie
adipose *Referring to fat. (adipose tissue)*	adiposo
adipsia *Absence of thirst which can be caused by SIADH, hydrocephalus or injury/tumor to/of the hypothalamus.*	adipsia
aditus *The entrance to an organ or part.*	ádito
adjust, to *To modify a plan.*	ajustar
adjustment *A modification of a plan.*	ajustamento
adjuvant *Term used to describe the medical treatment after initial therapy, as in adjuvant radiation therapy after initial chemotherapy.*	adjuvante
admission (to hospital)	admissão
adnexa *The appendages, for example, of the uterus are the ovaries, fallopian tubes and the ligaments of the uterus.*	anexo
adolescence	adolescência
adrenal *Referring to being near the kidney.*	adrenal
adrenal cortex *The outer layer of the adrenal gland.*	córtex adrenal
adrenal gland *A gland located on the superior aspect of both kidneys.*	glândula supra-renal
adrenal medulla *The innermost part of the adrenal gland.*	medula da glândula supra-renal
adrenalectomy *Excision of the adrenal gland.*	adrenalectomia
adrenaline (epinephrine) *A hormone secreted by the adrenal glands and a synthetic medication used for treatment of allergic reactions and cardiac arrest.*	adrenalina

English	Portuguese
adrenergic *That which is activated or transmitted by epinephrine.*	adrenérgico
adrenocorticotrophic hormone (ACTH) *A hormone that influences the cortex of the adrenal glands.*	hormônio adrenocorticotrópico
Adson maneuver *A test used to screen for thoracic outlet syndrome.*	manobra de Adson
advanced stage *A late period of a disease.*	estágio terminal
adventitia *Outermost.*	adventícia
adverse effect *In reference to medication use, it is an undesirable consequence of the drug.*	efeito adverso
advise, to *To give counsel.*	aconselhar
aerobe *An organism that grows in the presence of oxygen.*	aeróbio
aerodontalgia *The dental pain that occurs with low atmospheric pressure, like during airflight.*	aerodontalgia
aerophagy or aerophagia *A condition associated with hysteria in which one swallow repeatedly swallows air and then belches.*	aerofagia
afebrile *Absence of fever.*	apyretic; apirético
affect *The expression of emotions or feelings.*	afeto
affected	afetado
affective disorders *Manic-depressive psychosis.*	distúrbios afetivos
afferent loop syndrome *The obstruction of the duodenum or jejunum after gastrojejunostomy, resulting in duodenal distention.*	síndrome da alça aferente
afferent *Moving toward the center.*	aferente
affinity *To have a natural liking for.*	vizinhança
afibrinogenemia *Marked deficiency of fibrinogen in the blood.*	afribinogenemia
aflatoxin *A toxin produced by Aspergillus flavus.*	aflatoxina
after-load *Referring to the amount of pressure the heart needs to pump against. If one has left heart failure it is beneficial to reduce after-load.*	pós-carga
after-pains *The pain experienced after childbirth caused by uterine contractions.*	dores pós-parto; dores puerperais
after-taste *The sensation of a prolonged savor following eating/ drinking.*	paladar tardio
afterbirth *The tissue expelled after the birth of a child that includes the placenta and allied membranes.*	páreas secundinas
agar *Media used for bacterial cultures.*	ágar
age *Length of life.*	idade
agenesis *The absence of an organ. (cerebellar agenesis)*	agenesia
agglutination *The process of adherence of a mass.*	aglutinação
aggression *Violent or hostile behavior.*	agressão
aging *Becoming older.*	evelhecimento
agitation *A state of extreme emotional disturbance.*	agitação
aglutition *The inability to swallow.*	aglutição
agnathia *Congenital abnormality characterized by the absence of the mandible.*	agnatia
agnosia *A condition exhibited by the loss of sensory stimuli.*	agnosia
agonist *A synthetic compound that activates cells normally activated by natural chemicals.*	agonista
agony *Anguish or torment.*	agonia
agoraphobia *The fear of being in a large open space.*	agorafobia
agranulocytosis *A condition characterized by leukopenia and neutropenia.*	agranulocitose
agraphia *The inability to express one's thoughts in writing.*	agrafia

English	Portuguese
agreement *Accordance in opinion or feeling.*	acordo
ague *A term used to describe recurrent fever and shivering typically associated with malaria.*	ágüe
Aicardi syndrome *A rare genetic anomaly in which the corpus callosum is absent or insufficient. It is characterized by seizures, microphthalmos, coloboma and developmental delays.*	síndrome de Aicardi
AIDS *Acquired Immunodeficiency Syndrome*	SIDA (P), AIDS (B)
air	ar
air embolism *The blockage of an artery or vein by an air bubble.*	êmbolo de ar
air flow *The rate of air movement.*	fluxo de ar
air hunger *The sensation of shortness of breath.*	fome aérea
akathisia *A condition exhibited by motor restlessness and inability to sit quietly.*	acatisia
akinesia *An absence of movement or sparsity of movement.*	acinesia
akinesthesia *Lack of perception of movement.*	acinestesia
albinism *Congenital absence of pigment in the eyes, skin and hair.*	albinismo
albino *A person who lacks pigment in the eyes, skin and hair.*	albino
albumin *A protein that is soluble in water and coagulates if heated.*	albumina
albuminuria *The presence of albumin in the urine.*	albuminúria
alcohol *Ethanol or ethyl alcohol.*	álcool
alcoholic *A person with alcohol dependence.*	alcoólico
alcoholism *An addiction to alcohol.*	alcoolismo
aldehyde *A substance derived by oxidizing and containing a CHO group from alcohol.*	aldeído
aldosterone *A steroid secreted by the adrenal cortex that regulates electrolytes.*	aldosterona
aldosteronism *A condition characterized by the excessive secretion of aldosterone.*	aldosteronismo
alert *Being in a watchful, ready state.*	alerta
alexia *Inability to read due to a central brain lesion.*	alexia
algae *Nonflowering plants containing chlorophyll but without stems, roots, or leaves.*	alga
algid *cold*	frio
algophilia *Sexual perversion; getting pleasure in giving or receiving pain.*	algofilia
algorithm *Any procedure designed to solve a problem in a step-by-step or mechanical fashion.*	algoritmo
alimentary *Referring to the gastrointestinal tract.*	alimentar
alkali *A class of compounds that form soluble carbonates.*	álcali
alkaline *Referring to something with properties of an alkali.*	alcalino
alkalinuria *The urine in an alkaline state.*	alcalúria
alkaloid *Plant derived nitrogenous organic compound.*	alcalóide
alkalosis *A condition in which the pH is increased.*	alcalose
alkaptonuria *A condition exhibited by the urine turning dark upon standing because of the presence of alkapton bodies in it.*	alcaptonúria
allantois *A posterior portion of the hind-gut of an embryo.*	alantóide
allele *A type of a gene; in humans there are two alleles per chromosome pair.*	alelo
allergen *Compound that causes an allergic reaction.*	alérgeno
allergy *An immune response by the body to a compound it is hypersensitive to.*	alergia

English	Portuguese
alleviate, to	aliviar
allograft *A tissue transplant of from someone of the same species but different genotype.*	aloenxerto
allopathy *Treatment of disease with minute amounts of natural substances.*	alopatia
alopecia *The absence of hair in areas where it normally exists.*	alopecia
alpha wave *Electroencephalographic waves with a frequency of 8-13 per second.*	onda alfa
alpha-fetoprotein *A glycoprotein that has a high serum level in hepatocellular and nonseminomatous germ cell tumors.*	alfa-fetoprotéinas
alteration *The process of change or modification.*	alteraçõa
altitude sickness *A general term used for an illness that occurs at high altitude.*	náusea das alturas; doença de Acosta; doença das montanhas
alveolar *Referring to the alveolus.*	alveolar
alveolus *A small sac like structure commonly used for the pulmonary alveolus.*	alvéolo
Alzheimer's disease *A dementia of unknown cause or pathogenesis.*	doença de Alzheimer
amalgam *An alloy that includes mercury as one ingredient.*	amálgama
amalgamate,to *To make an amalgam by dissolving a metal in mercury.*	amalgamar
amastia *A development condition exhibited by the absence of breasts.*	amastia
amaurosis *Blindness that occurs without an ocular lesion but may include the optic nerve.*	amaurose
amaurosis fugax *This transient monocular blindness is considered a sign of an impending stroke.*	amaurose fugaz
amaurotic pupil *A pupil that will not respond to light when directly exposed but will respond when the other eye is exposed to light.*	pupila amaurótica
ambidextrous *Ability to use both hands equal ability.*	ambidextro
ambisexual *Referring to both sexes.*	ambissexual
amblyopia *Decreased vision without an ocular lesion.*	amblipoia
ambulation *Relating to walking.*	ambulatório
ambulatory electrocardiographic monitoring *A continuous recording of the electrocardiogram used to detect occult dysrhythmias.*	monitorar ECG ambulatorial
ameba *A one-celled protozoan.*	amebas
amebiasis *A condition in which one is infected with amebae, mostly commonly Entamoeba histolytica.*	amebíase
amebic liver abscess *A pus filled fluid collection within the liver caused by amoebe.*	abscesso amebiano de fígado
amebicide *A compound used to treat amebiasis.*	amebicida
ameboma *A mass caused by inflammation as seen in amebiasis.*	ameboma
amelia *A congenital anomaly exhibited by the absence of limbs.*	amelia
amelioration *The act of making something better or improvement.*	melhoria
amenorrhea *The absence of menses.*	amenorréia
amentia *The absence of mental ability.*	amentia
ametria *Obsolete term for congenital uterine agenesis.*	ametria
ametropia *Abnormal refractive ability of the eyes resulting in hypermetropia, myopia or astigmatism.*	ametropia
amino acid *A compound containing a carboxyl and an amino group.*	aminoácido

English	Portuguese
ammonia *A colorless alkaline gas.*	amônia
amnesia *The inability to remember past events.*	amnésia
amnesia, antegrade *The inability to remember events which occurred after the insult that caused the condition.*	amnésia anterógrada
amnesic stroke *Cerebral infarct exhibited by loss of memory.*	acidente vascular cerebral amnésico
amniocentesis *Transabdominal aspiration of amniotic fluid.*	amniocentese
amniography *X-ray of the gravid uterus after insertion of opaque dye.*	amniografia
amnion *The membrane lining the placenta which produces the amniotic fluid.*	âmnio
amniotic fluid *The fluid surrounding the fetus.*	fluido amniótico
amorphus *A fetus with no heart and no definitive shape.*	amorfo
amount *The total or the aggregate.*	soma
ampulla *The dilated end of a duct.*	ampola
ampulla chyli *Also called cisterna chyli; it is a dilated area of the thoracic duct that collects lymph from several areas.*	cisterna do quilo
amputation *Typically referring to the surgical removal of a limb.*	amputação
amygdala *Any almond shaped structure such as the tonsil*	amígdala
amylase *An enzyme involved in the hydrolysis of starch.*	amilase
amyloidosis *The accumulation of amyloid in body tissues.*	amiloidose
amyotonia *A condition associated with the lack of muscle tone.*	myatonia
amyotrophic lateral sclerosis *A progressive neurodegenerative disorder.*	esclerose lateral amiotrófica
amyotrophy *Atrophy of muscle tissue.*	amiotrofia
anabolism *The formation of molecules in organisms from simpler molecules.*	anabolismo
anacrotic *Referring to a prominent bulge on the ascending portion of a pulse recording.*	anacrótico
anaerobe *An organism that lives in the absence of oxygen.*	anaeróbio
anal *Near or referring to the anus.*	anal
anal fistula *An opening in the skin that tracts to the anal canal thus causing some fecal material to leak from the opening in the skin.*	fístula anal
analeptic *A medication used as a stimulant to the central nervous system.*	analéptico
analgesia *The absence of pain.*	analgesia
analgesic *A medication used to remove pain.*	analgésico
analogous *To resemble or be similar to.*	análogo
anaphase *A stage in mitosis following metaphase.*	anáfase
anaphoresis *Reduced activity of the sweat glands.*	anaforese
anaphylaxis *An exaggerated response to a foreign substance.*	anafilaxia
anaplasia *The loss of normal differentiation of tumor cells.*	anaplasia
anastomosis *Surgical formation of a connection between two previously separate parts.*	anastomose
anatomical chart *A pictorial diagram of part of the anatomy.*	gráfico anatômico
anatomical dead space *The area between the mouth and pulmonary alveoli.*	espaço morto anatômico
anatomical *Referring to the anatomy.*	anatômico
anatomical snuff-box *The area on the back of the hand near the base of the thumb that is between the extensor pollicus longus and extensor pollicus brevis.*	tabaqueira anatômico
anatomy *The study of body structure.*	anatomia

English	Portuguese
ancylostomiasis *A type of nematode parasite, also called hookworm.*	ancilostomíase
androgen *A compound that produces masculinizing characteristics.*	androgênio
androgynous *Referring to a female pseudohermaphroditism (a genetic female with masculine characteristics).*	andrógino
android pelvis *A pelvis shaped like a man's.*	pelve andróide
androsterone *A hormone excreted in the urine of men and women.*	androsterona
anemia *Lower than normal red blood cell count.*	anemia
anencephaly *The congenital absence of the cranial vault and cerebral hemispheres.*	anencefalia
aneroid *The absence of liquid.*	aneróide
anesthesia *Loss of sensation.*	anestesia
anesthetic *A chemical that produces anesthesia.*	anestésico
anesthetist *A person who administers anesthesia.*	anestesista
aneurysm *A condition exhibited by the dilatation of the walls of an artery or vein to form a blood-filled sac.*	aneurisma
angiectasia *Dilation of a blood or lymph vessel.*	angiectasia
angina pectoris *Exercise induced myocardial ischemia.*	angina do peito
angioedema *Also called angioneurotic edema, it is caused by a histamine reaction. It can produce welts in mild cases but in severe cases can cause swelling of the lips and tongue.*	edema angioneurótico
angiogram *Radiologic imaging of blood vessels.*	angiograma
angiography *Roentgenographic imaging of blood vessels.*	angiografia
angioma *A tumor comprised of blood or lymph vessels.*	angioma
angioneurotic *Caused by a neurosis affecting the blood vessels, like vasospasm.*	angioneurótico
angioneurotic edema *A condition exhibited by sudden edema of skin and mucous membranes.*	edema angioneurótico
angioplasty *Surgical alteration of blood vessels.*	angio-plastia
angiosarcoma *A sarcoma comprised of blood vessels.*	angiossarcoma
angiospasm *A spasm of a blood vessel.*	angiospasmo; vasoespasmo
angiotensin *A blood protein that increases aldosterone secretion.*	angiotensina
angiotensin converting enzyme inhibitors (ACEI) *A class of medicines that prevent conversion of angiotensin I to angiotensin II, a potent vasoconstrictor.*	inibidor da enzima que converte a angiotensina
angitis or angiitis *The inflammation of a lymph or blood vessel.*	angiite
anguish *Significant mental or physical pain.*	agonia
anhidrosis *A condition exhibited by reduced quantity of sweat.*	anidrose
anhidrotic *Something the reduces the quantity of sweat.*	anidrótico
anhydrous *Lacking water.*	anidro
aniseikonia *A condition in which the ocular image of an object is viewed differently by each eye.*	aniseiconia
anisocoria *Pupillary diameter inequality.*	anisocoria
anisocytosis *Variation in size of erythrocytes.*	anisocitose
anisomelia *Unequal size of arms or legs.*	anisomelia
anisometropia *Refractive power inequality between the two eyes.*	anisometropia
ankle *The area of the ankle joint.*	tornozelo, maléolo
ankle clonus *An abnormal response exhibited by alternating plantar- and dorsiflexion noted after the examiner rapidly dorsiflexes the foot.*	clono calcâneo

English	Portuguese
ankle edema or dependent edema *Extracellular fluid volume noted by swelling or pitting.*	edema de declive
ankle joint *The articulation of the tibia/fibula and talus.*	articulação talocrural
ankle support *A mechanical device or banding to support the ankle.*	suporte calcâneo
ankle swelling *Enlargement of the ankle region with or without pitting.*	tumefação de calcâneo
ankyloglossia *Limitation of tongue motion because of a short frenulum.*	anciloglossia
ankylosing spondylitis *A type of arthritis found in the spine that is exhibited by bony fusion.*	espondilite ancilosante
ankylosis *Abnormal immobility of a joint.*	ancilose
annular *Referring to a ring.*	anular, anelar
anomia *Inability to name or recognize familiar objects.*	anomia
anonychia *Congenital absence of fingernails or toenails.*	anoniquia
anoperineal *Referring to the anus and perineum.*	anoperíneo
anorchous *The absence of testicles.*	anorquia
anorectal *Referring to the anus and rectum.*	anorético
anorexia nervosa *A mental disorder characterized by the desire to avoid eating and to lose weight.*	anorexia nervosa
anorexia *The loss of appetite.*	anorexia
anorrectal abscess *A localized collection of pus in the anorrectal region.*	abscesso anorético
anosmia *Lack of the sense of smell.*	anosmia
anovulatory *Lack of ovulation.*	anovulatório
anovulatory cycle *A menstrual cycle in which no ovum is released.*	ciclo anovulatório
anoxemia *Reduction in blood oxygen concentration.*	anoxemia
anoxia *Reduced oxygen levels in body tissues.*	anoxia
antacid *A medication, usually with a calcium or magnesium base that binds with acid in the stomach.*	antiácido
antagonist *A muscle or agent that acts in counteract to effects of another muscle or agent.*	antagonista
antiemetic *A medication used to control nausea.*	antiemético
antemortem *Refers to: before death.*	antes da morte
antenatal *Refers to events before birth.*	antenatal
anterior root *A motor nerve root that is in the anterior part of the spinal cord between the anterior and lateral funiculi.*	raiz anterior
anterior *Toward the front.*	anterior
anterograde *Moving forward.*	anterógrado
anteroinferior *Toward the front and lower part.*	ântero-inferior
anterolateral *Toward the front and away from the midline.*	ântero-lateral
anteromedian *Toward the front and toward the midline.*	ântero-mediano
anteroposterior *From front to the back. (An AP x-ray has the beam directed from the front to the back.)*	ântero-posterior
anterosuperior *Toward the front and the upper part.*	ântero-superior
anteversion *The forward leaning of an organ.*	anteversão
anthelmintic *An agent used to destroy worms.*	antihelmíntico
anthracosis *Pneumoconiosis caused by coal dust.*	antracose
anthrax *An infectious disease caused by Bacillus anthracis; there are cutaneous, inhalation and gastrointestinal syndromes.*	antraz
anti-inflammatory agents *Medications used to reduce inflammation.*	anti-inflamatório

English	Portuguese
antibiotic *A medication that inhibits or kills microorganisms.*	antibiótico
antibody *A protein that combines with and counteracts foreign substances.*	anticorpo
anticholinergic *Parasympathetic blocker.*	anticolinérgico
anticholinesterase *Cholinesterase blocker.*	anticolinesterase
anticoagulant *Medication used to inhibit coagulation.*	anticoagulante
anticodon *A series of three nucleotides that form a unit of genetic code for transfer RNA.*	anticódon
anticonvulsant *Medication used to treat seizures.*	anticonvulsivante
antidepressant *Medication used to treat depression.*	antidepressor; antidepressivo
antidiuretic hormone *Vasopressin.*	hormônio antidiurético
antidote *A medication that neutralizes a toxin.*	antídoto
antigen *A foreign substance, like bacteria, that induces an immune response.*	antigénio (P), antígeno (B)
antiglobulin test (Coombs' test) *Test used to detect erythroblastosis fetalis.*	prova antiglobulina
antihemophilic factor *Also called factor VIII. A deficiency of the factor causes hemophilia.*	fator anti-hemofílico
antihistamine *Medication used to treat conditions exhibited by a histamine response*	anti-histamina
antilymphocyte *A serum globulin that has antibodies to lymphocytes.*	anti-linfocito
antilymphocyte globulin *The gamma globulin portion of antilymphocyte serum.*	globulina anti-linfocito
antimalarial *Medication used to treat malaria.*	antimalárico
antimetabolite *A substance that impedes metabolism.*	antimetabólito
antimigraine *Medication used to treat headaches.*	anti-hemicrânia
antimitotic *Impeding mitosis.*	antimitótico
antimycotic *Inhibition of fungal growth.*	antimicótico
antinuclear factor *Also called antinucleic antibody (ANA); it is found in conditions such as lupus and rheumatoid arthritis.*	anticorpo antenuclear
antiperistaltic *An agent that impedes normal peristalsis.*	antiperistáltico
antipruritic *Medication used to treat pruritus.*	antiprurítico
antipyretic *Medication used to treat fever.*	antipirético
antiseptic *A substance that inhibits microorganism growth.*	anti-séptico
antiserum *A substance that contains antibodies to specific antigens.*	anti-soro
antispasmodic *Medication used to treat muscle spasm.*	antiesposmódico
antithrombin *A substance that inhibits thrombin, thus decreasing the body's ability to coagulate.*	antitrombina
antithyroid *A substance inhibiting the effect of the thyroid.*	antitireóde
antitoxin *A substance that inhibits the effect of a toxin.*	antitoxina
antitussive *Medication used to diminish a cough.*	antitussivo
antivenin *An antitoxin formulated for various types of snake bites.*	antiveneno
antrotomy *To cut open the antrum.*	antrotomia
antrum *Referring to a cavity or chamber.*	antro
anuria *The lack of urine excretion.*	anúria
anus *The body opening distal to the rectum.*	ânus
anxiety *Nervousness or unease.*	ansiedade
anxiety neurosis *Abnormal presence of anxiety.*	ansiedade neurose
anxious *Experiencing nervousness or unease.*	ansioso

English	Portuguese
aorta *The large artery originating at the left ventricle and going to the pelvis where it bifurcates.*	aorta
aortic insufficiency *A dysfunction of the aortic valve allowing backflow of blood into the heart.*	insuficiência aórtica
aortic *Referring to the aorta.*	aórtica
aortic stenosis *Narrowing of the aortic orifice.*	estenose aórtica
aortic valve *The valve situated between the left ventricle and the aorta.*	válvula aórtica
apart *Separated by a distance.*	distância, à
apathy *Lack of interest in one's environment or indifference.*	apatia
aperistalsis *Lack of intestinal peristalsis.*	aperistaltismo
aperture *An opening or hole, as in the hole the light passes through in a camera.*	abertura
apex *The highest point of something.*	ápice; ápex
apex of heart *Normally found 8cm to the left of the midsternal line in the 5th intercostal space.*	ápex cardíaco
Apgar score *A scoring system for newborns that utilizes heart rate, respiratory effort, muscle tone, responsiveness and skin color.*	escore de Apgar
aphagia *The lack of eating.*	afagia
aphakia *The congenital absence of the lens of the eye.*	afacia; afaquia
aphasia *Diminished ability to communicate via speech or writing.*	afasia
aphid *A minute insect that feeds on plants.*	afídio
aphonia *The loss of voice.*	afonia
aphthous stomatitis *Grouped small lesions that occur on the tongue or in the mouth.*	estomatite aftosa
apicectomy *Removal of the apex of the petrous portion of the temporal bone.*	apicectomia
aplastic anemia *Bone marrow failure causing a decrease in all types of blood cells.*	anemia aplásica
apnea *Absence of respiration.*	apnéia
apocrine gland *A gland that releases some of its cytoplasm in secretions; an example is axillary sweat glands.*	glândula apôcrina
aponeurosis *A tendinous expansion that connects with muscle to move a part.*	aponeurose
apophysis *Generally a bony outgrowth that forms a process or tubercle.*	apófise
apoplexy *Extravasation of blood within an organ.*	apoplexia
appearance *The way someone looks or presents.*	aparência
appendectomy *Surgical excision of the appendix.*	apendectomia
appendicitis *Inflammation of the appendix.*	apendicite
appendix *An appendage of the cecum.*	apêndice
apperception *The ability to interpret sensory impressions.*	apercepção
application *The forms one fills out to obtain a grant.*	candidatura
applicator *A device used to apply a topical medication.*	aplicador
appointment *A previously scheduled time to see a person.*	encontro marcado
apprehensive *A fear that something unpleasant will happen.*	apreensivo
approval *Accepting something as satisfactory.*	aprovação
approximate *Nearly but not totally accurate.*	aproximado
approximate, to *To bring together, as in wound margins.*	aproximar
approximately *Nearly but not completely.*	aproximadamente

English	Portuguese
apraxia *The inability to carry out intentional movements when paralysis is not present.*	apraxia
apt *Suitable in the circumstances.*	adequado
aptitude *A natural talent for something.*	aptidão
aptyalism *Diminished or absence of saliva.*	aptialia
acquaint, to *To make someone familiar with something.*	conhecer
aqueous humor *The fluid between the cornea and lens, anterior to the globe.*	humor aquoso
aqueous *Use of water as a solvent or medium.*	aquoso
arachnodactyly *A condition exhibited by abnormally long and slender fingers.*	aracnodactilia
arachnoid *Refers to that which resembles a spider web.*	aracnóide
arbovirus *Virus that is transmitted by arthropods; responsible for diseases such as Yellow fever and dengue fever.*	arbovírus
arcuate nucleus *Small masses of gray matter found on the medulla oblongata.*	núcleo arqueado
arcus *Narrow opaque band.*	arco
areola *The pigmented skin surrounding a nipple.*	aréola
argininosuccinicaciduria *Presence of arginosuccinic acid in the urine; associated with mental retardation.*	argininssuccinicacidúria
argue, to *To debate or reason. (quarrel)*	arguir
Argyll Robertson symptom *Presence of small pupils that do not react to light but will constrict when the person focuses on a near object.*	sintoma Argyll Robertson
argyria *The greyish discoloration of the skin and conjunctiva.*	argiria
arm *One of two upper extremities.*	braço
armpit *A common term for axilla.*	sovaco
around *On every side of.*	cerca
arousal reaction *The change in brain wave patterns upon awakening.*	reação despertar
arrhenoblastoma *An ovarian tumor that results in masculine secondary sex characteristics.*	arrenoblastoma
arrhythmia *An abnormal heart rhythm.*	arritmia
arterial blood gas *Measurement of the arterial concentration of carbon dioxide and oxygen.*	gasimetria arterial
arterial *Referring to an artery.*	arterial
arteriectomy *Surgical excision of an artery.*	arteriectomia
arteriography *Roentgenography of an artery after infusion of contrast media.*	arteriografia
arterioplasty *Surgical repair of an artery.*	arterioplastia
arteriosclerosis *Hardening and thickening of arterial walls.*	arteriosclerose
arteriotomy *Creation of an opening in an artery.*	arteriotonia
arteriovenous malformation *A sac like structure created by the abnormal communication of an adjacent artery and vein.*	malformação arteriovenoso
arteritis *Inflammation of an artery.*	arterite
artery *Vessel that carries oxygenated blood from the heart to the periphery.*	artéria
arthralgia *Joint pain.*	artralgia
arthritis *Joint inflammation.*	artrite
arthrodesis *Surgical fusion of a joint.*	artrodese
arthrodynia *Joint pain.*	artrodinia
arthrography *Joint roentgenography.*	artrografia
arthroplasty *Plastic surgery involving a joint.*	artroplastia

English	Portuguese
arthroscopy *Viewing of the inside of a joint with a specially designed scope.*	artroscopia
arthrotomy *Surgical opening of a joint.*	artrotomia
articular *Referring to a joint.*	articular
artifact *An aberration from the normal.*	artefato
artificial *Not natural produced.*	artificial
arytenoid *Referring to the cartilage in the posterior larynx.*	aritenóide
asbestos *A heat resistant silicate material.*	asbesto
asbestosis *Lung disease caused by the inhalation of asbestos.*	asbestose
ascaricide *Agent that destroys ascaris.*	ascaricida
ascaris *A nematode from genus intestinal lumbricoid parasite, also called round worm.*	áscaris; lombriga
ascending colon *The portion of the colon between the cecum and the right colic flexure.*	cólon ascendente
ascertain, to *Synonym of "to determine".*	averiguar
ascites *Serous fluid in the abdominal cavity.*	ascite
ascorbic acid *Commonly known as vitamin C; a deficiency of this vitamin causes scurvy.*	ácido ascórbico
asepsis *Lack of infection.*	assepsia
aseptic *Being free of septic matter.*	asséptico
asexual *Without sex or sex organs.*	assexual
asleep *To be in a dormant or inactive state.*	adormecido
Asperger's syndrome *A condition characterized by disturbed social interaction; if was named after the Austrian scientist who first described it.*	sindrome de Asperger
aspermia *Absence of sperm.*	aspermia
asphyxia *A condition exhibited by a lack of oxygen and subsequent loss of consciousness or death.*	asfixia
aspiration biopsy *Removal of fluid from a cavity for pathologic analysis.*	biópsia por aspiração
aspiration pneumonia *Taking air or matter into the lungs.*	pneumonia por aspiração
aspirator *A device used to remove fluid from a cavity.*	aspirador
aspirin *Common name for acetylsalicylic acid.*	aspirina; ácido acetilsalicílico
assay *A procedure for measuring the activity of a biological sample.*	análise
assessment *An medical evaluation.*	avaliação
assistance *The act of helping.*	assistência
assisted ventilation *The act of helping one breathe through artificial means.*	assistência ventilação
asteatosis *A condition exhibited by diminished sebaceous secretion.*	asteatose
astereognosis *Lack of ability to recognize objects by touching them.*	estereognose
asterixis *Commonly known as a flapping tremor, it is characterized by involuntary jerking movements of the hands and is seen commonly in hepatic encephalopathy.*	asterixe
asthenia *Diminished strength and energy.*	astenia
asthenopia *Visual fatigue accompanied by ocular pain.*	astenopia
astragalus *Synonym of talus.*	astrágalo
astringent *An agent causing contraction of the skin.*	adstringente
astrocytoma *A tumor comprised of astrocytes.*	astrocitoma
astroglia *The neurologic tissue which is composed of astrocytes.*	astróglia

English	Portuguese
asymmetry *Lack of symmetry.*	assimetria
asymptomatic *The absence of symptoms.*	assintomático
asynclitism *Oblique presentation of the head during delivery.*	assinclitismo
at random *Occurring by chance alone.*	em aleatório
atavism *The inheritance of characteristics from remote rather than immediate ancestors.*	atavismo
ataxia *Lack of muscular coordination.*	ataxia
atelectasis *Incomplete expansion or collapse of a lung.*	atelectasia
atherogenic *Something that causes atheromatous lesions in arterial walls.*	aterogênico
atheroma *Degenerative arteriosclerosis.*	ateroma
athetosis *An involuntary symptom exhibited by continuous slow, writhing movements, mostly in the hands.*	atetose
athlete's foot *Common term for tinea pedis.*	micose do pé
atlas *The first cervical vertebra.*	atlas
atomizer *A device for propelling a fine mist.*	atomizador
atony *Absence of normal muscle tone.*	atonia
atresia *Closure of a body orifice as in atresia ani in which there is a congenital imperforate anus.*	atresia
atrial flutter *Sawtooth waves on an electrocardiogram with atrial rate of 250-330 per minute.*	agitação atrial
atrial natriuretic factor *A chemical secreted by the right atrium that promotes sodium excretion in the urine.*	ator natriurético atrial
atrial *Referring to the atrium.*	atrial
atrial septal defect *An abnormal communication between the atria of the heart.*	defeito septal atrial
atrio-ventricular block *An interruption of the electrical conduction at the atrio-ventricular node.*	bloqueio atrioventricular
atrioventricular bundle *Also called bundle of His.*	feixe de His
atrioventricular *Referring to the atrium and ventricle.*	atrioventricular
atrium *Referring to a chamber used as an entrance, as in the entrance to the heart.*	átrio
atrophic *Referring to atrophy.*	atrófico
atrophy *A diminution in the size of a part.*	atrofia
atropine *A parasympathetic agent derived from Atropa belladonna.*	atropina
attack *A fit or paroxysm.*	ataque
atypical *Not usual.*	atípico
audiogram *The recording of a one's hearing in decibels.*	audiograma
audiologist *A specialist in the field of hearing.*	audiologista
audiometer *A device used to measure hearing.*	audiômetro
auditory *Referring to hearing.*	auditivo
auditory agnosia *Caused by a temporal lobe lesion, it is characterized by inability to recognize sounds as words.*	agnosia do auditivo
aural *Referring to the ear.*	aural
auricle *The external portion of the ear.*	aurícula
auricular *Referring to the auricle.*	auricular
auriculotemporal *The area of the ear and temple.*	auriculotemporal
auscultation *The act of listening to sounds emanating from the body.*	ausculta; auscultação
autism *A mental condition exhibited by difficulty in forming relationships, communicating and uses abstract thought.*	autismo
autistic *Referring to autism.*	autista

English	Portuguese
autoantibody *An antibody that acts against the organism's own tissue.*	auto-anticorpo
autoantigen *A normal tissue constituent that prompts a cell-mediated response.*	auto-antígeno
autoclave *A device used for sterilization with the use of steam under pressure.*	autoclave
autogenous *Self-generated.*	autogênese
autograft *Grafting tissue from one part of person to another part of the same person.*	auto-enxerto
autohypnosis *Self-hypnosis.*	auto-hipnose
autoimmunization *The body's ability to promote an immune response without external resources.*	auto-imunização
autolysis *A state of self destruction of cells within a body.*	autolíse
autonomic nervous system *Responsible for regulation of cardiac muscle, smooth muscle and glandular activity.*	sistema nervoso autônomo
autopsy *Examination of a body post-mortem in an attempt to determine cause of death.*	autôpsia
autosomal *Referring to an autosome.*	autossômico
autotransfusion *The reinfusion of one's own blood.*	autotransfusão
availability *A person or thing that is available.*	disponibilidade
available *Attainable, obtainable.*	disponível
avascular *An area with no blood supply.*	avascular
avascular necrosis *Bone death caused by poor blood supply.*	necrose avascular
avian flu *A viral disease found in birds and fowl that can be transmitted to humans; it is exhibited by respiratory and gastrointestinal symptoms but can lead to encephalitis.*	influenza aviária
avian *Referring to birds.*	aviária
avitaminosis *A state of vitamin deficiency.*	avitaminose
avoidable *That which can be stopped or inhibited.*	evitável
awakening *The state of being conscious.*	despertar
away from *Separated from.*	fora de
axilla *The hollow beneath the arm.*	axila
axillary *Referring to the axilla.*	axilar
axis *The second cervical vertebra.*	eixo
axon *The structure along which nerve impulses are transmitted from the cell body to other cells.*	axônio
azo itch *A pruritus noted in people who use azo dyes.*	prurido do axo
azoospermia *The absence of spermatozoa in the semen.*	azoospermia
Azorean disease *A form of hereditary ataxia found in peoples of Azorean descent. Also called Machado-Joseph disease or Portuguese-Azorean disease.*	doença dos Açores
azotemia *Prerenal disease.*	azotemia
azoturia *An excess of urea in the urine.*	azotúria
Babinski's sign *A reflex that occurs when the plantar surface of the foot is stimulated. The great toe turns upward- normal in infancy but when it turns upward in an adult it means there is central nervous system injury.*	reflexo de Babinski; reflexo cutâneo-plantar
baby *A newborn.*	bebé (P); bebê (B)
baby-scale *A device used to weigh an infant.*	balança por bebé
bacillary *Referring to bacilli.*	bacilar
bacillus *A rod-shaped bacterium.*	bacilo
back pain *Discomfort on the dorsal surface of the torso.*	dor nas costas
bacteremia *The presence of bacteria in the blood.*	bacteriemia

English	Portuguese
bacteria *Plural for any organism of the order Eubacteriales.*	bactérias
bacterial *Referring to bacteria.*	bacteriano
bactericidal *An agent that destroys bacteria.*	bactericida
bacteriostatic *An agent that impedes bacterial growth.*	bacteriostático
bacteriuria *The presence of bacteria in the urine.*	bacteriúria
bagassosis *A pulmonary disorder contracted from inhalation of the waste of sugar cane (bagasse dust).*	bagaçose
Bainbridge reflex *Increase in heart rate due to increased pressure in the right atrium.*	reflexo de Bainbridge
Baker cyst *A synovial fluid collection in the popliteal fossa.*	cisto de Baker
balanitis *Inflammation of the glans of the penis.*	balanite
ballottement *Presence of movement of a floating object by palpation.*	baloteamento
balm *A topical medical preparation.*	bálsamo
bandage *A strip of gauze used to immobilize or support.*	bandagem; atadura
banding *The process of encircling with a thin piece of material.*	em bandas
barber's itch *Ringworm that is transmitted by contaminated shaving equipment.*	prurido do barbeiro
barium enema *Administration of barium into the rectum followed by roentgenography to check for rectal or colon abnormalities.*	enema de bário
Barretts's esophagus *A condition characterized by varying degrees of esophageal injury from gastric acid.*	esôfago de Barrett
Bartholin's cyst or abscess *This is a purulent fluid collection in the Bartholin cysts which are located in the perivaginal area.*	cisto de Bartholin
Bartter's syndrome *An autosomal recessive renal disorder with a defect in chloride reabsorption and secondary hyperaldosteronism.*	síndrome de Bartter
basal ganglia *Structures adjacent to the thalamus that are involved with coordination of movement.*	gânglio da base
basal *Referring to the base.*	basal
basilar *Referring to the base or lower segment.*	basilar
basilic vein *A vein in the hand that joins the brachial veins to form the axillary vein.*	veia basílica
basin *A small bowl used for washing.*	basia
basophil *A polymorphonuclear granulocyte.*	basófilo
bear, to *To endure or resist.*	suportar
bear, to *To give birth to a child.*	gravidez e parto
bearing down *As in during labor.*	esforço expulsivo de uma partuiente
beat *As in heart beat.*	batimento
Bechterew-Mendel reflex *Plantar flexion of the toes when the examiner percusses the dorsum of the foot; seen with pyramidal lesion.*	reflexo de Bechterew-Mendel
bed *A mattress resting on a frame.*	leito
bed rest *A medical order requiring one to stay in bed.*	repouso no leito
bedbug Cimex lectularius. *A small insect that is parasitic and hides in clothing or bedding.*	percevejo
bedpan *A metal or plastic vestibule one sits on while in bed to defecate.*	comadre; arrasterdeira
bedridden *Term used to indicate one is so ill they cannot get out of bed.*	acamado
bee sting *A piercing from a bee.*	picada de abelha
beforehand *In advance or previously.*	antemão

English	Portuguese
behavior disorder *An abnormal mental state.*	distúrbio de comportamento
Behçet syndrome *Characterized by recurrent oral and genital ulcers, uveitis, iridocyclitis and frequently arthritis.*	síndrome de Behçet
Bell's palsy *Unilateral facial paralysis related to dysfunction of the seventh cranial nerve.*	paralisia de Bell
below *Under.*	embaixo de
belt *A strap used to hold clothing up.*	cinto
benign *Not harmful.*	benigno
bereavement *The sorrow one feels with the loss of a loved one.*	duelo
berylliosis *A lung exhibited by granulomas and caused by inhalation of beryllium.*	beriliose
best *Optimal or ideal.*	melhor
betablocker *A substance that inhibits adrenergic stimulation. It is used to reduce pulse, blood pressure and to treat angina.*	bloqueador ß
beyond *On the farther side.*	ainda
bezoar *A concretion composed of either hair, vegetable/fruit fibers or hair and vegetable/fruit fibers that is found in the stomach.*	bezoar
Bezold-Jarisch reflex *A reflex in the vagus, originating in the heart, resulting in sinus bradycardia, hypotension and peripheral vasodilation.*	reflexo de Bezold-Jarisch
biased *Prejudiced.*	preconceituoso
biceps *A muscle with two heads usually referring to the biceps brachii which is used for forearm flexion.*	bíceps
biceps reflex *The biceps brachii tendon is hit with a reflex hammer and results in flexion of the forearm as a normal response. This assesses the C5-C6 region.*	reflexo bicipital
bicuspid *Having two points as in bicuspid valve or a premolar tooth.*	bicúspide
bifid *Presence of two branches.*	bífido
bifurcate ligament *A ligament on the dorsum of the foot that includes the calcaneonavicular and calcaneocuboid ligaments.*	ligamento bifurcado
bifurcate *When one branch divides into two branches.*	bifurcado
bilateral *Referring to both sides.*	bilateral
bile *An alkaline fluid secreted by the liver to aid digestion.*	bile
bile ducts *The structures that are conduits for passage of bile from the liver and gallbladder to the duodenum.*	ducto biliar
bile pigments *The golden brown or green-yellow color associated with bile.*	pigmento biliar
bile salts *Normally occurring salts of bile acids.*	sais biliares
Bilharzia *Historical name of a genus of flukes or nematodes now known as Schistosoma.*	Bilhárzia
biliary *Referring to bile, bile ducts or gallbladder.*	biliar
bilious *Something that contains bile.*	bilioso
bilirubin *A pigment found in bile that is responsible for the yellow color seen in patients with elevated serum levels of bilirubin.*	bilirrubina
biliuria *The presence of bile in the urine.*	bilúria
biliverdin *A green pigment formed by oxidation of bilirubin.*	biliverdina
bill *A financial statement that indicates how much one owes.*	fatura
Bill maneuver *During childbirth, use of forceps at midpelvis to help extract the head.*	manobra de Bill
bimanual *Use of two hands, as in bimanual pelvic examination in which the right hand touches the cervix uteri and the left hand presses above the mons pubis.*	bimanual

English	Portuguese
binaural *Referring to both ears.*	binauricular
binocular *Referring to both eyes.*	binocular
binovular *Derived from two different ova.*	binovular
bioassay *A laboratory test determination as compared to normal.*	bioensaio
bioavailability *The portion of a drug that is able to be utilized by the body after it is introduced to the body.*	biodisponibilidade
biochemistry *The study of chemistry and physiochemical processes in living organisms.*	bioquímica
biology *The study of living organisms.*	biologia
biopsy *The removal and examination of bodily tissues or fluids.*	biopsia
biotin *A vitamin involved in the synthesis of fatty acids and glucose.*	biotina
birth *The process of bearing offspring from the uterus.*	parto; nascimento
birth control *Any method of limiting contraception.*	contracepção
birth defect *A congenital anomaly.*	anomolia congênito
birth rate *The number of live births per 1000 of a given population per year.*	índice de natalidade
bistoury; scalpel *A surgical knife.*	bisturi
bitemporal hemianopsia *A visual defect seen commonly in pituitary tumors in which the visual defect is in the temporal portion of each eye.*	hemianopsia bitemporal
bitter (taste) *Having a harsh, unpleasant taste.*	amargo
black *Referring to the color, as in the color of coal.*	preto
black fly *From the family Simuliidae, a gnat that can cause disease in humans; also called buffalo fly.*	mosca preto
black stools *Common term for melena.*	melena
blackout *Common term for loss of consciousness.*	escurecimento; blecaute
blackwater fever *A term used to describe the fever associated with malaria when the urine is reddish-black.*	febre hemoglobinúrica
bladder, urinary *Vestibule for urine prior to being expelled via the urethra.*	vesícula urinária
blast injury *Trauma from a wave of air pressure.*	lesão de rajada
blastomycosis *Infection caused by organisms of genus Blastomyces.*	blastomicose
bleach *A solution that includes sodium hypochlorite.*	água sanitária
bleeding *Loss of blood.*	sangria
bleeding time *The time of bleeding after a controlled standardized puncture of the earlobe.*	tempo de sangramento
blemish *A small mark on one's skin.*	defeito; mancha
blennorrhea *Discharge from the mucous membranes, usually referring to gonorrhea.*	blenorragia
blepharitis *Inflammation of the eyelids.*	blefarite
blepharospasm *A spasm of the orbicularis oculi muscle that causes closure of the eyelid.*	blefaroespasmo
blind *Absence of sight.*	cego
blind loop syndrome *A condition in which there is a non-functional section of the bowel that is thought to be responsible for malabsorption and Vitamin B12 deficiency.*	síndrome da alça cega
blind spot *An area of insensitivity to light located at the point of entry of the optic nerve on the retina.*	pouco visível
blindness *Absence of visual perception.*	cegueira
blinking *To open and close the eyelid rapidly.*	piscar
blister *Common term for bulla.*	vesícula; empola

English	Portuguese
bloated *Sensation of having an abnormally large amount of air in the viscera.*	inchado
Boerhaave Syndrome *Rupture of the esophagus from vigorous vomiting, with resultant mediastinitis.*	síndrome de Boerhaave
blood *Plasma containing erythrocytes, leukocytes and platelets.*	sangue
blood alcohol level *A quantitative measurement of the amount of alcohol in the blood.*	alcoolémia
blood bank *An area where blood products are stored for later use.*	banco de sangue
blood brain barrier *A matrix of capillaries that move blood between the blood and brain, as well as, limiting some substances from passing.*	barreira hematocerebral
blood cells *A common term that does not differentiate between erythrocyte or leukocyte.*	célula sangüínea
blood clot *A mass of coagulated blood.*	coágulo sangüíneo
blood grouping *Testing blood to determine which type should be used for transfusion.*	tipagem sangüínea
blood pressure *Written as the measurement in mmHg at the time of systole of the left ventricle over the time of diastole.*	pressão arterial
blood sedimentation rate (ESR) *The settling time of erythrocytes in a prepared sample. This is a measure of the abnormal concentration of substances that are associated with pathological states.*	velocidade de sedimentação de hemácias
blood stream *Common term or the arterial or venous systems.*	corrente sangüínea
blood tubing *(used for infusion of blood)*	cano sangüínea
blood type *Determined and listed in the ABO system.*	tipo sangüíneo
blood volume *The amount of blood cells/plasma in the circulatory system.*	volume sangüíneo
blue *A color between green and violet.*	azul
blue diaper syndrome *A disorder of tryptophan absorption. Excess tryptophan is metabolized to indicans in the bowel, excreted in the urine and oxidized in the diaper to indigo, thus the blue diaper.*	síndrome de fralda azul
blunt *Having a flat or rounded end.*	cego
blurred vision *Low visual acuity.*	visão turva
blurt out, to *To speak without considering the repercussions.*	desvendar um segredo
blush, to *To have an increased volume of blood flow to one's face causing a red tint to the skin.*	rubor
body surface area *Dubois formula is: (weight in kilograms) to the 0.425th power x (height in centimeters) to the 0.725th power x 0.007184.*	corpo superfícies área; fórmula de Dubois
body weight *Relative mass as measured in kilograms or pounds.*	peso (corpo)
bolus *A fluid bolus is a phrase used for rapid infusion of fluid.*	bolo
bone *Skeletal tissue formed by osteoblasts.*	osso
bone graft *The transfer of bone to aid in the healing of a complex fracture.*	enxerto ósseo
bone marrow *The soft material filling the cavity of bones.*	medula óssea
bone marrow puncture *The aspiration of marrow to look for pressure of disease.*	poncionar medula óssea
bone scan *Bone imaging using technetium 99m (99mTc) diphosphate.*	escaneamento ósseo
bonesetter *A person who sets bones without being a physician.*	endireita
border *Margin.*	margem
born, to be *Being present as a result of birth.*	nascer

English	Portuguese
bottle *A container used for the storage of liquids.*	garrafa
bougienage *Passage of a bougie through a body orifice with the goal of increasing the diameter of the orifice.*	passagem de uma vela
brace, to *Application of a splint.*	atar
brace *A splint.*	suporte; órtose
brachial artery *A continuation of the axillary artery and branches into the radial and ulnar among others.*	artéria braquial
brachial plexus *A cluster of nerves coming off the last four cervical and first thoracic spinal nerves form the nerve supply the the chest and arms.*	plexo braquial
brachial plexus neuropathy *Characterized by acute arm or shoulder pain followed by focal muscle weakness.*	neuropatia plexo braquial
brachial *Referring to the arm.*	braquial
brachium cerebelli *Synonym of pedunculus cerebellaris superior (upper portion the cerebellum).*	pedúnculo cerebelar superior
Bracht maneuver *Delivery of a fetus in a breech position.*	manobra de Bracht
brachycephaly *The presence of a short broad skull.*	braquicefalia
bradycardia *Lower than normal cardiac rate measured in beats per minute.*	bradicardia
bradykinin *A peptide that causes contraction of smooth muscle and dilation of blood vessels.*	bradicinina
brain *A common term for cerebrum.*	cérebro
brain death *Cessation of cerebral functioning.*	morte cerebral
brain stem *An organ that consists of the medulla oblongata, pons and midbrain.*	tronco cerebral
brainstem herniation *Movement of the brainstem into the incisura because of increased intracranial pressure.*	herniação tronco cerebral
branchial *Referring to or resembling the gills of a fish.*	branquial
break *A common term for a fracture in a bone.*	fratura
breast *Mammary tissue including the areola.*	peito; mama
breast feeding *The process of giving milk to a baby via the nipple.*	alimentação mamária
breath *One respiration.*	respiração; fôlego
breath sounds *The noise heard upon auscultation with a stethoscope.*	sons respiratórios
breath test (for alcohol) *A check of alcohol level by testing exhaled air.*	bafômetro
breech birth *Delivery with the feet or buttocks coming first.*	parto nádegas
breech presentation *Position of the feet or buttocks near the cervix.*	apresentação de nádegas
bregma *Located at the convergence of the coronal and sagittal sutures.*	bregma
bright *Giving out a lot of light.*	brilhante
bring, to *To carry or transport something.*	trazer
brisk *Rapid or fast.*	rápido
broad ligament of uterus *Supports the uterus on both sides.*	ligamento largo
Brodie's knee *Also referred to as chronic hypertrophic synovitis of the knee.*	joelho de Brodie
broken (arm) *Fracture of the arm.*	braço fraturado
bromidrosis *Foul smelling perspiration.*	bromidrose
bromism *Poisoning caused by excessive intake of bromine.*	bromismo
bronchial carcinoma *A general term for a malignancy of the bronchi.*	carcinoma bronquiolar
bronchial *Referring to the bronchus.*	bronquiolar

English	Portuguese
bronchiectasis *The presence of abnormally wide bronchi or branches.*	bronquiectasia
bronchiole *A small branch that a bronchus divides into.*	bronquílo
bronchiolitis *Inflammation of the pulmonary bronchioles.*	bronquiolite
bronchitis *Inflammation of the mucous membranes of the bronchioles that causes bronchospasm and cough.*	bronquite
bronchogenic *Referring to the bronchi.*	broncogênico
bronchography *Roentgenography of the bronchi after administration of contrast media.*	broncografia
bronchopneumonia *Pneumonia that starts in the distal bronchioles.*	broncopneumonia
bronchoscopy *Use of a scope to visualize the bronchi.*	broncoscopia
bronchospasm *Bronchial smooth muscle spasm.*	broncospasmo
bronchus *The major air channels that bifurcate from the distal trachea.*	brônquio
brow presentation *The term used to describe which part of the body (forehead) is being delivered first in childbirth.*	apresentação de fronte
brown *Coffee-colored.*	castanho
Brown-Séquard syndrome *Unilateral spinal cord lesions, proprioception loss and weakness occur ipsilateral to the lesion, while pain and temperature loss occur contralateral.*	síndrome de Brown-Séquard
brucellosis *A gram-negative bacteria in cattle that causes persistent fever in humans.*	brucelose
Brudzinski sign *Involuntary flexion of the knees and hips after flexion of the neck while supine; seen in meningitis.*	sinal de Brudzinski
bruise *Common term for ecchymosis.*	contusão
bruit *An abnormal sound heard through a stethoscope indicating turbulent blood flow.*	ruído
brush *Implement used for cleaning or for taking a tissue sample.*	escova
brush biopsy *The process of tissue sampling using a brush.*	biopsia por escova
bubo *An inflamed, swollen lymph node in the axilla or inguinal region.*	bubão
bubonic plague *A form of plague exhibited by the formation of buboes.*	peste bubônica
buccal *Referring to the cheek.*	bucal
buccinator *A thin, flat muscle in the cheek wall.*	bucinador
buccinator muscle *Pulls the mouth posteriorly.*	músculo bucinador
Budd-Chiari syndrome *Hepatomegaly, severe portal hypertension and ascites related to thrombosis of the hepatic vein.*	síndrome de Budd-Chiari
bug *Insect.*	bicho
bulbar palsy *Paralysis due to changes in the motor center of the medulla oblongata.*	paralisia bulbar
bulbocavernosus reflex *Brisk contraction of the ischiocavernosus and bulbocavernosus muscles when the glans penis is compressed.*	reflexo bulbocavernoso
bulge *A protuberance on a flat surface.*	bojo
bulimia *Pathologic increase in hunger.*	bulimia
bulky *Voluminous or substantial.*	volumoso
bulla *A large cutaneous serous filled vesicle.*	bolha
bullous pemphigoid *A benign disease of the aged characterized by large bullae forming on the torso and extremities.*	penfigóide bulhosa
Bumke's pupil *Dilation of the pupil in response to anxiety.*	pupila de Bumke

English	Portuguese
bundle branch block *A cardiac dysrhythmia produced by a blockage of a branch of the bundle of His.*	bloqueio de ramo
bundle of His *The atrial contraction rhythm is facilitated by this bundle to the ventricles.*	feixe de His
bunion *Swelling of the bursa of the metatarsal head of the first metatarsal.*	joanete
burn *An injury caused by exposure to heat.*	queimadura
burr or bur *A rotary cutting instrument.*	trépano
burr hole *A treatment of subdural hematoma that involves drilling a hole into the cranium to release the hematoma.*	buraco trépano
bursitis *Inflammation of the bursa.*	bursite
burst, to *To rupture.*	arrebentar
buttocks *The bilateral region covering the gluteal muscles.*	nádegas
Buzzard maneuver *Testing of the patellar reflex while the client firmly touches the floor with their toes in a sitting position.*	manobra de Buzzard
bypass *An alternate route, typically referring to an arterial bypass.*	desvio
byssinosis *A disease caused by inhalation of cotton dust; a type of pneumoconiosis.*	bissinose
cachexia *Generalized weakness and severe wasting.*	caquexia
cadaver *A dead body.*	cadáver
caduceus *An ancient herald's wand with two serpents twined around that is a symbol of the medical arts.*	caduceu
caisson disease *Decompression sickness.*	doença do caixão
calcaneal spur *A bony protrusion on the calcaneus.*	esporão calcâneo
calcaneus *Commonly called the heel bone.*	calcâneo
calcareous *Referring to something containing lime or calcium.*	calcário
calciferol *It is formed when egesterol is exposed to ultraviolet light; a D vitamin.*	calciferol
calcification *Deposition of calcium salts causing hardening of an organic tissue.*	calcificação
calcitonin *A thyroid hormone that lowers serum calcium levels.*	calcitonino
calcium *A chemical element that is an essential component in teeth and bone.*	cálcio
calcium channel blocker *A medication used to treat angina, supraventricular arrhythmias and hypertension; it works by blocking calcium influx into myocytes and vascular smooth muscle cells.*	bloqueadores do canal de cálcio
calculus *A stone of minerals that can lead to the blockage of the bile duct or ureters.*	cálculo
calf *Muscles of the posterior portion of the lower leg.*	panturrilha; barriga da perna
calibrate, to *To adjust an instrument using a standard.*	calibrar
calibration *The process of calibrating an instrument.*	calibração
callosity *Callus; thickened hardened skin.*	calosidade
callus *Thickened hardened skin.*	calo
calorie *A unit of heat.*	caloria
calvaria *The portion of the skull that is composed of the superior aspects of the occipital, parietal and frontal bones.*	calvária
calyx *A cup shaped organ or cavity.*	cálice
canaliculus *A term for various small channels.*	canalículo
cancel, to *To stop or revoke.*	cancelar
cancellous *A bony mesh-like structure with many pores.*	gradeado

English	Portuguese
cancer; carcinoma *A disease of uncontrolled abnormal cell growth.*	cancro (P) câncer (B)
cancroid *A tumor occurring in the stomach, small or large bowel.*	cancróide
cancrum oris *Gangrenous stomatitis.*	estomatite gangrenosa
candle *A cylindrical piece of wax with a central wick.*	vela
canine teeth *Located between the incisors and premolars.*	dentes canino
canker sore *An ulceration, usually of the mouth or lips.*	afta
cannabis *A plant from the Cannibidaceae family that is known for its psychotropic effects.*	canabis
cannula *A tube inserted into the body.*	cánula
cantering rhythm *Gallop rhythm.*	ritmo de galope
capillary *A vessel that connects arterioles to venules.*	capilar
capillary fragility test *Application of a blood pressure cuff high enough to restrict venous return and after five minutes count the number or petechiae produced.*	prova da fragilidade capilar
capillary nevus *A growth of skin that involves the capillaries.*	nevo capilar
capitate bone *The bone at the base of the palm that articulates with the third metacarpal.*	osso capitato
Caplan nodules *These are pulmonary nodules noted in people with rheumatoid arthritis who were exposed to coal dust.*	nódulos de Caplan
capsule *A membranous sheath that covers an organ or structure.*	cápsula
capsulitis *Inflammation of a capsule.*	capsulite
capsulotomy *Incision of a capsule as in with eye surgery.*	capsulotomia
caput *The head.*	cabeça
caput succedaneum *Edema that occurs in the scalp of an infant during child-birth.*	cabeça sucedânea
carbohydrate *A group of organic compounds including sugar and starch.*	carbroidratos
carbon dioxide gas *A gas expelled during exhalation.*	dióxido de carbono
carbon monoxide poisoning *This tasteless, odorless gas causes constitutional symptoms but can lead to death upon inhalation.*	intoxicação pelo monóxido de carbono
carboxyhemoglobin *A compound formed from hemoglobin when it is exposed to carbon monoxide.*	carboxiemoglobina
carcinogenic *That which causes cancer.*	carcingênico
carcinoid *A tumor occurring in the stomach, intestine and colon.*	carcinóide
carcinoma *A malignant growth.*	carcinoma
carcinomatosis *Dissemination of cancer throughout the body.*	carcinmatose
cardia *The superior aspect of the stomach at the opening of the esophagus.*	parte cardial do estômago, que circunda a junção esofagogástrica
cardiac *Referring to the heart.*	cardíaco
cardiac arrest *Cessation of function of the heart.*	parada cardíaca
cardiac failure *Decreased cardiac output of the heart.*	insuficiência cardíaca congestiva
cardiac output *Amount of blood pumped by the heart in liters per minute.*	débito cardíaco
cardiac pacing *Electromechanical stimulation of the heart.*	estimulação cardíaco
cardiology *A specialty of medical practice involve treatment and prevention of heart disease.*	cardiologia
cardiomyopathy *Chronic cardiac muscle disease.*	cardiomiopatia
cardiopulmonary resuscitation *Use of artificial means to support respiration and circulation.*	ressuscitação cardiopulmonar

English	Portuguese
cardiovascular *Referring to the heart or circulatory system.*	cardiovascular
carditis *Inflammation of the heart.*	cardite
caregiver *A person who provides care to another.*	dador de cuidado
caries *Referring to decay or death of a tooth.*	cárie
carina *The protrusion of the lowest tracheal cartilage.*	carina
carneous *Synonym of fleshy.*	carnoso
carotene *A hydrocarbon that can be converted to vitamin A.*	caroteno
carotid body *Carotid artery receptors that are sensitive to blood chemistry changes.*	corpo carotídeo
carotid bruit *An abnormal noise heard over the carotid artery that may be a sign of stenosis or aortic valvular disease.*	ruído carótido
carotid sinus reflex *Bradycardia as a result of pressure on the carotid sinus.*	reflexo do seio carótico
carotid sinus syncope *Dizziness and syncope that results from hyperactivity of the carotid sinus reflex.*	síncope do seio carótico
carotid *Referring to the large artery on each side of the neck.*	carotídeo
carpal tunnel syndrome *Paresthesia that results from compression of the median nerve.*	síndrome do túnel do carpo
carpometacarpal *Referring to the carpus and metacarpus.*	carpometacárpico
carpopedal spasm *A spasm of the carpus and the foot.*	espasmo carpopedal
carpus *The joint between the hand and wrist.*	carpo
caruncle *A small fleshy protuberance.*	carúncula
casein *The principal protein in milk, a phospholipid.*	caseína
Casoni's test *Hydatid fluid is injected intradermally; subsequent formation of a larger papule indicates hydatid disease.*	teste de Casoni
cast; plaster cast *Use of plaster of paris to immobilize an extremity.*	molde de gesso
castor bean *A bean that can yield the poisonous compound ricin.*	mamona
castration *Excision of the gonads.*	castração
casualty *A person who is killed or seriously injured.*	acidente
cat cry syndrome *A hereditary congenital disorder exhibited by microcephaly, hypertelorism, and cognitive deficits.*	síndrome do miado do gato; cri-du-chat síndrome
cat scratch fever *An infectious disease characterized by local inflammation a the site of the scratch, local lymph adenopathy and fever.*	doença da arranhadura do gato
catabolism *The reduction of complex molecules to more simple ones in living organisms.*	catabolismo
catalepsy *A condition exhibited by rigidity and the person maintains the same position if he is moved by another.*	catalepsia
cataphoresis *The use of an electric field to move charged particles in fluid.*	cataforese
cataplexy *A condition exhibited by rigidity and immobility.*	cataplexia
cataract *An opacity of an eye lens or the capsule.*	catarata
catarrh *Inflammation of a mucous membrane.*	catarro
catatonia *Seen in schizophrenia, it is a state of stupor or excitability and abnormal movements.*	catatonia
catch a cold *To come down with a viral upper respiratory tract infection.*	pegar faringite (B); apanhar uma constipação (P)
catharsis *The act of cleansing or purging, usually referring to thought.*	catarse
cathartic *To be cleansed or evacuated, referring to thought or the cleansing of the bowels.*	carético

English	Portuguese
catheter *A flexible tube inserted into the body.*	cateter; sonda
cat's eye pupil *A pupil in the shape of an oval.*	pupila de gato
cauda equina syndrome *Neurologic condition manifested by pain, paresthesia and weakness but no bowel/bladder dysfunction.*	síndrome da cauda eqüina
caudal *Referring to a cauda.*	caudal
caudate *Referring to the caudate nucleus.*	caudato
causative *Something that induces an effect.*	causativo
caustic *Abrasive or corrosive.*	cáustico
cautery *Application of an electric current to cut something.*	cautério
cavernous hemangioma *A tumor composed of connective tissue with blood filled areas.*	hemangioma cavernoso
cavernous sinus *Large venous sinus located adjacent to the sphenoid bone and posterior to the petrosal sinuses.*	seio cavernoso
cavernous sinus thrombosis *A blood clot in the base of the brain.*	trombose de seio cavernoso
cavity *Pouch or chamber.*	cavidade
cecum *The portion of the bowel between the ileum and and the ascending colon.*	ceco
celiac *Referring to the abdominal cavity.*	celíaco
cell body *The portion of the cell containing the nucleus.*	corpo celular
cell membrane *The semipermeable structure surrounding the cytoplasm of a cell.*	membrana celular
cell *The smallest functional unit of an organism.*	célula
cell wall *The peripheral border of the cell.*	parede celular
cellulitis *Infection characterized by diffuse, subcutaneous inflammation.*	celulite
cellulose *A polysaccharide that occurs naturally in fibrous products.*	celulose
center *A point equidistant from all sides.*	centro
centigrade *A scale with 100 gradations, usually referring to a temperature scale.*	centígrado
centimeter *One hundredth of a meter.*	centímetro
central nervous system (CNS) *The brain and spinal cord.*	sistema nervoso central (SNC)
centrifuge *Machine used to separate substances of different weights.*	centrífuga
centripetal *The movement toward the center.*	centrípeto
cephalic *Towards the head.*	cefálico
cercaria *Larval trematode worm that live in a molluscan.*	cercária
cerebellum *The part of the brain in the posterior portion of the skull that controls muscle coordination and movement.*	cerebelo
cerebral malaria *A severe form of malaria manifested by seizures and a decreased level of consciousness.*	malária cerebral
cerebral palsy *A condition exhibited by motor incoordination and speech changes that is the result of brain injury occurring ante-, intra- or post- partum.*	paralisia cerebral
cerebral *Referring to the cerebrum.*	cerebral
cerebration *Operating activity of the cerebrum.*	cerebração
cerebrospinal fluid (CSF) *The fluid between the pia mater and arachnoid membrane.*	fluido cerebroespinhal
cerebrovascular accident (stroke) *A decrease in level of consciousness and paralysis caused by a cerebrovascular thrombosis, hemorrhage or vasospasm.*	acidente vascular cerebral (AVC)

English	Portuguese
cerumen *Waxy substance found normally in the external ear canals.*	cerume; cerúmen
cerumen impaction *External ear canal full of wax resulting in hearing loss until the impaction is removed.*	impactação cerúmen
Cervical insufficiency (formerly incompetent cervix) *Painless changes in the cervix that result in recurrent second semester pregnancy loss.*	cérvix incompotente
cervical pleura *The dome-like cap of the pleura.*	pleura cervical; cúpula da pleura
cervical *Referring to the neck or the cervix.*	cervical
cervicectomy *Excision of the cervix uteri.*	cervicectomia
cervicitis *Inflammation of the cervix.*	cervicite
cervix uteri *The narrow end of the uterus.*	colo uterino
cesarean section *Incision of the abdominal and uterine walls in order to deliver a fetus when natural delivery is not possible.*	cesariana
cestode *A class of parasitic flatworms.*	cestóide
chancre *The initial ulcer that is the source of entry for a pathogen.*	cancro
chancroid *A sexually transmitted disease caused by Haemophilus ducreyi that is exhibited by ulcers without indurated margins.*	cancróide
check for, to	controlar por
cheek *Lateral facial tissue.*	bochecha
chelation *The process used to bind a compound with metal typically used in the treatment of poisoning.*	quelação
cheilitis *Inflammation of the lip.*	quilite
chemoreceptor *A sense organ that responds to stimuli.*	quimiorrecptor
chemosis *Swelling of conjunctival tissue adjacent to the cornea.*	bocejo
chemotaxis *The response of an organism to chemical agents.*	quimiotaxia
chemotherapy *Use of medication (chemical agents) in the treatment of disease. This term is commonly used to refer to the treatment of cancer patients with medication.*	quimioterapia
chest *Thorax.*	tórax
chest leads *Leads going from the skin to an electrocardiographic device.*	derivção padronizada; derivção indireta
chest wall *Thoracic wall.*	parede torácica
chest x-ray *Roentography of the thorax.*	radiografia de tórax
chew, to *Masticate.*	mastigar
Cheyne-Stokes respirations *A breathing pattern characterized by alternating apnea with hyperpnea.*	respiração de Cheyne-Stokes
chiasma *The optic chiasma is the area inferior to the hypothalamus where the optic nerves cross.*	quiasma
chicken pox, varicella *A viral disease characterized by extremely pruritus blisters over the entire body.*	varicela; catapora
chigger *A parasitic mite of the genus Trombicula.*	bicho-do-pé
child *A person aged 1 to 8 years old.*	criança; menino
childbirth *Parturition; the process of labor and delivery of an infant.*	parto
childhood *The time between infancy and puberty.*	infância
chill *Sensation of coldness.*	calafrio
chimera *A mixture of genetically distinct tissues.*	quimera
chin *Mentum; the anterior projection of the lower jaw.*	mento; queixo
chiropodist *A doctor trained in the treatment of feet.*	quiropodista
chiropractic *Referring to the medical practice of adjusting malaligned joints.*	quiropráctico

English	Portuguese
chiropractor *A medical practitioner who is involved with the treatment of disease by manipulating malaligned joints.*	quioprráctica
chlamydiosis *A disease caused by the species Chlamydia.*	clamidiose
chloasma *Brown or black macula that occur on the face during pregnancy or when there is ovarian dysfunction.*	cloasma
chloroform *A colorless, sweet smelling liquid formerly used as a general anesthetic.*	clorofórmio
chloroma *A malignant tumor associated with myelogenous leukemia.*	cloroma
choanae *The two openings between the nasal cavity and the nasopharynx.*	coana
choanal atresia *A congenital condition characterized by blockage of the nasal passages by tissue.*	atresia das coanas
choice *Selection or decision.*	seleção
choke, to *To retch, cough or fight for breath.*	sufocar-se; asfixiar
cholagogue *A compound used to stimulate flow of bile from the liver.*	cholagogo
cholangiogram *Radiologic imaging of the gallbladder and bile ducts.*	colangiograma
cholangitis *Inflammation of the bile ducts.*	colangite
cholecystectomy *Surgical excision of the gallbladder.*	colecistectomia
cholecystenterostomy *Creation of a surgical anastomosis between the intestine and the gallbladder.*	colecistenterotomia
cholecystitis *Inflammation of the gallbladder.*	colecistite
cholecystolithiasis *The presence of gallstones in the gallbladder.*	colecistolitíase
choledocholithotomy *Creation of an incision in the bile duct for the purpose of removing a stone.*	coledocolitotomia
cholelithiasis *Presence or creation of gallstones.*	colelitíase
cholemia *Bile or bile products in the blood.*	colemia
cholera *An infectious disease exhibited by vomiting and diarrhea and caused by Vibrio cholerae.*	cólera
cholestatic hepatitis *Liver inflammation caused by obstruction of bile flow from the liver to the duodenum.*	hepatite colestática
cholesteatoma *A cystic mass that has a lining made of keratinizing material and cholesterol.*	colesteatoma
cholesterol *A compound or its derivatives are found in cell membranes and precursors to hormones but high levels can cause atherosclerosis.*	colesterol
cholinergic *Referring to the stimulation, activation or transmission of acetylcholine.*	colinérgico
cholinesterase *An esterase used to cleave acetylcholine into choline and acetic acid.*	colinesterase
choluria *Term indicating the presence of bile in the urine.*	coluria
chondralgia *Cartilaginous pain.*	condralgia
chondritis *Cartilaginous inflammation.*	condrite
chondroma *Cartilaginous hyperplastic growth.*	condroma
chondromalacia *Excessive softening of the cartilages.*	condromalacia
chondromalacia of the patella *Softening of the articular cartilage of the patella.*	rotúla condromalacia
chondrosarcoma *Cartilaginous tumor which exhibits rapid growth.*	condrossarcoma
chorda *A cord or sinew.*	corda
chordee *Downward bending of the penis.*	corda venérea

English	Portuguese
chorditis *Inflammation of a vocal or spermatic cord.*	cordite
chorea *Involuntary, continuous rapid, jerking movements.*	coréia
chorionic villus *Cord-like projections of a fertilized ovum.*	vilosidades coriônicas
choroid *Similar to the chorion (fertilized ovum or zygote)*	coróide
choroiditis *Inflammation of the choroid.*	coroidite
choroidocyclitis *Inflammation of the ciliary processes and choroid.*	coroidociclite
chromatin *A desocyribose nucleic acid that carries the genes of inheritance.*	cromtina
chromosome *A structure in the nucleus of living cells that carries genetic information.*	cromossoma
chronic *When referring to an illness, it means recurring or persistent.*	crônico
chyle *A combination of lymph fluid and fat that enters the blood via the thoracic duct.*	quilo
chylomicron *A one micron particle of emulsified fat.*	quilomícron
chylous *Referring to chyle.*	quiloso
chyme *The gruel produced by gastric digestion.*	quimo
cicatricial *Referring to cicatrix.*	cicatricial
cicatrix (scar) *New tissue in a healed wound.*	cicatriz
cilia *The hairs growing on the eyelid or a motile extension of a cell surface.*	plural de cilium
ciliary body *The connection between the iris and the choroid.*	corpo ciliar
cinchonism *The toxic effects induced by ingestion of cinchona bark; it is exhibited by tinnitus, deafness and cognitive changes.*	cinchonismo
circadian *Referring to a 24 hour period.*	circadiano
circadian rhythm *Naturally recurring fluctuations in a 24 hour period.*	ritmo circadiano
circumcision *Surgical excision of the foreskin.*	circuncisão
circumference *The distance around an object or part.*	circunferência
circumflex nerve *The axillary nerve that has an origin in the posterior branch of the brachial plexus.*	nervo circunflexo
circumscribed *To have well defined borders.*	circunscrito
cirrhosis *A liver disease characterized by destruction of liver cells and increased connective tissue.*	cirrose
cirsoid *Similar to a tortuous vein, artery or lymph vessel.*	cirsóide
cisternal puncture *A trans-occipitoatlantoid ligament puncture of the cisterna magna so CSF can be obtained.*	punção cisternal
clasp *Holding onto something with one's hand.*	abraço
clasp knife reflex *An abnormal response seen in the setting of a pyramidal tract lesion in which there is a rapid decrease in resistance during passive movement of a joint.*	espacticidade em faca de mola
claudication *Intermittent claudication is a phrase used to describe pain experienced in the leg from arterial insufficiency.*	claudicação
claustrophobia *An unreasonable fear of being in an enclosed environment.*	claustrofobia
clavicle *A bone that articulates with the sternum and scapula.*	clavícula
clavus *A corn or horny protrusion.*	calosidade
clawhand *A hand deformity caused by ulnar nerve palsy exhibited by the hyperextension of the metacarpophalangeal joints and flexion of the interphalangeal articulations.*	mão em garra
clean catch urine specimen *A urine specimen obtained by having a patient cleanse the perineal area prior to voiding in a collection device.*	espécime urinárais meso-corrente

English	Portuguese
clear *Lucid.*	lúcido
clear *Transparent.*	claro
clear one's throat, to *To cough lightly in attempt to speak more clearly.*	carraspear
clearance *The process of removing something.*	depuração
cleavage *A sharp division or demarcation.*	clivagem
cleft lip *A congenital abnormal opening of the lip.*	lábio leporino; lábio fendido
cleft palate *A congenital abnormal opening in the palate.*	fenda palatina
cleidocranial dysostosis *A congenital condition exhibited by abnormal ossification of the cranial bones and absence of clavicles.*	disostose cleidocraniana
cleidotomy *A procedure used in difficult deliveries in which the clavicle is broken to facilitate childbirth.*	cleidotomia
click *A sound heard by the sudden closure of a heart valve.*	estalido
clinic *A building where patients are evaluated.*	clínica
clinical record *The ongoing medical summary.*	fichário
clinical examination *Physical assessment data.*	exame clínico
clitoris *A small erectile body in the anterosuperior aspect of the vulva.*	clitóris
clockwise *Movement in the same direction as a normal clock.*	sentido horário
clonic *Referring to a spasm that alternates in rigidity and relaxation.*	clônico
closed	fechado
closed reduction *The realignment of a fracture without use of surgery.*	redução fechada (de fraturas)
clot *A thrombus or embolus.*	coágulo
clubbing *Increase in the mass of the soft tissue of the terminal phalanges.*	baqueteamento
cluster headache *A unilateral, severe, recurrent headache.*	cefaléia em cacho
cnemial *Referring to the shin.*	cnemial
coagulation *The formation of a clot.*	coagulação
coarctation of the aorta *A stricture, as in narrowing of the aorta.*	coarctação aórtica
coated tablet *A pill covered with a substance to slow absorption or reduce gastric irritation.*	comprimido com revestimento entérico
cobalt *A metal that with causes polycythemia with increased ingestion.*	cobalto
cocaine *A highly addictive opiate derivative.*	cocáina
cocaine addiction *Physical habituation to cocaine.*	dependência cocáina
coccus *A spherical shaped bacterium.*	coco
coccydynia *Coccygeal pain.*	coccidinia
coccyx *The small bone formed by the natural fusion of rudimentary vertebrae.*	cóccix
cochlea *The essential organ of hearing which is in a spiral form.*	cóclea
cock-up splint *A splint used to maintain the wrist in dorsiflexion; used for carpal tunnel syndrome.*	suporte por túnel do carpo
cockroach *A beetle-like insect with long legs and antennae.*	barata
cod *A large marine fish, also called codfish.*	bacalhau
codeine *A morphine derived analgesic.*	codéina
codon *A series of three nucleotides that form a unit of genetic code.*	códon
coffee-ground emesis *Bloody vomitus with appearance of ground coffee.*	vômito em borra de café

English	Portuguese
cogwheel rigidity *As in cogwheel rigidity which is a jerky passive movement after there was increased tone.*	rigidez em roda dentada
cognition *The process of acquiring thought or understanding.*	cognição
cognitive disorders *Any disease process that involves altered cognition.*	distúrbio de cognição
coitus *Sexual intercourse between members of the opposite sex.*	coito
cold *Having a sense of being cold.*	frio (temperatura baixa)
cold sore *A perioral blister caused by herpes simplex.*	herpes simples
cold *Viral upper respiratory tract infection.*	coriza (B); constipação (P)
colectomy *Surgical removal of part of the colon.*	colectomia
colic *Acute abdominal pain.*	cólico
colitis *Inflammation of the colon.*	colite
collagen *The principal supportive protein bone, skin, tendon and cartilage.*	colágeno
collapse *A physical or mental breakdown.*	desabamento
collarbone *Common term for the clavicle.*	clavícula
collodion *A product of the breakdown of colloid.*	colódio
colloid *A solution used for infusion, such as albumin or hetastarch, that are more likely to remain in the intravascular space than crystalloids.*	colóide
coloboma *A congenital defect that involves a fissure of the eye.*	coloboma
colon *The portion of the large intestine that goes from the cecum to the rectum.*	cólon
colonoscopy *Inspection the color, ideally to the cecum, with a lighted scope.*	colonoscopia
color blindness *The inability to distinguish colors.*	cegueira para cores; daltônico
color chart *A card used to check for color blindness.*	gráficos coloridos de Ruess
color of conjunctiva *A point of assessment to check for pallor.*	cores de conjunctiva
colostomy bag *A pouch attached to the skin with a mild adhesive that collects stool emitted from a colostomy.*	bolsa de colostomia
colostomy *Surgically creating an opening in the colon that is extended to outside the abdominal wall.*	colostomia
colostrum *The fluid secreted by the mammary glands a few days around parturition.*	colostro
colpitis; *vaginitis Inflammation of the vagina.*	colpite
colpocele *A hernia into the vagina.*	colpocele
colporrhaphy *A surgical procedure that involves suturing the vagina.*	colporrafia
colposcope *A scope used to visualize the vagina.*	colposcópio
colposcopy *Use of a scope to visualize the vagina and cervix.*	colposcopia
coma *A state of unconsciousness.*	coma
comatose *Referring to a coma.*	comatose
comedone *The medical term (singular) for blackheads.*	comedão
commensal *Living in or on another organism without being a detriment.*	comensal
comment *A remark providing an opinion.*	comentário
common *That which is usual.*	comum
compatible *To coexist without problems.*	compatível
compendium *A concise summary about a subject.*	compêndio
complaint *Grievance.*	queixa
complement fixation test *A laboratory test for the presence of an antibody in the serum that involves inactivation of the complement in the serum.*	prova da fixação de complemento

English	Portuguese
complete blood count *An assay that includes white blood cell, red blood cell, platelet count, hemoglobin, hematocrit and white blood cell differential.*	contagem sangüínea completa
compliance *The act of going along with a plan.*	complacência
comply, to *Adhere to.*	aceder
compound *A substance formed by covalent union of two or more atoms.*	composto
compound fracture *Open fracture.*	fratura aberta
comprehension *Understanding.*	compreensão
compression *Squeezing together.*	compressão
concavity *The state of being concave.*	concavidade
concentration *The quantity of a substance per unit volume.*	concentração
concentric *Referring to circles or arcs that share the same center.*	concêntrico
conception *The act of an egg being fertilized by sperm.*	concepção
concha *A part of the body that is spiral shaped. Nasal concha are the small bones in the sides of the nasal cavity.*	concha
concretion *A hard solid mass.*	concreção
concussion *Head trauma resulting in temporary loss of consciousness.*	concussão
condom *A covering for the penis or the vagina (female condom) used during sexual intercourse that is meant to reduce the chance of pregnancy or infection.*	preservativo
condyle *A rounded protrusion of a bone.*	côndilo
condyloma *A warty papule near the anus or vulva.*	condiloma
cone *A light sensitive cell in the retina.*	cone
confabulation *The fabrication of experiences to compensate for memory loss.*	confabulação
confidence *Self-assurance.*	confiánca
confinement *As in confined to bed.*	confinatmento
conflict *Dispute or disagreement.*	conflito
confusion *Disorientation.*	confusão
congenital *A disease or anomaly present from birth.*	congênito
congenital heart disease *A cardiac disorder present prior to birth.*	doença fetalis cardíaca
congenital syphilis *Passed to the child in utero, the child may have failure to thrive, fever and a flattened bridge of the nose.*	sífilis congênito
congestive	congestivo
congestive heart failure *A diminished cardiac output leading to passive engorgement.*	insuficiência cardíca congestiva
conjugate diameter *A pelvic inlet measurement used to determine whether a woman is capable of delivering a fetus vaginally.*	diametro conjugado
conjunctiva *The membrane that lines the eyelid.*	conjuntiva
conjunctival reflex *Closure of the eyes in response to irritation of the conjunctiva.*	reflexo conjuntiva
conjunctivitis *Inflammation of the conjunctiva.*	conjuntivite
consanguinity *The relationship by blood.*	consangüinidade
conscious *Being award and being able to respond to one's surroundings.*	consciência
consensual light reflex *Constriction of the pupil of one eye in sync with the other pupil upon exposure to light.*	reflexo luminoso consensual
conservative *Control rather than elimination of a disease.*	conservador
consistent *Compatible with something or congruous with.*	consistente

English	Portuguese
consolidation *An area of fixed secretions in the lung.*	consolidação
constipation *A condition exhibited by difficulty in having a bowel movement due to hard stools.*	constipação (B); prisão de ventre (P); obstipação
constriction *Circumferential tightening.*	constrição
contact *The touching of two bodies or a person who has been exposed to a contagious disease.*	contato; contacto
contact lens *A lens that fits over the cornea to correct refractive errors.*	lentes de contacto
contagious *Description of a disease that can be spread by direct or indirect contact.*	contagioso
contaminate, to *To make impure by exposing to an polluted agent.*	contaminar
content *What something is made up of.*	matéria
contraceptive *A device or medication used to prevent pregnancy.*	contraceptivo
contradictory *Two elements that are inconsistent.*	contraditório
contraindication *A situation in which two elements are inconsistent.*	contradição
contusion *An area of broken capillaries in the skin causing discoloration; commonly called a bruise.*	contusão
convenient *Opportune or well-timed.*	conveniente
conversion reaction *When referring to a psychiatric condition it is the exhibition of physical symptoms as a manifestation of mental disease.*	reação de conversão
convex *Having an exterior curved the outside of a sphere.*	convexo
convulsion *An involuntary series of tonic and clonic movements.*	convulsão
cool *Chilly or cold.*	fresco; frio
cope, to *To deal with a difficult situation.*	lidar com
copper *A chemical element with atomic number of 29.*	cobre
copra itch *A pruritus noted in people working with copra (dried kernel from a coconut).*	prurida da copra
copulation *Sexual relations.*	cópula
cor pulmonale *Heart disease that is secondary to lung disease.*	coração pulmonar
coracoid *A prominence on the scapula to which the biceps is attached.*	coracóide
cord compression *Pressure being applied to the spinal cord.*	compressão de cordão espinhal
cord presentation *The presence of the umbilical cord at the cervix during active labor.*	prolapso do cordão umbilical
core *Central part of a structure.*	núcleo
cornea *The transparent segment located at the anterior part of the eye.*	córnea
corneal *Referring to the cornea.*	corneano
corneal reflex *Closure of the eyelids when the cornea is touched lightly with a soft material. Also called the lid reflex.*	reflexo corneano
corneal transplant *Surgical replacement of a cornea with a donor cornea.*	transplante corneal
coronal suture *The line of intersection of the frontal bone and the two parietal bones.*	sutura coronal
coronary angiography *Roentgenographic visualization of the coronary vessels after injection of dye.*	angiografia coronário
coronary occlusion *A blockage in a coronary artery.*	oclusão coronaria
coronary vessel *Referring to a coronary artery.*	vaso cororário
coroner *A person who investigates sudden or suspicious deaths.*	médico legista
coronoid *Crown-shaped.*	coronóide

English	Portuguese
corpulence *Fatness.*	corpulência
corpus callosum *A point of connection between the two cerebral hemispheres.*	corpo caloso
corpus luteum *A structure that is discharged from an ovary; it degenerates if it is not impregnated.*	corpo lúteo
corpuscle *A red or white blood cell.*	corpúsculo
cortex *An external layer.*	córtex
cortical *Referring to the cortex.*	cortical
corticosteroid *A hormone developed in the adrenal cortex.*	corticosteróide
corticotropin *A hormone of the adrenal cortex.*	corticoropina
cortisol *An adrenal cortical hormone, also called hydrocortisone.*	cortisol
cortisone *An adrenal cortical hormone responsible for carbohydrate regulation.*	cortisona
coryza *An acute condition exhibited by copious nasal discharge.*	coriza
cost *The fee or penalty.*	preço
costochondritis *Inflammation of the rib and or its cartilage.*	costocondrite
cotton wool *Raw cotton.*	algodão
cotton wool spots *Condition characterized by blue or white discoloration on the retina related to nerve ischemia.*	mancha algodonosas
cough *Forceful expulsion of air from the lungs.*	tosse
coughing fit *An episode of prolonged, forceful coughing.*	tosse prolongado
count, to *To determine a number.*	contar
cowpox; vaccinia *A viral disease of cows that was used for an original smallpox vaccine.*	varíola bovina
cow's milk	leite de vaca
coxalgia *Pain in the hip.*	coxodinia
crab louse *Phthirus pubis is formal name for a louse that infests pubic hair and causes intense itching.*	piolho caranguejo; piolho pubiano
crack one's knuckles *Moving the fingers side to side or with flexion in such a manner to cause a popping or crackling sound.*	estourar nó dos dedos
crackles or rales *A crackling noised noted while auscultating the lungs.*	estalido
cradle *A bed for an infant.*	berço
cramp *A painful contraction of muscles.*	grampo
cranial mononeuropathy III *Dysfunction of the third cranial nerve causes double vision and eyelid drooping.*	mononeuropatia cranial III
cranial mononeuropathy VI *A disorder of the sixth cranial nerve causes double vision.*	mononeuropatia cranial VI
cranial *Referring to the skull.*	cranial; craniano
cranioclast *An instrument used to crush a fetal skull.*	cranioclasto
craniopharyngioma *A tumor that originates in the hypophyseal stalk.*	craniofaringioma
craniosynostosis *Closure of the sutures of the skull that occurs prematurely.*	craniossinostose
craniotabes *Softening of the skull bones causing widened sutures; this occurs in rickets.*	craniotabe
craniotomy *Surgical creation of a hole in the skull.*	craniotomia
cranium *The skeleton of the head.*	crânio
craving *An unusually strong urge for something.*	desejo
craw-craw *A pruritic papular skin eruption sometimes caused by Onchocerca.*	kra-kra
creatine *A compound involved with muscle contraction.*	creatina

English	Portuguese
creatinine *A compound excreted in the urine that is produced by the metabolism of creatine.*	creatinina
Credé's maneuver *Manual pressure over the bladder to assist in expression of urine in an atonic bladder.*	manobra de Credé
cremasteric reflex *Retraction of the testicle and scrotum upon stroking of the ipsilateral inner thigh.*	reflexo cremastérico
crenotherapy *A form of treatment from mineral springs.*	crenoterapia
crepitus *A noise heard when one auscultates the lungs that is similar to the sound of rubbing hair between one's fingers. It is also considered the sound of two broken bones rubbing together.*	crepitação
cretinism *A chronic condition caused by diminished thyroid hormone secretion.*	cretinismo
crevice *A narrow opening.*	fenda
cribriform *Like a sieve; the olfactory nerves pass through the cribriform plate of the ethmoid bone.*	cribriforme
cricoid cartilage *The ring-shaped cartilage of the larynx.*	cartilago cricóide
cripple *A person with a physical disability; not used in polite society.*	aleijado
crisis *A turning point in the treatment of a disease.*	crise
Crohn's disease *An inflammatory bowel disease.*	doença de Crohn
cross-infection *Transfer of infection between individuals, each with a different organism.*	infecção cruzada
cross-matching (blood) *Evaluation of blood to determine compatibility between the donor and recipient prior to transfusion.*	reação cruzada
cross-section *A transverse section through a specimen or structure.*	corte transversal
croup *An acute laryngeal condition that is accompanied by a hoarse, barking cough.*	crupe
cruciform *Shaped like a cross.*	cruciforme
crural; femoral *Referring to the femur or leg.*	crural
crush syndrome *Rhabdomyolysis occurring as a result of muscle injury from mechanical stress.*	síndrome de esmagamento
crust *Dried serous exudate covering a wound.*	crosta
crutch *Long metal or wooden stick used for support while walking.*	muleta
cryesthesia *Abnormal sensitivity to cold.*	criestesia
cryosurgery *The application of extreme cold to destroy tissue.*	criocirurgia
cryotherapy *The use of cold for therapeutic purposes.*	crioterapia
cryptococcal meningitis *A meningeal infection associated with AIDS.*	meningite criptocócica
cryptorchism *A condition characterized by the failure of the testes to descend into the scrotum.*	criptorquismo
cryptosporidiosis *A parasitic related diarrhea seen in AIDS.*	criptosporidiose
crystalloid *A substance that can pass through a semipermeable membrane; not a colloid.*	cristalóide
crystalluria *The presence of crystals in the urine.*	cristalúria
CSF *Abbreviation for cerebrospinal fluid.*	FCE fluido cerebroespinhal
CT scan *Computerized axial tomography.*	TC tomografia computadorizada
cubital fossa *The bend at the elbow.*	fossa cubital
cuffed endotracheal tube *A cannula that has an balloon on the tip that can be inflated with air and placed into the trachea.*	tubo endotraqueal
culdoscopy *Examination of the female pelvic viscera with a scope inserted through the posterior vaginal fornix.*	culdoscopia

English	Portuguese
culture *The growth of bacteria in artificial medium.*	cultura
culture broth *A medium used to grow bacteria.*	meio cultura
cumulative effect *A consequence of successive additions.*	efeito cumulativo
cuneiform *The three bones between the navicular bone and the metatarsals.*	cuneiforme
curare *A toxic botanical substance used at one time in poison darts in South America. Curare derivatives have been used in general anesthesia.*	curare
curative *A remedy capable of healing completely.*	curativo
cure *A remedy for a medical illness.*	cura
curettage *Removal of tissues from a cavity.*	curetagem
curette *The instrument used during a curettage.*	cureta
current *Flow or stream.*	corrente
currently *Presently.*	circulante
Cushing's syndrome *Characterized by truncal obesity, moon face, acne, abdominal striae, hypertension, decreased carbohydrate tolerance, protein catabolism, psychiatric disturbances, and osteoporosis.*	síndrome de Cushing
cushion *A pillow or stuffed pad used to sit on.*	almofada
cut *An incision.*	dissecção
cutaneous *Referring to the skin.*	cutâneo
cuticle *The dead skin at the base of the toenail or fingernail, also called the eponychium.*	cutícula
cyanocobalamin *Also called B12; used to treat pernicious and other macrocytic anemias.*	cianocobalmino
cyanosis *Bluish discoloration of the skin and mucous membranes.*	cianose
cyclical vomiting *Periods of recurrent vomiting with no apparent pathologic cause and the person has a normal state of health between the episodes.*	vômito cíclico
cyclitis *Inflammation of the ciliary body.*	ciclite
cyclodialysis *The surgical creation of a communication between the anterior chamber of the eye and the suprachorodial space for the purpose of treating glaucoma.*	ciclodiálise
cycloplegia *Paralysis of the ciliary muscle.*	cicloplegia
cyclothymia *Manic-depressive tendencies.*	ciclotimia
cyclotomy *Surgically creating an opening in the ciliary body.*	ciclotomia
cystadenoma *Adenoma associated with cysts of neoplastic origin.*	cistadenoma
cystectomy *Surgical removal of a cyst or the bladder.*	cistectomia
cystic *Referring to a cyst.*	cístico
cystic duct *The duct connecting the gallbladder to the common bile duct.*	ducto cístico
cystic fibrosis *A congenital disorder exhibited by abnormal thick mucous which leads to problems in the intestines, pancreas and lungs.*	fibrose cística
cysticercosis *The state of being infected with a type of tapeworm.*	cisticerose
cystinosis *A congenital disorder of increased cystine that leads to renal insufficiency, rickets and dwarfism.*	cistinose
cystinuria *The presence of cystine in the urine.*	cistinúria
cystitis *Inflammation of the urinary bladder.*	cistite
cystocele *Protrusion of the urinary bladder through the vaginal wall.*	cistocele

English	Portuguese
cystography Roentgenographic visualization of the urinary bladder after insertion of contrast media.	cistografia
cystolithiasis Presence of a calculus in the urinary bladder.	cistolitíase
cystoscope A device used to visualized the urinary bladder.	cistoscopio
cystoscopy Direct visualization of the urinary bladder with a cystoscope.	cistoscopia
cytology The study of cells, their function and structure.	citologia
cytoplasm The protoplasm of the cell except for the nucleus.	citoplasma
cytotoxic Referring to being harmful to cells.	citotóxico
cytotoxin That which is harmful to cells.	citotoxina
dacryoadenitis Inflammation of the lacrimal gland.	dacrioadenite
dacryocystitis Inflammation of a lacrimal sac.	dacriocistite
dacryocystorhinostomy Surgical reaction of a communication between the lacrimal sac and nasal cavity.	dacriocistorrinostomia
dacryolith A stone in the lacrimal sac or duct.	dacriólito
dandruff Dead skin found in the hair.	caspa
dark adaptation Adjustment to low light by reflex dilation of the pupil.	adaptação á escuridão
date of admission Beginning date of hospitalization.	data de admissão
date of birth	data de nascimento
daughter	filha
De Quervain tenosynovitis Inflammation of the tendons of the wrist including the abductor pollicis longus and extensor pollicis brevis.	tonossinovite de De Quervain
dead Deceased.	morto
dead space The area in the respiratory tract where air is not exchanged.	espaço morto
deadline Cutoff date.	último prazo
deaf Absence of the sense of hearing.	surdo
deaf-mute Inability to hear or speak.	surdo-mudo
deafness Having impaired hearing.	surdez
death The action of dying.	morte
debility Physical weakness.	debilidade
debridement Trimming the dead tissue adjacent to a wound.	debridamento
decade Ten years.	década
decapitate, to The physical separation of the head from the body.	decapitação
decerebrate rigidity Rigid extension of the arms which is an abnormal posture associated with increased intracranial pressure.	rigidez descerebrada
decerebrate The removal of the brain.	descerebrar
decibel A unit used in the measurement of sound.	decibel
decidua The mucous membrane lining the uterus during pregnancy.	decídua
deciduous teeth The first teeth.	dentes decíduo
decline As in a decrease in status or health.	declínio
decompensation The inability of an organ to respond to functional overload.	descompensação
decompression The surgical procedure relieving pressure on a part.	descompressão
decrease Becoming smaller or fewer.	decréscimo
decubitus ulcer A wound caused by laying in one position for too long; also referred to as a pressure ulcer.	úlcera de decúbito

English	Portuguese
decussation *An area of intersection.*	decussação
deep *Having significant depth.*	profundo
deep tendon reflex *Reflexes exhibited by the stretching of a tendon.*	reflexo profundo tendinoso
deep vein thrombosis (DVT) *A blood clot that forms within a vein, typically in the lower extremities.*	trombose venosa profunda (TPV)
deer tick *Ixodes scapularis.*	carrapato das patas pretas
defecation *The discharge of feces from the rectum.*	defecação
defect *A shortcoming or imperfection.*	defeito
defibrillator *A device used to convert an abnormal cardiac rhythm (ventricular fibrillation) into a normal rhythm with use of electrical stimulation.*	desfibrilação
deficiency *Insufficiency or deficit.*	deficiência
deformity *A malformation or imperfection.*	deformidade
deglutition *The process of swallowing.*	deglutição
dehydration *The status of having a decrease in total body water.*	desidratação
delirium *An acute mental state exhibited by altered thought processes and restlessness.*	delírio
delirium tremens *A condition seen when alcohol is withdrawn which is exhibited by restlessness, hallucinations and tremors.*	delírio por supressão álcool
delivery *The process of giving birth.*	parto; nascimento
deltoid *A term referring to "three". The deltoid muscle has its origin at three areas: clavicle, acromion, and spine of the scapula.*	deltóide
delusion *A belief that is contradictory to rational thought.*	delírio; ilusão
delusional *Referring to a delusion.*	delirante
demanding *Requiring a lot of skill or requiring a lot of others.*	exigente
demarcation *Having a fixed boundary.*	demarcação
dementia *A chronic brain disorder exhibited by memory loss, personality changes and faulty reasoning.*	demência
demography *The study of the structure of human populations.*	demografia
demulcent *Something that relieves irritation or inflammation.*	demulcente
demyelinating disease *A condition characterized by the loss of myelin.*	doença desmielinizante
dendrite *Impulses are transmitted along a dendrite to a nerve cell body.*	dendrito
denervation *The removal of nerve supply.*	desnervação
dengue *A mosquito-borne viral disease exhibited by fever and joint pain.*	dengue
density *The denseness of an object.*	densidade
dental *Referring to teeth.*	dental
dental calculus *Calcium phosphate and carbonate adhered to the teeth.*	cálculo dentário
dental caries *Decay of teeth.*	cárie dentária
dentatum *Also referred to as dentate nucleus of cerebellum.*	dentado
dentist *A professional capable of treating diseases of the teeth and gums.*	dentista
dentition *The natural teeth.*	dentição
denture *A frame that holds artificial teeth.*	dentadura
deny, to *To reject or repudiate.*	negar
deoxyribonucleic acid (DNA) *The carrier of genetic information.*	ácido desoxirribonucléico
depilatory *An agent used to remove hair.*	depilatório

English	Portuguese
depressed *Melancholy.*	deprimido
depressed skull fracture *Concave fracture deformity of the skull.*	fratura do crânio com afundamento
depression *A medical condition exhibited by profound despondency.*	depressão
deprivation *The lack of a necessity.*	privação
dermatitis *Non-specific inflammation of the skin.*	dermatite
dermatography *A description of the skin.*	dermatografia
dermatologist *A physician specializing in dermatology.*	dermatologiststa
dermatology *The medical profession involving the treatment of skin conditions.*	dermatologia
dermatome *The area of sensation of the skin supplied by a single posterior spinal root.*	dermátomo
dermatomycosis *An infection of the skin by Trichophyton, Microsporum or Epidermophyton fungi.*	dermatomicose
dermatomyositis *Inflammation of the skin, subcutaneous tissue and adjacent muscle.*	dermatomiosite
dermatophyte *A fungal parasite living on the skin.*	dermatófito
dermatosis *Any skin disease.*	dermatose
dermis *The "true skin" that lies beneath the epidermis.*	pele
dermographia *A raised, pale line with hyperemic borders is elicited upon scratching the skin with a dull instrument, in this condition.*	dermografia
dermoid cyst *An abnormal growth containing hair follicles, skin and sebaceous glands.*	cisto dermóide
descending *Moving toward the inferior portion.*	descendente
desensitize, to *To gradually expose a person to an offending agent to prevent an abnormal response upon a secondary exposure.*	dessensibilizar
desiccation *The act of drying up.*	dessecação
desmoid *A tumor typically found in the abdomen which contains. muscle and connective tissue.*	desmóide
despite *Notwithstanding.*	despeito
desquamation *The shedding of skin in flakes or sheets.*	descamação
deterioration *Worsening in one's medical condition.*	deterioração
detoxification *The process of removing toxins from the body.*	detoxicação
detrimental *Harmful.*	maligno
detritus *Particulate matter produced by the decomposition of an organic substance.*	detrito
detrusor urinae *Smooth muscle fibers that extend from the urinary bladder to the pubis.*	detrusor da urina
deuteranomaly *Abnormal color vision sometimes called "green weakness".*	deuteranomalia
deviated septum *Characterized by deviation of the nasal septum.*	septo desviado
deviation *Away from the norm.*	desvio
dexter; *right; straight; erect*	destro
dextran *A high glucose polymer used as a plasma substitute.*	dextrana
dextrocardia *Location of the heart in the right hemithorax.*	dextrocardia
dhobie itch *So called because the contact dermatitis is caused by the soap used by laundry workers in India who are called "dhobie".*	tinha crural

English	Portuguese
diabetes insipidus *Caused by a deficiency in vasopressin, it is exhibited by great thirst and large volume urine output (and normal blood sugar).*	diabete insípido
diabetes mellitus *A disease exhibited by a deficiency of the pancreatic hormone insulin.*	diabete melito
diabetic *A person who has diabetes mellitus.*	diabético
diabetic neuropathy *Pain and burning initially in the feet, associated with diabetes mellitus.*	neuropatia diabético
diagnostic *A specific symptom or characteristic.*	diagnóstico
diapedesis *The outward passage of blood elements through an intact vessel wall.*	diapedese
diaper *Undergarment worn to absorb urine in incontinent persons.*	fralda
diaper rash *Macular rash in the inguinal/perineal region related to exposure to urine.*	erupção cutâneo das fraldas
diaphoretic *Exhibited by profuse perspiration.*	diaforético
diaphragm *The muscular separation between the thoracic and abdominal cavities.*	diafragma
diaphragmatic hernia *Protrusion of visceral contents through the diaphragm.*	hérnia diafragmática
diaphysis *The central part of a long bone.*	diáfise
diarrhea *Increase in frequency and a loose consistency of the stools.*	diarréia
diarthrosis *An articulation allowing free movement.*	diartrose
diastase *Amylase.*	diastase
diastole *The period of dilatation of the heart; between the first and second heart sounds.*	diástole
diathermy *The use of heat produced from high-frequency electric currents to medically or surgically treat someone.*	diatermia
diathesis *A medical tendency to develop a specific condition.*	diátese
die, to *To stop living, to expire.*	morrer
diet *The kinds of food a person eats.*	dieta
dietitian *A professional who works with diet and nutrition.*	médico especialista em dietas
differential *A term used to refer to the various options for diagnoses.*	diferencial
differential diagnosis *A list of possible alternative diagnoses for a patient who is ill.*	diagnóstico diferencial
differential leukocyte count *The percentage of different types of leukocytes.*	célula sangüínea branca diferential
digestion *The process of enzymatic breakdown of food in the alimentary canal.*	digestão
digit *Finger.*	dígito
digitalis *Cardiac medication derived from the leaf of Digitalis purpurea.*	digital
dilatation *The process of becoming wider or larger.*	dilatação
dilator *An instrument that dilates.*	dilatador
dilution *The process of making a weaker solution.*	diluição
dimercaprol *A medication used as a binding agent for heavy metal poisoning.*	dimercaprol
dioptre *Referring to refraction or transmitted and refracted light.*	dioptria
dioxide *A compound containing two oxygen atoms.*	dióxido
diphtheria *A contagious bacterial disease characterized by a grey membrane on the pharynx along with respiratory or cutaneous symptoms; caused by Corynebacterium diphtheriae.*	difteria

English	Portuguese
diplegia *The paralysis of both arms or both legs.*	diplegia
diplococcus *A bacterium that occurs in pairs including pneumococcus and Neisseria gonorrhoeae and Neisseria meningitidis.*	diplococos
diploid *A nucleus containing two complete sets of chromosomes.*	diplóide
diplopia *Double vision.*	diplopia
dipsomania *Twins that are joined at some part of their bodies.*	dipsomania
dirty *Unclean.*	sujo
disability *Decreased or impaired mental or physical ability.*	incapacidade
disaccharide *A type of sugar that yields two monosaccharides upon hydrolysis.*	dissacarídeo
disappearance *An instance of something/someone gone missing.*	desaparecimento
disarticulation *The separation or amputation of a joint.*	desarticulação
discharge, ear *Otic secretions.*	descarga ótico
discharge, nasal *Nasal secretions.*	descarga rinal
discharge, postpartum vaginal *The secretions noted after delivery.*	pós-descarga
discharge, vaginal *Vaginal secretions.*	descarga vaginal; corrimento vaginal
discharge date *The day a patient is released from the hospital.*	data de alta
discomfort *A feeling of physical or mental unease.*	desconforto
discrete *Separate and distinct.*	discreto
disease *Malady or disorder.*	doença
disease outcome *The response obtained from treatment.*	resultado
disequilibrium *The absence of stability.*	desequilíbrio
disinfectant *A substance that kills bacteria.*	desinfetante
dislocation *The displacement of a bone when referring to an articulation.*	deslocação
disorder *Impairment.*	distúrbio
disorientation *Mental confusion.*	desorientação
displacement *Movement from normal position.*	deslocamento
disrobe, to *To remove clothing.*	despojar
dissecting aneurysm *A condition in which blood is present between the layers of an artery.*	aneurisma dissecante
dissection *Autopsy or postmortem exam.*	dissecção
dissemination *To be spread or dispersed widely.*	disseminação
dissolution *Disintegration.*	dissolução
distal *Situated away from the center of the body.*	distal
distended bladder *Urinary bladder filled beyond the normal capacity.*	bexiga distensão
distension *Swollen.*	distensão
distichiasis *Presence of two rows of eyelashes on one eyelid which are turned inward toward the globe.*	distiquíase
distribution *The manner in which something is shared or spread out.*	distribuição
diuresis *Increased excretion of urine.*	diurese
diuretic *Medication which causes an increased excretion of urine.*	diurético
diurnal *Occurring during the day.*	diurno
diverticulitis *Inflammation of the diverticulum.*	diverticulite
diverticulosis *Presence of diverticulum.*	diverticulose

English	Portuguese
diverticulum A sac or pouch created by herniation of a mucous membrane in the alimentary canal.	divertículo
diver A person who swims in deep water.	mergulhador
dizygotic twins Twins from two separate zygotes (non-identical twins).	gêmeos dizigóticos
dizziness Sensation of losing one's balance.	vertigem
DNA Deoxyribonucleic acid. The hereditary material in humans and almost all other organisms.	ADN ácido desoxirribonucléico
DNR Do not resuscitate. The term used to indicate a person should not have life sustaining measures taken if they were to have cardiopulmonary arrest.	não ressuscitar
donor Referring to a person who donates tissue or an organ.	doador
dopa reaction A dopa-oxidase reaction, changing dopa into melanin.	reação dopa
dopamine An intermediate product in the creation of norepinephrine.	dopamina
dorsal Referring to the back or back surface.	dorsal
dorsal root A description of the site of ganglion found on the dorsal root of each spinal nerve.	raiz dorsal
dorsiflexion Backward bending of the foot or hand.	dorsiflexão
dorsum The back part.	dorso
dosage The amount and frequency a medication is given.	dosagem
dose The quantity of a medication.	dose
dose, maintenance The chronic dose given after the initial bolus.	dosa de manutenção
dosing interval The number of times per unit a medication is given.	dose freqüência
double Twice the size, quantity or strength.	duplo
douche Cleansing of a canal; unless otherwise specified it refers to cleansing of the vaginal canal.	ducha
Douglas' pouch A recess in the peritoneum between the rectum and the uterus. Also called the rectouterine pouch.	bolsa de Douglas
down In a lower position.	desanimado
Down's syndrome A congenital chromosomal defect (trisomy 21) that causes diminished intellectual function, short stature and a broad face.	síndrome de Down
drainage tube A cannula used to allow outflow of fluids.	sonda de drenagem
drape The fabric used as a sterile covering in the OR.	campo
drastic Having significant effect.	drástico
dream The thoughts or images occurring during sleep.	sonho
dressing The gauze applied to a wound.	curativo
dribble, to To slowly, drip-by-drip, release urine for example.	gotejar
drill Cylindrical metal tool uses for creating a hole in bone in surgery.	broca
drink, to To imbibe.	beber
drinking water Water clean enough to ingest orally.	água potável
drop A single bit of fluid as in a drop seen while giving IV fluids.	glóbulo líquido, um
drop by drop Expression meaning little by little.	gota a gota
drop foot gait A gait characterized by dragging the foot, as there is no ankle dorsiflexion; usually associated with steppage gait.	marcha em passos altos
drop foot The symptom in a person with a nerve injury causing impaired ankle dorsiflexion.	pé em gota; pé caído

English	Portuguese
dropper *A device used to administer medicines one drop at a time.*	conta-gotas
drops per minute *Refers to iv fluid rate.*	gotas por minuto
drowning *The process of dying from submerging in and inhaling water.*	afogamento
drowsiness *Sleepiness.*	sonolência
drug *A medication, sometimes with negative connotation.*	droga
drug dependence *Addiction to a substance.*	abuso de substâncias
drug eruption *A diffuse rash caused by a medication.*	erupção por drogas
drug reaction *Typically refers to an adverse effect of medication.*	reação por drogas
drunk *Inebriated.*	inebriação
dry *Absence of moisture.*	seco
dry cough *A cough without sputum production.*	tosse seca
dual diagnosis *Term used to describe the presence of alcohol/ drug addiction associated with a psychiatric diagnosis such as depression.*	abuso de substâncias e diagnóstico psiquiátrico
duct *Hollow tubular tissue used to carry fluid from a secretory organ.*	ducto
ductus arteriosus *A fetal artery that communicates between the pulmonary artery and the descending aorta.*	ducto de Botallo
dumping syndrome *Characterized by rapid bowel evacuation after eating in patients with prior gastric surgery.*	síndrome do esvaziamento rápido
duodenal *Referring to the duodenum.*	duodenal
duodenal ulcer *A defect in the lining of the first portion of the small bowel, typically caused by H. pylori.*	úlcera duodenal
duodenectomy *Excision of the duodenum.*	duodenectomia
duodenitis *Inflammation of the duodenum.*	duodenite
duodenum *The portion of the small bowel between the stomach and jejunum.*	duodeno
duplication *The process of duplicating something.*	duplicação
Dupuytren's contracture *A disease of the palmar fascia causing a flexion contracture of the fourth and fifth fingers.*	contratura de Dupuytren
dura mater *The outermost covering of the brain and spinal cord.*	dura-máter
dust *Dry earthen particles found on the ground and surfaces.*	pó
dwarf *Abnormally small person.*	anão
dysaphia *Altered sense of touch.*	disafia
dysarthria *Difficulty in articulation of speech.*	disartria
dysbarism *Condition caused by a change in pressure, noted most commonly among scuba divers.*	disbarismo
dyschezia *Pain experienced during defecation.*	disquezia
dyschondroplasia *The formation of cartilaginous and bony tumors near the epiphyses.*	discondroplasia
dyscoria *A discordance in pupillary reaction.*	discoria
dyscrasia *An abnormal condition, mostly referring to the blood.*	discrasia
dysdiadocokinesia *The inability to arrest one motor response and substitute its opposite.*	disdiadococinesia
dysentery *A severe form of diarrhea with blood and mucous in the stool.*	disenteria
dysesthesia *1. Impairment of the sense of touch. 2. The presence of persistent pain upon receiving a light touch.*	disestesia
dysfunction *Abnormal function in a gland or body organ.*	disfunção
dyshidrosis *Disregulation of sweating*	disodrose

English	Portuguese
dyshidrotic eczema *A dermatitis characterized by vescicobullous lesions.*	eczema disodrotica
dyskinesia *Abnormal movement.*	discinesia
dyslalia *The absence of comprehensible speech articulation.*	dislalia
dyslexia *Difficulty in learning or reading written language with no effect on intelligence.*	dislexia
dysmenorrhea *Pain during menstruation.*	dismenorréia
dyspareunia *Pain during sexual intercourse.*	dispareunia
dyspepsia *Indigestion.*	dispepsia
dysphagia *Difficulty in swallowing.*	disfagia
dysphasia *Difficulty in speaking caused by cerebral dysfunction.*	disfasia
dysplasia *The increase in organ size due to an increase in the number of abnormal cell types.*	displasia
dyspnea *Difficult breathing.*	dispnéia
dystocia *Difficult birth caused by fetal position, narrow pelvis or lack of opening of the cervix.*	distocia
dysuria *Difficulty or pain upon urination.*	disúria
ear *The organ of hearing and balance.*	orelha; ouvido
ear infection *General term referring to otitis media or otitis externa.*	infecção orelha
ear, external *Auris externa.*	ouvido externo
ear, inner *Auris interna.*	ouvido interno
ear, middle *Auris media.*	ouvido médio
ear-drum *Common term for tympanic membrane.*	tímpano
earache *Pain associated with the ear.*	otalgia
earlobe *The soft, fleshy inferior portion of the pinna.*	lóbulo da oelha
eat, to *To consume food.*	comer
eating disorder *General term for pathologic eating habits.*	distúrbio alimentar
ecchondroma *Hyperplastic growth of cartilage on the surface of other cartilage.*	econdroma
ecchymosis *Skin discoloration caused by bleeding beneath the epidermis.*	equimose
Echinococcus *A tapeworm of the family Taeniidae that can cause hydatid cysts.*	equinococo
echocardiography *The use of ultrasound waves to visualize the heart and its structures.*	ecocardiografia
echolalia *The meaningless repetition of the words spoken by another person.*	ecolalia
eclampsia *A maternal condition characterized by convulsions and hypertension that can lead to maternal and fetal death.*	eclâmpsia
ecmnesia *Memory loss for recent events but retained memory of remote events.*	ecmnésia
ectasia *Expansion or distension.*	ectasia
ectoderm *The outermost layer of the three layers of the embryo.*	ectoderma
ectopic *Abnormal position.*	ectópico
ectopic pregnancy *A pregnancy that is not intrauterine.*	gravidez ectópica
ectrodactylia *A congenital anomaly exhibited by absence of one digit or part of a digit.*	ectrodactilia
ectropion *Eversion of the eyelid, usually the lower lid.*	ectrópio
eczema *A medical condition exhibited by pruritic, red, scaly patches on the scalp, cheeks and extensor surfaces.*	eczema
edema *Extravascular fluid accumulation.*	edema

English	Portuguese
edematous *Referring to the presence of edema.*	edematoso
education *Instruction or guidance.*	educação
effector *An organ that responds to a stimulus.*	efetor
efficacious *Effective.*	eficaz
effort *Attempt or endeavor.*	esforço
effusion *The accumulation of fluid in a body cavity.*	efusão
egg	ovo
egocentric *Thinking of self without considering the feelings or thoughts of others.*	egocêntrico
ehrlichiosis *A tickborne infectious disease.*	erliquiose
ejaculation *The emission of semen at the moment of sexual climax in a male.*	ejaculação
elastic bandage *A stretch gauze used for compression of an extremity.*	bandagem elástico
elastin *A connective tissue-based glycoprotein.*	elastina
elbow *The joint between the humerus and radius/ulna.(right elbow, left elbow)*	cotovelo (cotovelo direito, cotovelo esquerdo)
elderly *Advanced in years.*	idosos
elective *Non-urgent and not life-saving.*	electivo
electrocardiogram *Display of a person's heart beat that can be used in the diagnosis of cardiac disorders.*	eletrocardograma
electroconvulsive therapy (ECT) *The electrical stimulation of the brain to treat mental disorders.*	terapia eletroconvulsiva
electrode *A device used to facilitate conduction of electricity to or from a body.*	eletrodo
electroencephalogram (EEG) *A display of brain waves used in the diagnosis of brain disorders, especially epilepsy.*	eletroencefalograma
electrolyte *The ionized constituents including potassium, sodium, chloride and others.*	eletrólito
electromyography *The display of the electrical activity of muscle.*	eletromiografia
electron microscope *A device that uses electron beams and lenses to give high magnification.*	microscópio eletrônico
electrophoresis *The movement of charged particles in a fluid that is under the influence of an electric field. This is used in testing for various maladies in the form of serum protein electrophoresis.*	eletroforese
elephantiasis *A condition caused by nematode parasites leading to lymphatic obstruction and limb or scrotal swelling.*	elefantíase
elixir *A medical solution.*	elixir
emaciation *Abnormally thin and weak.*	emaciação
embolectomy *The removal of an embolus.*	embolectomia
embolus *A blood clot, air bubble or fatty deposit that cause obstruction of a vessel.*	êmbolo
embryo *The term used to describe a fertilized ovum in the first 8 weeks of development.*	embrião
embryology *The study of the embryo.*	embriologia
emergence *Coming into prominence.*	emersão
emergency *An urgent, life-threatening situation.*	emergência
emergency room *A ward used for initial treatment of critical patients.*	sala de emergência
emesis *Vomiting.*	êmese
emesis basin *A small bowl used to catch vomitus.*	bacia rasa de desenho curvo
emetic *An agent that induces vomiting.*	emético

English	Portuguese
emmetropia *The normal correlation between eye refraction and the axial length of the eyeball.*	emetropia
emollient *Having softening or soothing qualities.*	emoliente
emotion *An intense feeling.*	emoção
empathy *To be concerned for and share the feelings of another.*	emaptia
emphysema *Abnormal enlargement of the airspaces distal to the terminal bronchioles.*	enfisema
empty *Containing nothing.*	vazio
empty sella syndrome *Compressed or flattened pituitary related to herniating arachnoid, surgery or radiotherapy.*	síndrome sela vazia
empyema *A collection of purulent material in a body cavity, usually referring to a thoracic empyema.*	empiema
emulsion *The dispersion of one liquid into another, but it is not dissolved.*	emulsão
enarthrosis *The type of joint in which a spherical bone is set into the socket of another bone.*	enartrose
encephalic *Referring to the brain.*	encefálico
encephalitis *Inflammation of the brain.*	encefalite
encephalocele *The protrusion of the brain through a defect in the skull.*	encefalocele
encephalography *Roentgenography of the brain.*	encefalografia
encephalomacia *Abnormal softness of the brain.*	encefalomalacia
encephalomyelitis *Inflammation of the brain and spinal cord.*	encefalomielite
encephalopathy *Degeneration of cerebral function.*	encefalopatia
enchondroma *An abnormal increase in cartilage growth on the inside of bone or of other cartilage.*	encondroma
encopresis *Involuntary defecation.*	encoprese
end organ *The encapsulated end of a sensory nerve.*	órgão terminal
end point *The last stage of a process.*	ponto terminal
end stage *Terminal stage. End stage cancer means there is no cure possible and death is imminent.*	estágio final
endarteritis *Tunica intima inflammation.*	endarterite
endemic *When a disease is commonly found in a location or in a people group.*	endêmico
endocarditis *Inflammation of the endocardium.*	endocardite
endocervicitis *Inflammation of the mucosal lining of the cervix.*	endocervicite
endocrine gland *A gland that secrete hormones and other substances into the blood.*	glândula endócrino
endocrine *Referring to glands that secrete hormones and other chemicals into the blood.*	endócrino
endocrinology *The study of endocrine glands and hormones.*	endcrinologia
endoderm *The innermost layer of the embryonic germ cell layers.*	endoderma
endogenous *Originating from within.*	endogênico
endolymph *The fluid collection the labyrinth of the ear.*	endolinfa
endometrioma *An isolated benign mass containing endometrial tissue.*	endometrioma
endometriosis *Presence of uterine mucosal tissue in the pelvis in abnormal locations.*	endometriose
endometritis *Inflammation of the endometrium.*	endometritie
endometrium *The mucous membrane lining of the uterus.*	endométrio
endoneurium *The tissue in a peripheral nerve that separates the individual nerve fibers.*	endoneuro

English	Portuguese
endoplasmic reticulum *A framework of tubules within the cytoplasm of eukaryotic cells.*	retículo endoplasmático
endorphin *Hormone secreted that activates the body's opiate receptors and acts as an analgesic.*	endorfina
endoscope *A device used to view the interior of a hollow organ (sigmoidoscope, gastroscope)*	endoscópio
endothelioma *A mass that propagates from the endothelium of blood vessels, lymphatics or serous cavities.*	endotelioma
endotracheal *Within the trachea.*	endotraqueal
endow, to *To supply or provide for.*	doar
enema *A procedure involving insertion of fluid into the rectum.*	enema
enkephalin *Peptide found in the brain that has similar effects as the endorphins.*	encefalinas
enlargement *Becoming bigger.*	aumento
enophthalmos *Posterior displacement of the eyeball in the orbit.*	enoftalmia
enormous *Very large.*	enorme
enostosis *The abnormal bony growth inside a bone or on the cortex.*	enostose
ensure, to *To make certain of.*	assegurar
ENT *Abbreviation for ears, nose and throat.*	ONG ouvido, nariz, e garganta
enteral feeding *Nutrition supplied via the alimentary canal.*	nutrição entérico
enterectomy *Surgical resection of part of the intestine.*	enterectomia
enteric *Referring to the intestines.*	entérico
enteritis *Inflammation of the intestines.*	enterite
enterobiasis *An infection caused by worms from the genus Enterobius.*	enterobíase
enterococcus *A gram positive cocci that occurs naturally in the intestine but is pathogenic elsewhere in the body.*	enterococo
enterolith *A calculus of the intestine.*	enterólito
enteroptosis *Inferior displacement of the intestines in the abdomen.*	enteroptose
enterotomy *A surgical opening of the intestines.*	enterotomia
entrapment neuropathy *Weakness or numbness caused by compression of a peripheral nerve.*	neuropatia de encarceramento
enucleation *Surgical removal of a globe.*	enucleação
enuresis *Involuntary urination.*	enurese
enzyme *A compound that acts as a catalyst for reactions within cells as assists with digestion outside of cells.*	enzima
eosinophil *A cell with eosin stain used to designate a type of leukocyte that is elevated during allergic reactions.*	eosinófilo
eosinophilia *An increased number of eosinophils in the blood.*	eosinofilia
ependyma *The glial lined covering of the cerebral ventricles and the central portion of the spinal cord.*	epêndima
ependymoma *A tumor composed of cells that line the ventricles of the brain.*	ependimoma
ephedrine *A chemical used to treat asthma because it expands bronchial passages and used to control spinal anesthesia associated shock because it constricts blood vessels.*	efedrina
ephemeral fever *A fever lasting no more than 24-48 hours.*	febre efêmera
epiblepharon *A condition exhibited by the eyelashes pressing against the eyeball.*	epibléfaro
epicardium *The serous membranous, innermost lining of the pericardium.*	epicárdio

English	Portuguese
epicondyle *A protrusion at the distal end of the humerus.*	epicôndilo
epicondylitis *Inflammation of the epicondyle.*	epicondilite
epicranium *The skin, fibrous layer (aponeurosis), and muscles lining the scalp.*	epicrânio
epidemic *Ubiquitous development of an infectious disease.*	epidemia
epidemiology *The study of the incidence, development and control of disease.*	epidemiologia
epidermis *The skin cells overlying the dermis.*	epiderme
epidermophytosis *A fungal skin infection caused by an organism from the genus Epidermophyton.*	epidermofitose
epididymitis *Inflammation of the duct that moves sperm from the testis to the vas deferens.*	epididimite
epididymo-orchitis *Inflammation of the epididymis and the testis.*	epididimorquite
epidural *The space around the dura of the spinal cord.*	epidural
epidural anesthesia *Medication into this space produces analgesia for surgical procedures.*	anestesia epidural
epidural hematoma *Formation of a collection of blood outside the dural layer of the brain; usually caused by trauma.*	hematoma epidural
epigastrium *The section of the abdomen that overlies the stomach.*	epigástrio
epiglottis *Tissue at the base of the tongue that covers the trachea when one swallows.*	epiglote
epilation *Removal of hair and the roots.*	depliação
epilepsy *A condition associated with abnormal brain activity and exhibited by sudden, recurrent convulsions, sensory disturbances and loss of consciousness.*	epilepsia
epileptic seizure *A convulsion related to abnormal brain activity (as opposed to being precipitated by hypoglycemia.)*	convulsão
epileptiform *Being similar to epilepsy.*	epileptiforme
epileptogenic *That which induces seizures.*	epileptogênico
epinephrine *A hormone secreted by the adrenal gland.*	epinefrina
epiphysis cerebri *A small structure situated on the mesencephalon between the two sections of the thalamus.*	epífise cerebral;corpus da glândula; corpo pineal
epiphysitis *Inflammation of the end of a long bone that is separated from the shaft by a cartilaginous disc.*	epifisite
episcleritis *Inflammation of the tissue lying above the sclera.*	episclerite
episiotomy *A surgical incision of the vagina used to aid childbirth.*	episiotomia
epispadias *A congenital condition characterized by the urethral meatus being at the superior aspect of the penis*	epispadia
epistaxis *Bleeding emanating from the nose.*	epistaxe
epithelial *Referring to the epithelium.*	epitelial
epithelial cast *Debris found in the urine composed of columnar renal epithelium.*	cilindro epitelial
epithelioma *A malignant tumor composed of epithelial cells.*	epitelioma
epithelium *The tissue lining the skin and the gastrointestinal tract that is derived from the embryonic ectoderm and endoderm..*	epitélio
epitrochlea *The medial condyle of the humerus.*	epitroclear
equal *The same or uniform.*	igual
equilibrium *When opposing forces are in balance.*	equilíbrio
equipment *Apparatus or instrument.*	equipamento
ergometer *A device that measures energy expenditure.*	ergômetro

English	Portuguese
ergonomics *The study of workplace design that focuses on reducing work-related injuries.*	ergonomia
ergosterol *A compound converted to vitamin D2 upon exposure to ultraviolet light.*	ergosterol
erosion *The gradual destruction of surface tissue.*	erosão
error *Mistake or inaccuracy.*	erro
eructation *Belch or burp.*	eructação
erysipelas *An acute infection caused by Streptococcus pyogenes that causes fever along with swelling and inflammation. The infection frequently effects the face or one leg.*	rosa; erisipila
erythema mutliforme *A skin condition exhibited by purpuric lesions and bullae usually on the distal parts of extremities but can affect the face and trunk.*	eritema multiforme
erythema nodosum *The presence of red or purple nodules on the pretibial area.*	eritema nodoso
erythroblast *A nucleus containing immature erythrocyte.*	eritatoblasto
erythroblastosis fetalis *A hemolytic disease of the newborn.*	eritroblastose fetal
erythrocyanosis *A condition exhibited by purple patches with asymmetric swelling, pruritus and burning.*	eritrocianose
erythrocyte *Called a red blood cell, it transports oxygen and carbon dioxide to and from the tissues.*	eritrócito
erythrocytopenia *Low level of erythrocytes in the blood stream.*	eritrocitopenia
erythrocytosis *A higher than normal level of erythrocytes in the blood stream.*	eritrocitose
erythropoiesis *The production of red blood cells.*	eritropoiese
eschar *Dry, hard, dead tissue commonly seen with a chronic pressure ulcer or anthrax.*	escara
eserine *Physostigmine.*	eserina
esophageal *Referring to the esophagus.*	esofágico
esophagectomy *Surgical removal of the esophagus.*	esofagectomia
esophagitis *Inflammation of the esophagus.*	esofagite
esophagoscopy *Visual inspection the esophagus utilizing a scope.*	esofagoscopia
esophagus *The muscular tube that connects the throat to the stomach.*	esôfago(B), esófago (P)
esotropia *Medial deviation of the eyes at primary gaze.*	esotropia
essential *Crucial or necessary.*	essencial
estrogen *A hormone involved with developing and maintaining female sexual characteristics.*	estrogênio
ethanol *Synonym for ethyl alcohol.*	etanol
ethmoid bone *A bone at the root of the nose which has perforations for the olfactory nerves to transit.*	osso etmóide
etiology *The underlying cause of a problem.*	etiologia
eunuch *A man who has been castrated.*	eunuco
euthanasia *Killing someone painlessly who is thought to have a terminal condition.*	eutanásia
evacuation *The emptying of an organ of fluids or gas.*	evacuação
evaluation *Assessment or evaluation.*	avaliação
eventration *Protrusion of the intestines from the abdomen.*	eventração
eversion *To turn outward.*	eversão
every *Each or all possible.*	cada
every day *Each day.*	cada dio
every other day *On alternate days.*	um dia sim
evident *Obvious.*	evidente

English	Portuguese
evisceration *The removal of bowels from the body.*	evisceração
evoked potential *Electrical impulses that can be noted after stimulation of sensory organs.*	potencial evocado
evulsion *Forcible extraction.*	evulsão
exacerbation *Worsening of an existing problem.*	exacerbação
examination *Assessment or evaluation.*	exame
exanthema *A rash that accompanies a disease or fever.*	exantema
excess *Surplus or overabundance.*	excesso
exchange transfusion *Treatment of hyperbilirubinemia in neonates.*	tranfusão de troca
excipient *An inactive substance used to deliver an active substance.*	excipiente
excisional biopsy *Surgical removal of tissue for pathologic examination.*	biópsia excisional
excoriation *Superficial loss of skin.*	excoriação
excrement *Feces.*	excremento; fezes
excreta *Fecal material.*	excreções
exenteration *Complete surgical removal of an organ.*	exenteração
exercise-induced dyspnea	dispnéia por esforço
exercised induce angina *Chest pain noted during exertion related to coronary artery disease.*	angina por esforço
exfoliation *The shedding of scales.*	descamação
exhumation *To remove a dead body from a grave.*	exhumar
exogenous *Referring to external factors.*	exógeno
exomphalos *Umbilical hernia.*	exoftalmia; exoftalmo
exostosis *A bony prominence growing from the surface of a bone.*	exostose
exotoxin *A toxin released from a living cell.*	exotoxina
exotropia *A type of strabismus that is characterized by the eyes turned outward.*	exotropia
expansion *Enlargement or increase in size.*	expansão
expect, to *To suppose or presume.*	esperar
expectorant *A substance that promotes the secretion of sputum.*	expectorante
expectoration *The presence of sputum that has been coughed out.*	expectoração
expiration date *The date when a medication should no longer be used.*	data de expiracão
expiratory *Referring to exhalation of air from the lungs.*	expiratório
expiratory reserve volume *Amount of air left in the lung after a maximal exhalation, in liters.*	volume de reserva expiratório
exploratory laparotomy *Abdominal surgery with the intent of examining the abdominal contents.*	laparotomia exploratório
expulsion *Evacuation or elimination.*	expulsão
expulsion of placenta *Passage of the placenta out the cervix after childbirth.*	expulsão placentário
extend, to *To expand or stretch out.*	estender
extension *Going from a bent to straight position.*	extensão
extensor plantar response *Great toe extension indicating a positive Babinski sign.*	reflexo plantar
extensor *Referring to the extension of an extremity or part of an extremity.*	extensor
external ear canal *Auditory canal.*	ouvido externo
external *Outside of the body.*	externo

English	Portuguese
extirpate, to *To totally destroy.*	extirpar
extracapsular *Situated outside a capsule.*	extracapsular
extracellular *Outside the cell.*	extracelular
extract *A substance in a concentrated form.*	extrato
extrapyramidal tract *Motor nerves that are not part of the pyramidal tract.*	trato extrapiramidal
extrasystole *Either a premature atrial or ventricular contraction.*	extra-sístole
extravasation *Referring to a situation in which blood or fluid goes out of a vessel it is normally flowing into.*	extravasamento
extremity *Refers to one arm or one leg.*	extremidade
extrinsic *Coming from outside or external sources.*	extrínseco
extubation *The removal of a tube that was in a body orifice.*	extubação
exudate *The fluid, cells, and debris found in the tissues or a cavity (like pleural space) during inflammation.*	exsudato
eye drops *Liquid applied to eyes for various medical problems.*	gotas oftalmológicas
eyebrow *Supercilium.*	sobrancelha
eyeglasses *Eye wear used for cosmetic or prescription purposes.*	óculos
eyeground *The fundus that is visualized with an ophthalmoscope.*	fundo do olho
eyelash *Each of the short hairs on the eyelid.*	cílio; pestana
eyelid *Palpebra.*	pálpebra
eyesight *A person's ability to see.*	visão; capacidade de ver
face *Anterior aspect of the head from the forehead to the chin.*	face
face presentation *Referring to the part of the body coming out of the cervix first during childbirth.*	apresentação facial
facet *A small flat surface of a bone.*	faceta
facial nerve *Cranial nerve VII that supplies the face and tongue.*	nervo facial (VII)
facial paralysis *Lack of movement or sensation in the distribution of the facial nerve.*	paralisia facial
facial reflex or bulbomimic reflex *Pressure on the eyeballs causes contraction of facial muscles on the side contralateral to the side of the lesion in the patient in a coma. In coma from a metabolic problem the reflex is present bilaterally.*	reflexo facial
facies *A facial expression that is typical for a particular disease.*	expressão (facial)
faint *Weak and dizzy.*	desmaio; síncope
fair *Equitable.*	feira
falciform *Referring to something that is curved. The falciform ligament attaches the liver to the diaphragm.*	falciforme
fallopian tubes *Either of a pair of long narrow ducts located in a female's abdominal cavity that transport the male sperm cells to the egg.*	trompa de Falópio; tubo de Falópio
Fallot, tetrology of *Congenital cardiac defects including ventricular septal defect, pulmonic valve stenosis or infundibular stenosis, and dextroposition of the aorta.*	tétrade de Fallot
falx cerebri *A fold in the dura that separates the two cerebral hemispheres.*	foice do cérebro
familial *Referring to the family*	familial
family	família
family history *A review of past medical history of related persons.*	médico antecedente de família
family planning *Birth control.*	controle de natalidade

English	Portuguese
Fanconi's syndrome *An idiopathic refractory anemia exhibited by pancytopenia, bone marrow hypoplasia and congenital anomalies.*	síndrome de Fanconi
faradism *The gradual increasing and decreasing of the amplitude of electricity.*	faradismo
farmer's lung *Coined because farmers are susceptible to this disease by inhaling fungi from hay; also called Aspergillosis.*	pulmão dos fazendeiros
fart, to *Slang term for releasing flatus.*	peidar
fascia *The fibrous sheath enclosing a muscle or organ.*	fáscia
fascicle *A bundle of nerve or muscle fibers.*	fascículo
fasciculation *Involuntary contraction of muscle fibers.*	fasciculação
fasciitis *Inflammation of a fascia.*	fasciíte
fasciotomy *Incision into a fascia.*	fasciotomia
fasting *Absence of caloric intake for a specified period.*	jejum
fat *A greasy or oiling substance naturally occurring in the body.*	godura
fat embolism *A deposit of fat that obstructs a vessel.*	embolia gordurosa
fatal *Lethal.*	fatal
fatigue *Tiredness and exhaustion.*	fadiga
fatty *Greasy or oily.*	gorduroso
fatty acid *A carboxylic acid occurring as a an ester in fats and oils.*	ácido graxo
favus *Tinea capitis caused by Trichopyton schoenleini.*	favo
fear *Fright or trepidation.*	medo
febrile *Presence of an supraphysiologic temperature.*	febril
fecal impaction *The presence of hard excrement in the rectum that requires manual removal.*	impactação fecal
feces *Excrement.*	fecal
fecundity *The capability of producing offspring quickly and frequently.*	fecundidade
feeble-minded *Antiquated term used to describe a person unable to make seemingly simple decisions because of a cognitive impairment.*	fraco de espírito
feeding behavior *How a child is tolerating breast or cup feeding.*	comportamento alimentação
feel better, to *To have improved health symptomatically.*	sentir-se melhor
feel, to *To perceive or discern.*	sentir
Felty syndrome *Rheumatoid arthritis with leukopenia and splenomegaly.*	síndrome de Felty
female *Feminine.*	fêmea
feminine pad *Gauze specially designed to absorb menstrual flow.*	tampão
femoral artery *Continuation of the external iliac to the popliteal artery.*	artéria femoral
femoral nerve *Supplies the motor function of the quadriceps and the sensation over the anterior and medial thigh.*	nervo femoral
femoral triangle *An area that is bordered by the sartorius muscle, the adductor longus muscle and the inguinal ligament.*	triângulo femoral
femur *The long bone in the thigh.*	fêmur
fenestration *Usually referring to a surgical window.*	fenestração
fertility *The ability of a person to contribute to contraception.*	fertilidade
fertilization *The melding of male and female gametes to form a zygote.*	fertilização
fester, to *To become infected.*	infeccionar

English	Portuguese
festinating gait *Walking with increased speed involuntarily; often seen in Parkinson's disease.*	marcha festinante
fetal alcohol syndrome *A condition caused by alcohol use by the mother during pregnancy and exhibited by poor intrauterine growth, decreased muscle tone, delayed development and widened palpebral fissures.*	síndrome alcoólica fetal
fetal distress *Term used to describe an abnormal heart rate or rhythm in a fetus indicating the need for urgent childbirth.*	desconforto fetal
fetal heart tone *Refers to the cardiac rate and pattern of the fetus.*	tons cardíacos fetal
fetal monitor *Device used to monitor fetal heart rate and rhythm.*	monitor fetal
fetal movements *Sensations by the mother of fetal activity.*	movimento fetal
fetal position *Refers to how the fetus lies within the uterus.*	posição fetal
fetal *Referring to the fetus.*	fetal
fetichism *The glorification of an inanimate object.*	fetichismo
fetor *A foul odor.*	fedor
fetus *Medical term for the infant prior to birth.*	feto
fever *A temperature above the normal range.*	febre
fibrillation *Uncoordinated, ineffective contraction as in atrial fibrillation.*	fibrilação
fibrin *An insoluble protein formed when fibrinogen is acted upon by thrombin.*	fibrina
fibroadenoma *A benign breast mass composed of fibrous and glandular tissue.*	fibroadenoma
fibroblast *A collagen producing cell in connective tissue.*	fibroblasto
fibrochondritis *The inflammation of a structure composed of cartilage and fibrous tissue.*	fibrocodrite
fibroelastosis *The abnormal increase in growth of fibrous and elastic tissue.*	fibroelastose
fibroid *A benign mass, typically uterine, composed of fibrous and muscle tissue.*	fibróide
fibromyoma *A mass containing fibrous and muscle tissue.*	fibromioma
fibrosarcoma *A sarcoma composed primarily of malignant fibroblasts.*	fibrossarcoma
fibrosis *Connective tissue that is scarred and thickened after injury.*	fibrose
fibrositis *Fibrous connective tissue that is inflamed.*	fibrosite
fibula *The smaller of two bones in the lower leg.*	fíbula; perônia
Fifth disease *Erythema infectiosum is a viral disease caused by parovirus B19.*	quinta doença
filaria *A parasitic nematode worm that is transmitted by flies and mosquitos causing filariasis.*	filária
file *Patient record or folder.*	pasta de documentos
filiform *Threadlike.*	filiforme
filum terminale *The thin structure at the end of the conus medullaris which connects the spinal cord with the coccyx.*	filamento terminal
fimbria *A slender projection at the end of the fallopian tube near the ovary.*	fímbria
finger *Any of the five digits on the hand.*	dedo
finger agnosia *The inability to distinguish which finger is being touched.*	agnosia digital
finger nose test *A test for dysmetria in which a person reaches out to touch their own nose with an extended finger with their eyes closed.*	testo de dedo-nariz

English	Portuguese
fingerstick device *A device used to project a lancet into the skin so a drop of blood can be obtained for analysis.*	dispositivo lanceta
fingertip *Distal aspect of a finger.*	ponto do dedo
fingernail *Thin horny plate over the dorsal aspect of the end of finger.*	unha
finger-thumb reflex *Opposition and adduction of the thumb with flexion at the MCP joint and extension at the interphalangeal joint when there is flexion of the 3rd, 4th, and 5th finger. This is present normally and absent with with pyramidal lesions.*	reflexo do polegar
Finkelstein test *Pain elicited with thumb flexion and wrist flexion is indicative of De Quervain tenosynovitis.*	testo de Finkelstein
firm *Hard or unyielding.*	firma
first aid *The initial treatment after an injury.*	primeiros socorros
fish *A cold-blooded vertebrate with gills and fins.*	peixe; pescado
fissure *A general term for a cleft or deep groove. An anal fissure, for example, is a small ulcer adjacent to the anus.*	fissura
fist *When a person has their fingers clenched tightly to the palm.*	punho
fistula *An abnormal communication between two organs or an organ and the skin, as in rectovaginal fistula.*	fístula
fixation *1. An obsessive interest. 2. The securing of a body part.*	fixação
flaccid *Limp. A term applied to an extremity one cannot move actively.*	flácido
flagellation *1. The protrusion found on flagella. 2. Massage administered by tapping a body part with fingers.*	flagelação
flagellum *A slender appendage that allows protozoa to swim.*	flagelo
flail chest *The term used when one has multiple rib fractures causing a segment of the chest wall to move incongruently with the rest of the chest wall.*	tórax móvel
flame photometer *A device used to measure the intensity of light.*	fotômetro de chama
flap *A term used to describe a piece of tissue partially excised and placed over an adjacent surface.*	flape
flare-up *A sudden worsening one's condition.*	exacerbação
flask *A narrow-necked container.*	frasco
flat *Level or even; without bulges.*	chato
flatfoot *Common term for pes planus.*	pé chato
flatten, to *To make even.*	alisar
flatulence *The gas expulsed from the anus.*	flatulência
flatus *Term for air that is expelled from the anus.*	flato
flatworm *A class of worms that includes parasitic flukes and tapeworms.*	verme plano
flea *A small wingless insect that feeds on blood of mammals.*	pulga
flesh *The tissue between the skin and bones.*	carne
flexor *A muscle that bends an extremity or part of an extremity.*	flexor
flexure *The action of bending.*	flexura
flight of ideas *Streams of unrelated ideas noted in a manic phase.*	fuga de idéias
floating *Buoyant or suspended.*	flutuante
flow *Movement in a continuous stream.*	fluência
fluid intake *The amount of oral consumption plus the amount of intravenous fluids administered.*	consumo de fluido
fluke *Parasitic nematode worm; an example is Schistosoma.*	trematódeo
fluoresceine *A fluorane dye used to check for corneal ulcers.*	fluoresceína

English	Portuguese
fluorescent antibody test (FTA test)	testo de anticorpos fluorescentes
fluorescent screen *A screen used to view x-rays.*	fluorescência tela
fluoridation *The addition of fluorine to something.*	fluoretação
fluorine *A chemical that causes severe burns if exposed to the skin.*	flúor
fluoroscopy *The continuous viewing of roentgenographic images with a fluorescent screen.*	fluoroscopia
flush, to *Term used to describe an irrigation procedure, as in flushing an NG tube.*	jato de água
flushing *Transient erythema due to heat, stress or disease.*	rubor
flutter *Used to describe a cardiac rhythm disturbance, as in atrial flutter.*	agitação
foam *A mass of small bubbles in a liquid.*	espuma
Foley catheter *A drainage tube placed in the urinary bladder via the urethra.*	sonda de Foley
folic acid *Also called pteroylglutamic acid; a deficiency can cause megaloblastic anemia.*	ácido fólico
follicle stimulating hormone (FSH) *An anterior pituitary gland hormone responsible for production of sperm or ova.*	hormônio folículo-estimulante
follicular *Referring to a small secretory gland.*	folicular
fontanelle or fontanel *The space between the bones in the skull that are separate at birth.*	fontanela
food *Nutrition.*	alimento
food intake *Quantitative record of nutritional intake.*	consumo de alimento
food poisoning *Poisoning where the active agent is in the food.*	intoxicação alimentar
foot *The lower extremity distal to the ankle.*	pé
foot and mouth disease *A contagious viral disease exhibited by oral and digital vesicles.*	doença do pé e boca; fata contagiosa
foot drop *Caused by palsy of the nerve controlling foot dorsiflexion.*	pé caído
foramen *An opening in a bone.*	forame
foramen magnum *The hole in the skull that the spinal cord passes through.*	forame magno
foramen ovale *A hole in the atrial septal wall in a fetus.*	forame oval
forced vital capacity *Vital capacity measured as the patient is exhaling as rapidly as possible.*	capacidade vital forçada (CVF)
forced expiratory volume per second (FEV1) *The amount of air exhaled with maximal effort, measured in liters, over one second.*	volume expiratório forçado (VRE)
forceps *A surgical instrument, commonly called tweezers.*	fórceps; pinça
forearm *Segment of the arm from the elbow to wrist.*	antebraço
forearm crutch *A long stick with a place for a hand-grip to aid in ambulation when there is lower extremity weakness.*	muleta de antebraço
forebrain *The part of the brain that includes the thalamus, hypothalamus and cerebral hemispheres.*	cérebro anterior
forehead *Section of the face from the hairline to the eyebrows.*	fronte
foreign body *Term used to describe an object found in a body orifice that is not part of the body.*	corpo estranho
forensic *Referring to the scientific method of studying crime.*	forense
foreskin *Also called prepuce, the skin that naturally covers the glans but can be rolled back.*	prepúcio
former *Prior.*	formador
formulary *A list of medicines that are permissible to prescribe.*	formulário
fornix *A vaulted structure.*	fórnice

English	Portuguese
forwards *Towards the front.*	adiante
fossa *A shallow depression.*	fossa
fourchette *The fork shaped fold of skin where the labia minora meet superior to the perineum.*	fúrcula
fovea *The area on the retina where the visual acuity is optimal.*	fóvea
Foville's syndrome *Caused by a lesion within the pons, there is ipsilateral facial and abducens nerve paralysis and contralateral hemiplegia.*	síndrome de Foville
fracture *A broken bone.*	fratura
fracture, avulsion *A broken bone associated with a ligament or tendon pulling a piece of the bone away.*	fratura por avulsão
fracture, closed *A broken bone where there is no break in the skin.*	fratura fechada
fracture, comminuted *A broken bone where one segment overrides the other.*	fratura cominutiva
fracture, depressed *The presence of concavity associated with a fracture as in a depressed skull fracture.*	fratura afundamento
fracture, greenstick *A spiral fracture.*	fratura em galho verde
fracture, open *A fracture in which there is a break in the skin and bone is exposed.*	fratura aberta
fracture, pathologic *A fracture due at least in part to another condition, such as a fracture at a location where there is bone cancer.*	fratura patológico
fracture, stress *A fracture associated with overuse.*	fratura por estresse
fragilitas ossium *A condition exhibited by excessively brittle bones. Also called osteogenesis imperfecta.*	fragilidade ósseo
framboesia; yaws *An endemic tropical disease caused by Treponema pertenue.*	framboesia
free *Lacking or absent.*	livre
free from *Without or clear of.*	de fora
freezing (as in ambient temperature) *Below 0 Celsius.*	cogelação
fremitus *A vibration that is appreciated with palpation.*	frêmito
frenulum *The tissue that connects the inferior portion of the tongue to the base of the mouth.*	frênulo
frequency *Rate of occurrence.*	freqüência
friable *Easily reduced to powder.*	friável
friction *Grating or rasping.*	fricção
friction rub *A noise heard during cardiac auscultation in patients with pericarditis, for example.*	atrito de fricção
frog *A tailless amphibian that is short with long hind legs for jumping.*	rã
frog in the throat, to have *An expression describing hoarseness.*	rouquidão
frontal *Referring to the anterior aspect, as in frontal lobe.*	frontal
frontal sinus *A paranasal sinus on both sides of the lower part of the frontal bone.*	seio frontal
frost itch *A pruritus noted when exposed to cold weather.*	prurido de inverno
frostbite *Local tissue destruction after exposure to cold.*	geladura
froth *Covered with a mass of small bubbles.*	espuma
froth at the mouth, to *To have a mass of saliva with small bubbles in it coming out of the mouth.*	espumar por boca
frozen *Past participle of to freeze. Freeze: turn a liquid into a solid.*	gelado

English	Portuguese
frozen shoulder *Common term for adhesive capsulitis.*	ombro congelado; capsulite adesiva
fructosuria *Presence of fructose in the urine.*	frutosúria
FTA test *Fluorescent treponemal antibody test for syphilis.*	testo de absorção de anticorpo treponêmico fluorescente
full-term *A normal length pregnancy.*	período de gestação
fulminant *Sudden and severe.*	fulminante
function *An activity natural to a person or thing.*	função
fundus oculi *Portion of the interior eyeball in the posterior aspect which can be viewed by an ophthalmoscope.*	fundo de olho
fundus of the stomach *Referring to the part of the stomach above the cardiac notch.*	fundo gástrico
fungicide *An agent that destroys fungus.*	fungicida
fungus *A spore-producing organism that feeds on organic matter.*	fungo
funiculus of the spinal cord *The white matter of the spinal cord that is further defined by location.*	funículo da medula espinhal
funiculus, lateral *The lateral white column of the spinal cord between the anterior and posterior nerve roots.*	funículo lateral
funiculitis *Inflammation of the funiculi.*	funiculite
funnel chest *Anterior thorax funnel shaped depression, also called pectus excavatum.*	tórax em funil
furuncle *A painful erythematous nodule with a central core.*	furúnculo
furunculosis *The presence of multiple furuncles.*	furunculose
fusiform *Spindle-shaped.*	fusiforme
gag reflex *Contraction of the pharynx muscles when the back of the pharynx is stimulated by touch.*	reflexo de ânsia
gait *The way one walks.*	marcha; andadura
galactocele *A milk-filled cyst in the mammary gland.*	galactocele
galactorrhea *Excessive production of milk.*	galactorréia
galactose *A sugar that is a constituent of lactose.*	galactose
galactosemie *1. Galactose in the blood. 2. A congenital condition exhibited by impaired carbohydrate metabolism.*	galactosemia
gallbladder *The organ adjacent to the liver that stores bile and secretes it into the duodenum.*	vesícula biliar
gallop *An abnormal heart sound.*	galope
gallstone *Calculus produced in the bile duct or gallbladder.*	colélito
galvanism *The use of electric currents for medical treatment.*	galvanismo
galvanometer *A device used to measure small electric currents.*	galvanômetro
gamete *A germ cell that is able to unite with another germ cell of the opposite gender to form a zygote.*	gameta
gamma globulin *A blood serum protein with little electrophoretic mobility.*	gamaglobulina
gamma ray *A type of electromagnetic radiation.*	raios gama
ganglionectomy *The removal of a benign swelling on a tendon sheath.*	ganglionectomia
gangrene *Tissue death from either impaired blood flow or an infection.*	gangrena
gaping *Wide open.*	aberto
gargle, to *To rinse one's mouth out and exhale through the liquid.*	gargarejar
gargoylism *A congenital defect, also known as Hurler syndrome, it is characterized by skeletal anomalies, mental retardation and gargoyle-like facial features.*	gargulismo

English	Portuguese
gas gangrene *A life and limb threatening disorder caused associated with tissue death and caused by an anaerobic bacterium in the genus of Clostridium.*	gangrena gasosa
gastrectomy *Complete or partial surgical resection of the stomach.*	gastrectomia
gastric lavage *Instillation and removal of large quantities of saline into the stomach in order to treat poisoning.*	lavagem do estômago;
gastric *Referring to the stomach.*	gástrico
gastric secretions *Fluids secreted from gastric mucosa.*	secreção do estômago
gastrin *Hormones that stimulates gastric secretions.*	gastrina
gastritis *Inflammation of the stomach.*	gastrite
gastrocele *Protrusion of part of the stomach in the form of a hernia.*	gastrocele
gastrocnemius *A large muscle in the lower leg, responsible for ankle plantar flexion, that is attached to the distal femur and achilles tendon.*	gastrocnêmio
gastrocolic reflex *Peristalsis of the colon produced by food entering the stomach.*	reflexo gastrocólico
gastroduodenal ulcer *A lesion in the mucosal lining of the stomach or duodenum.*	úlcera gastroduodenal
gastroenteritis *A bacterial or viral infection that leads to vomiting and diarrhea.*	gastroenterite
gastroenterostomy *A surgical opening in the stomach or intestine.*	gastroenterostomia
gastrointestinal tract *The alimentary canal from the distal esophagus to the cecum.*	trato gastrointestinal
gastrojejunostomy *A surgical procedure that directly connects the stomach to the jejunum.*	gastrojejunostomia
gastropexy *Securing the stomach to the abdominal wall.*	gastropexia
gastroscopy *Use of an endoscope to directly visualize the stomach.*	gastroscopia
gastrostomy *A surgical creation of an opening in the stomach.*	gastrostomia
gauge *The size or thickness of something. An 18gauge needle.*	calibrador
gauze *A fabric used for dressing changes.*	gaze
gavage syringe *A syringe used for irrigation.*	seringa de gavagem
gavage *The instillation of food into the stomach with use of a tube.*	gavagem
gavage tube *A tube used for instillation of liquids into the stomach.*	sonda de gavagem
gaze *Steady, intent look.*	fitar
gel *A jellylike substance.*	gel; gelatina
gene *A unit of heredity that is passed on from parent to child.*	gene
general *Common or expected.*	comum
general appearance *The overall look of a patient.*	aparecimento global
genetic counseling *A discussion of the concerns related to genetic testing.*	consulta genético
genetic *Referring to genes or heredity.*	genético
geniculate *Bent at a sharp angle.*	geniculado
geniculate body *Protrusions on the thalamus that relay visual and auditory signals to the brain.*	corpo geniculado
geniculate ganglion *The sensory ganglion of the facial nerve.*	gânglio geniculado
geniculate neuralgia *Severe intermittent pain in the external ear and deep in the ear.*	neuralgia geniculada

English	Portuguese
genital ambiguity *A disorder of sexual development in which the genitalia are not sufficiently developed to tell clearly if the person is male or female.*	genitália ambigua
genital herpes *A sexually transmitted infection caused by herpes simplex.*	herpes genital
genital wart *The common term for Condylomata acuminata.*	verruga genital
genitalia *Genitals.*	genitália
genitourinary *Referring to the urinary system through the organs or urine excretion.*	genitourinário
genome *A full set of genetic information for an organism.*	genoma
gentian violet *An antiseptic derived from rosaniline.*	violeta de genciana
genu valgum *A condition exhibited by the knees turning inward, commonly referred to as knock-knee.*	joelho valgo
genu varum *A condition exhibited by the knees turning outward, commonly referred to as bowleg.*	joelho varo; perna arqueada
GERD gastroesophageal reflux disease *A condition characterized by gastric contents being regurgitated into the esophagus or mouth.*	gastroesofagopatia por refluxo (GEPR)
geriatrics *The study of the health of old people.*	geriatria
germ *Microorganism.*	germe
German measles *(rubella) A contagious viral infection.*	sarampo alemão
gerontology *The study of old persons.*	gerontologia
Gerstmann syndrome *Finger agnosia, agraphia and acalculia caused by a lesion between the occipital region and angular gyrus.*	síndrome de Gerstmann
gestation *The development of a fetus from conception until birth.*	gestação; gravidez
giant *Huge or massive.*	gigante
giardiasis *A flagellate protozoa, Giardia lamblia, that causes diarrhea.*	giardíase
giddiness *A tendency to fall or dizziness.*	vertigem
gingival *Referring to the gums.*	gengival
gingivitis *Inflammation of the gums.*	gengivite
ginglymus *A joint that allows movement in one direction only.*	gínglimo
glabella *The area of the forehead above and between the eyebrows.*	glabela
glance *A brief look at something.*	golpe de vista
glans penis *The distal aspect of the penis.*	glande peniana
glare *An angry stare.*	ofuscamento
Glasgow coma scale *A scale used to grade one's level of consciousness with a score of 3 being totally unresponsive and a score of 15 being normal.*	escala de Glasgow do coma
glaucoma *A condition characterized by increased intraocular pressure.*	glaucoma
glenoid *Referring to the fossa that is a shallow depression, such as the hollow of the scapula where the humeral head sets.*	glenóide
glioma *A neural malignant tumor of glial cells.*	glioma
gliomyoma *A mass with gliomatous and myomatous characteristics.*	gliomiome
globus pallidus *A portion of the lentiform nucleus in the brain.*	globo pálido
glomerulonephritis *Inflammation of the renal glomeruli, usually from hemolytic streptococcus.*	glomerulonefrite
glomerulus *A grouping of capillaries where waste is filtered from the blood.*	glomérulo

English	Portuguese
glomus tumor *A reddish-blue painful papule that occurs on the distal aspects of the digits.*	tumor glômico
glossal *Referring to the tongue.*	glossal
glossectomy *Surgical resection of the whole or part of the tongue.*	glossectomia
glossitis *Inflammation of the tongue.*	glossite
glossodynia *Tongue pain.*	glossodinia
glossopharyngeal *The name for cranial nerve IX that supplies the tongue and pharynx.*	glossofaríngeo
glottis *Essentially the vocal structure, including the true vocal cords and the opening between them.*	glote
glove *A covering for hand protection.*	luva
glove anesthesia *Absence of sensation of the hand and wrist.*	anestesia em luva
glucagon *A pancreatic enzyme responsible for breakdown of glycogen to glucose.*	glucagon
glucose tolerance test *The oral administration of a carbohydrate load and then evaluation of the blood sugar at timed intervals.*	prova de tolerância à glícose
glue *Plastic cements*	cola
glue sniffing addiction *Habituation of plastic cement fumes inhalation which includes toluene, xylene and benzene.*	dependência do inalação de cola
gluteal *Referring to the gluteus.*	glúteo
gluteal fold *The horizontal crease between the buttock and upper thigh.*	dobra glútea
gluteal or gluteus muscle *A paired set of three muscles, the gluteus maximus, medius and minimus, that all have origins in the ilium and insertions in the femur. (buttocks)*	músculo glúteo
gluteal reflex *After the skin of the buttocks are stimulated the gluteal muscles contract.*	refexo glúteo
glycemia *The amount of glucose in the blood.*	glicemia
glycerin *A byproduct in the manufacture of soap that is used as a laxative.*	glicerina
glycogen *A compound that stores glucose and when it undergoes hydrolysis forms glucose.*	glicogênio
glycogenesis *The production of glycogen from glucose.*	gliocogênese
glycolysis *The production of energy and pyruvic acid when glucose is broken down by enzymes.*	glicólise
glycoprotein *A protein that has a carbohydrate attached to its polypeptide chain.*	glicoproteína
glycosuria *Presence of glucose in the urine.*	glicosúria
gnathic *Referring to the jaws.*	gnático
gnosia *Ability to recognize things and people.*	gnose
goblet cell *Aids in the secretion of respiratory and intestinal mucous.*	célula calciforme
goggles *Close fitting, protective eyeglasses.*	óculos de proteção
goiter *Swelling of the thyroid gland.*	bócio
gold *Precious metal with atomic number of 79.*	ouro
gonad *A testis or an ovary.*	gônada
gonadal dysgenesis *The lack of complete development of the gonads.*	disgenesia gonadal
gonadotrophin *Pituitary hormone that promotes gonadal activity.*	gonadotrofina
gonococcus *A diploccocal bacteria that is the causative agent in gonorrhea, formally Neisseria gonorrhoeae.*	gonococo

English	Portuguese
gonorrhea *A sexually transmitted disease that is exhibited by purulent discharge from the vagina or penis.*	gonorréia
gonorrheal arthritis *A type of arthritis caused by the gram negative diplococcus Neisseria gonorrhoeae.*	artrite gonorréica
gonorrheal ophthalmia *An acute purulent conjunctivitis that can occur in neonates within 2-5 days of birth.*	oftalmia gonorréica
Goodpasture' syndrome *Glomerulonephritis, preceded by hemoptysis. The nephritis can quickly progress to death from renal failure.*	síndrome de Goodpasture
goose bumps *Cutis anserina.*	pele de ganso
gouge *A chisel with a concave blade used in surgery.*	goiva
gout *Monosodium urate crystal deposition disease.*	gota
gown *A sterile gown used during surgical procedures.*	vestido estéril
grade *A level of rank or quality.*	cagegoria
Graefe's sign *Also called lid lag, a sign characterized by the upper eyelid not closing over the globe. This is seen commonly in exophthalmic goiter.*	sinal de Graefe
graft *A piece of tissue surgically transplanted.*	enxerto
gram *A unit of mass, 1/1000th of a kilogram.*	grama
granular layer *A deep layer of the cerebellum.*	camada granular
granulation tissue *Vascular connective tissue forming granular protrusions on the surface of a healing wound.*	tecido de granulação
granulocyte *A white blood cell with cytoplasmic secretory granules.*	granulócito
granuloma *A mass of granulation tissue.*	granuloma
grasp reflex *Flexion of the fingers or toes when stimulated.*	reflexo da apreensão
Graves' disease *A form of hyperthyroidism exhibited by a goiter and exophthalmos.*	doença de Graves; doença de Basedow ou Parry
gravida *Pregnant.*	grávida
gray matter *The section of the brain and spinal cord composed of branching dendrites and nerve cell bodies.*	substância cinzenta do sistema nervoso
greater than normal *Above normal.*	supra-normal
grief *Deep sorrow.*	aflição
grip strength *Quantitative measurement of the force of a hand grip.*	aperto de mão
groan *A deep inarticulate sound made due to pain or despair.*	gemido
groggy *Drowsy.*	instável
groin pull *A muscle strain in the inguinal region.*	lesão de virilha
groin *The genital region.*	virilha
gross *Distended; not well defined.*	grosa
ground itch *Marked pruritus caused by a hookworm larvae, known otherwise as cutaneous larva migrans.*	prurido do solo
growth *The increase in physical size.*	crescimento
growth hormone-releasing factor *Released by the hypothalamus, it induces the release of somatotropin.*	fator de liberação do hormônio do crescimento
grunting *A low guttural sound used to describe a person with profound respiratory difficulty.*	gemente
guaiac *A substance derived from guaiacum trees used to test for trace amounts of blood, in stool for instance.*	guáiaco
guarding *A symptom used to describe a patient resisting an examination because of severe pain; often seen in patients with peritonitis.*	defesa
Guillain-Barré syndrome *An acute autoimmune disorder that causes nerve inflammation subsequently muscle weakness.*	síndrome de Guillain-Barré

English	Portuguese
guinea worm *A parasitic nematode worm that, in cases of infection, lives under the skin, formally called Dracunculus medinensis.*	verme da Guiné
gum *Gingiva.*	gengiva
gum (chewing gum)	goma de mascar
gumboil *Swelling noted on the gingiva over a dental abscess.*	parúlide
gumma *A soft granulomatous tumor of the skin or cardiovascular system seen in tertiary syphilis.*	goma; sifiloma
gunshot wound *An penetrating injury sustained from a bullet.*	ferida de bala
gustatory agnosia *The loss of the sense of taste.*	agnosia gustativo
gustatory *Referring to sense of taste.*	gustativo
guttural *Having a harsh quality; coming from the back of the throat.*	guteral
gynecology *The branch of medicine associated with the reproductive system of women.*	ginecologia
gynecomastia *Enlargement of the breasts.*	ginecomastia
gyrus *Convolutions of the brain where there is infolding.*	giro
habit *A custom or inclination.*	hábito
hair (of body)	cabelo de corpo
hair (of head)	cabelo da cabeça
hair cell *Epithelial cells with hairlike projections.*	célula pilosas
hair follicle *Tubelike invagination of the epidermis that the hair shaft develops from.*	folículo piloso
hairy *A profuse amount of hair.*	hirsuto
hairy tongue *Lingua villosa, a benign condition associated with antibiotic used caused by candida albicans infection.*	língua pilosa
half *Divided in two.*	metade
half-life *The time a drug decreases its effect in half over time.*	meia-vida
halitosis *Foul odor emanating from the mouth.*	halitose
hallucination *A perception that is not based on reality.*	alucinação
hallucinogen *A substance that elicits hallucinations.*	alucinógeno
hallux valgus *Also called bunion, it is the lateral deviation of the great toe.*	hálux valgo
hallux varus *Medial deviation of the great toe.*	hálux varo
hamartoma *A nodule of superfluous tissue.*	hamartoma
hamate bone; uncinate bone *The medial bone in the distal row of carpal bones adjacent to the fifth metacarpal.*	hamato; uncinado
Hamman-Rich syndrome *Idiopathic pulmonary fibrosis.*	síndrome de Hamman-Rich
hammer toe *A condition characterized by extension of the proximal phalanx and flexion of the second and distal phalanges.*	artelho em martelo
Hampton maneuver *Rolling a patient during gastrointestinal fluoroscopy in order to obtain an air contrast of the antrum and duodenum.*	manobra de Hampton
hamstrings *Tendons of the posterior thigh.*	jarrete
hand *The upper extremity distal to the wrist.*	mão
hangnail *A loose piece of skin attached near the medial or lateral nail fold.*	unheiro
Hanhart's syndrome *Also referred to as micrognathia with peromelia. There is hypoplasia of the mandible, malformed or missing teeth, birdlike face and severe upper extremity deformities.*	síndrome de Hanhart
Hansen's disease *Leprosy*	doença de Hansen

English	Portuguese
haploid *Either a single set of chromosomes or a set of nonhomologous chromosomes.*	haplóide
hapten *The molecular component that determines immunologic specificity.*	hapteno
hard *Rigid or very firm.*	duro
hard of hearing *Decreased sense of hearing.*	ser surdo
harmless *Safe or benign.*	inofensivo
hay fever *An allergy exhibited by pruritus of the eyes and nose, rhinorrhea and excessive lacrimal secretion.*	febre de feno
hazy *Cloudy.*	nebuloso
head	cabeça
head trauma *Any injury to the brain.*	lesão da cabeça
headache *Cephalgia.*	cefaléia; cefalalgia
healing *The process of becoming healthy again.*	curador
health *The state of being free of illness.*	saúde
health center *A physical location where patients are treated.*	clínica
healthy *In good health.*	sadio
hearing *Auditory perception.*	audição
hearing aid *A device that fits in the ear used to amplify sound.*	auxílio auditivo
heart *Muscular organ that pumps blood thru the circulatory system.*	coração
heart beat *A single contraction of the heart.*	batimento cardíaco
heart block *An alteration in the cardiac electrical conduction system.*	bloqueio cardíaco
heartburn *Synonym of pyrosis.*	azia
heart lung machine *Device used during cardiac surgery to replace the function of the heart and lungs while surgery is performed.*	máquina coração-pulmão
heart murmur *An abnormal heart sound usually related to valvular disease.*	sopro cardíaco
heart rate *Number or cardiac contractions per minute.*	freqüência cardíaca
heat *The quality of being hot.*	calor
heat exhaustion *A condition that occurs secondary to prolonged exposure to high ambient temperature; it is exhibited by subnormal temperature, dizziness and nausea.*	exaustão de calor
heat stroke *A condition caused by excessive exposure to high ambient temperature; it is exhibited by dry skin, thirst, vertigo, muscle cramps and nausea. The three forms are heat exhaustion, heat cramps and sunstroke.*	insolação
heavy *Possessing great weight.*	pessoa
hebephrenia *A type of schizophrenia exhibited by hallucinations and inappropriate laughter.*	hebefrenia
Heberden's node *Hard nodules formed at the distal interphalangeal joints in osteoarthritis.*	nodos de Herberden
hedonism *Devoting oneself to being happy.*	hedonismo
heel *Proximal portion of the plantar aspect of the foot.*	calcanhar
heel-shin test (heel to knee to toe test) *A test of position sense and coordination; one moves the heel of one foot from the knee on the other foot down to the foot.*	testo de calcanhar-canela
height *Distance between the bottom of the foot and top of the head.*	altura
Heimlich maneuver *A forceful upward thrust to the diaphragm to dislodge an airway obstruction.*	manobra de Heimlich
heliotherapy *Treatment of disease with sunlight.*	helioaeroterapia

English	Portuguese
helium *An inert gas that is the lightest of the noble gases.*	hélio
helminth *A fluke, tapeworm or nematode.*	helminto
helminthiasis *Being infected by a helminth.*	helmintíase
hemagglutinin *An antibody that facilitates the agglutination of blood.*	hemaglutinina
hemangioma *A benign tumor composed of blood vessels.*	hemangioma
hemarthrosis *Presence of intra-articular blood.*	hemartrose
hematemesis *Vomiting blood.*	hematêmese
hematin *The insoluble iron protoporphyrin component of hemoglobin.*	hematina
hematocele *A mass or area of swelling caused by the accumulation of blood.*	hematocele
hematochezia *Presence of blood in the excrement.*	hematoquezia
hematocrit *The measurement of the volume of red blood cells compared to the total volume of blood; recorded in percent.*	hematócrito
hematoma *A mass containing blood.*	hematoma
hematometra *The accretion of blood in the uterus.*	hematométria
hematomyelia *Accumulation of blood in the spinal cord.*	hematomielia
hematoporphyrin *A derivative of heme that does not contain iron.*	hematoporfirina
hematosalpinx *Presence of blood in the fallopian tube.*	hematossalpinge
hematuria *The presence of blood in the urine.*	hematúria
heme *A constituent of hemoglobin that is an insoluble iron protoporphyrin.*	heme
hemeralopia *Night blindness.*	hemeralopia
hemianopsia *Blindness over half the field of vision.*	hemianopsia; hemianopia
hemiballismus *Severe motor restlessness unilaterally, usually from a subthalamic lesion.*	hemibalismo
hemicolectomy *Surgical removal of part of the colon.*	hemicolectomia
hemicrania *1. Pain on one side of the head. 2. Incomplete anencephaly.*	hemicrânia
hemiparesis *Unilateral muscle weakness (half the body).*	hemiparesia
hemiplegia *Paralysis of one side of the body.*	hemiplegia
hemisphere *Referring to either the right or left portion of the cerebrum.*	hemisfera
hemizygote *A cell with only one set of genes.*	hemizigoto
hemochromatosis *A hereditary condition exhibited by iron deposition in the tissue and leading to liver disease, bronze discoloration of the skin and diabetes.*	hemocromatose
hemoconcentration *Decrease in the total fluid content of the blood, leading at times to a falsely elevated hematocrit.*	hemoconcentração
hemocytometer *A device used for counting cells from a blood sample.*	hemocitômetro
hemodialysis *The process of filtering blood outside the body to remove toxins normally excreted by functioning kidneys.*	hemodiálise
hemoglobin *An iron containing protein used for the transport of oxygen in blood.*	hemoglobina
hemoglobinuria *Presence of free hemoglobin in the urine.*	hemoglobinúria
hemolysis *Breakdown of hemoglobin.*	hemólise
hemolytic *Something that causes hemolysis.*	hemolítico
hemolytic anemia *Reduced number of erythrocytes due to shortened survival and inability of the bone marrow to compensate.*	anemia hemolítico

English	Portuguese
hemopericardium *Abnormal presence of blood in the pericardium.*	hemopericárdio
hemoperitoneum *Abnormal presence of blood in the peritoneum.*	hemoperitôneo
hemophilia *A hereditary bleeding disorder characterized by hemarthroses and deep tissue bleeding as a result of absence of a coagulation factor such as factor VIII.*	hemofilia
hemophiliac *A person with hemophilia.*	hemofílico
hemophilic arthropathy *The permanent joint disease caused by recurrent bleeding into the joint.*	artropatia hemofílico
hemophthalmia *Bleeding within the eye.*	hemoftalmia
hemopneumothorax *Accumulation of blood and air in the pleural space.*	hemopneumotórax
hemopoiesis *The production of blood cells from stem cells.*	hemopoiese
hemopoietic Referring to *a hormone secreted by the kidneys that stimulates the bone marrow to produce erythrocytes.*	hemopoiético
hemoptysis *Expectoration of blood.*	hemoptise
hemorrhage *Bleeding from a damaged blood vessel.*	hemorragia
hemorrhoidectomy *Surgical excision of a hemorrhoid.*	hemorroidectomia
hemorrhoids *Engorgement of the veins in the anus or rectum.*	hemorróidas
hemostasis *The control of bleeding.*	hemostasia
hemothrorax *The abnormal presence of blood in the pleural cavity.*	hemotórax
hence *Thus.*	daqui
Henoch purpura *Exhibited by vomiting, diarrhea, abdominal pain and hematuria; a non-thrombocytopenic purpura.*	púrpura de Henoch
Henri, syndrome of *Congenital anomaly exhibited by different sized external orifices of the nostrils.*	síndrome de Henri
heparin *A polysaccharide that occurs naturally in the liver and is used as a medication to induce a hypocoagulable state.*	heparina
hepatectomy *Partial or complete surgical resection of the liver.*	hepatectomia
hepatic duct *The right and left hepatic ducts join the cystic duct to form the common bile duct.*	ducto hepático
hepatic flexure of the colon *The junction of the ascending and transverse portion of the colon.*	flexura direita do cólon
hepatic *Referring to the liver.*	hepático
hepatitis *Inflammation of the liver.*	hepatite
hepatocyte *A liver cell.*	hepatócito
hepatojugular reflex *The presence of jugular venous distension with compression of the abdomen for at least 10 seconds.*	refluxo hepatojugular
hepatoma *A tumor of the liver.*	hepatoma
hepatomegaly *Enlargement of the liver.*	hepatomegalia
hepatosplenomegaly *Enlargement of the spleen and the liver.*	hepatosplenomegalia
hereditary spherocytosis *A familial hemolytic disease exhibited by abnormally thick erythrocytes.*	esferocitose hereditária
hereditary *That which is transmitted genetically*	hereditário
hermaphrodite *A person possessing gonadal characteristics of both sexes.*	hermafrodita
hernia, femoral *A bulge in the upper thigh/groin region because of bowel protruding through the muscle. Also called crural hernia.*	hérnia femoral
hernia, incarcerated *An irreducible hernia.*	hérnia encarcerada
hernia, inguinal *Protrusion of abdominal-cavity contents through the inguinal canal.*	hérnia inguinal

English	Portuguese
hernia, lumbar *Defect in the lumbar muscles or the posterior fascia, below the 12th rib and above the iliac crest.*	hérnia lombar
hernia, umbilical *Protrusion of abdominal contents at the umbilicus.*	hérnia umbilical
herniated disc *Prolapse of the nucleus pulposus into the spinal cord.*	disco herniado
herniorrhaphy *The surgical repair of a hernia.*	herniorrafia
heroin *A morphine derivative that is highly addictive.*	heroína
herpangina *An infectious disease caused by Coxsackie virus exhibited by vesicular lesion on the soft palate.*	herpangina
herpes *A skin condition exhibited by formation of clustered vesicular lesions; herpes simplex is at times referred to, albeit incompletely, as herpes.*	herpes
herpes zoster; shingles *A unilateral vesicular rash along one dermatome and caused by inflammation of a posterior nerve root by "the chicken pox virus".*	herpes zóster; zona
herpetic *Referring to herpes.*	herpético
herpetiform *Something that is characteristic of herpes.*	herpetiforme
heterochromia iridis or syndrome of Eric *Congenital anomaly in which the iris of each eye is of a different color.*	íris da heterocromia; síndrome de Eric
heterogenous *That which originates outside the organism.*	heterogêneo
heterotropia *Synonym of strabismus.*	heterotopia
heterozygous *Having different alleles concerning a certain trait.*	heterozigoto
hiatus hernia *Protrusion of part of the stomach through the esophageal hiatus of the diaphragm.*	hérnia do hiato
hiccup *Involuntary spasm of the diaphragm with sudden closure of the glottis; this causes a characteristic cough.*	soluço
hidradenitis *Inflammation of a sweat gland. When there is purulent discharge it is called hidradenitis suppurativa.*	hidradenite
hidrosis *The production and secretion of sweat.*	hidrose
high *Elevated.*	elevado
high blood pressure *Elevated arterial blood pressure.*	hipertensão
high cholesterol *Elevated serum cholesterol.*	hipercolesterolemia
hilar *Referring to a hilus.*	hilar
Hillis-Müller maneuver *A procedure to determine the descent of the head during active labor.*	manobra de Hillis-Müller
hilum or hilus *A depression where blood vessels and nerve fibers enter an organ.*	hilo
hindbrain *The brainstem which includes the pons, medulla oblongata and cerebellum.*	metencéfalo
hip *The lateral eminence of the pelvis from the waist to the thigh; it is formed by the iliac crest and greater trochanter.*	quadril
hip joint *The lateral eminence of the pelvis from the waist to the thigh; it is formed by the iliac crest and greater trochanter.*	articulação coxofemoral
hip replacement *Both joint surfaces are replaced by high density material such as plastic or metal.*	artroplastia do quadril
hippocampus *The area at the base of the cerebral ventricles thought to be the center of memory and emotion.*	hipcampo
Hippocratic oath *An vow taken by doctors, indicating they will treat people properly.*	juramento de Hipócrates
hirsutism *Abnormal growth on hair on a person's face and body.*	hirsutismo
histamine *A chemical responsible for the reaction exhibited when a person has an allergic reaction.*	histamina

English	Portuguese
histidine *An amino acid precursor to histamine.*	histidina
histiocyte *A phagocytic cell found in connective tissue.*	histiócito
histochemistry *Study of intracellular distribution of chemicals, reaction sites and enzymes.*	histioquímica
histology *The study of the structure and composition of minute structures.*	histologia
histoplasmosis *A fungal pulmonary infection from bat and bird excrement.*	histoplasmose; doença de Darling
HIV *Abbreviation for human immunodeficiency virus.*	vírus da imunodeficiência humana
hoarse *A rough, harsh sounding voice.*	rouco
Hodgkin's disease *Also called Hodgkin's lymphoma, it is a cancer that begins in the lymphocytes.*	doença de Hodgkin
hollow *An indentation.*	cavidade
homeless *Having nowhere to live.*	desabrigado
homeopathy *A treatment of disease by use of minute doses of toxic substances that would normally be harmful.*	homeopatia
homeostasis *The tendency of an organism to maintain a stable and uniform state.*	homeostase
homicide *When one person kills another.*	homicído
homograft *A graft of tissue from the same species as the recipient.*	homoenxerto
homolateral *Ipsilateral.*	homolateral
homologous *Referring to something derived from the same species but different genotype.*	homólogo
homosexual *A person sexually attracted to someone of the same gender.*	homossexual
homozygous *Having identical alleles for a particular trait.*	homozigoto
hookworm *A parasitic infection of the family Strongylidae that can cause anemia.*	ancilóstomo duodenal
hordeolum *Inflammation of the sebaceous gland of the eye.*	hordéolo
hormone *A substance produced in the body that effects a specific organ.*	hormônio
horn *A keratinized outgrowth.*	chifre
Horner syndrome *A lesion of the cervical sympathetic chain causes ipsilateral myosis, ptosis and facial anhidrosis.*	síndrome de Horner; ptose simpática
horseshoe kidney *Anomalous renal development.*	rim em ferradura
hospital *Acute care medical/surgical facility.*	hospital
hospital discharge *To leave the hospital.*	alta da hospital
hot *Very warm.*	quente
hot flash *A symptom of menopause manifested as a sudden sensation of fever.*	rubor climatérico
housemaid's knee *Also referred to as prepatellar bursitis.*	joelho da dona-de-casa
HPV human papillomavirus *The virus that causes genital warts.*	vírus do papiloma humano
Hueter's maneuver *The application of downward and forward pressure on the tongue while passing an gastric tube.*	manobra de Hueter
human *Homo sapien.*	humano
humerus *The long bone in the upper arm.*	úmero
humor, aqueous *The gelatinous fluid circulating between the cornea and lens.*	humor aquoso
humor, vitreous *The fluid circulating between the lens and retina.*	humor vítreo
hunchback *Synonym of kyphosis.*	corcunda

English	Portuguese
hunger *A sense of discomfort caused by a lack of food.*	fome
Huntington's chorea *A neurodegenerative disease characterized initially by behavioral changes and later by a movement disorder. Called Huntington's disease now.*	doença de Huntington
Hutchinson's mask *The sensation the face is covered in cobwebs, associated with tabes dorsalis.*	máscara de Hutchinson
Hutchinson's pupil *Dilation of a pupil related to third nerve palsy on the side of the lesion as seen in herniation.*	pupila de Hutchinson
hyaline *Having a glassy, transparent appearance.*	hialina
hyaloid *Transparent.*	hialóide
hybrid *An animal or plant produced from two different species.*	híbrido
hydatid cyst *A cyst produced by and containing tapeworm larvae.*	cisto hidático
hydatiform *Referring to a hydatid cyst.*	hidatiforme
hydrarthrosis *An accumulation of water-like fluid in a joint cavity.*	hidrartrose
hydration *Used to describe fluid balance.*	hidratação
hydrocele *The accumulation of fluid in a body sac.*	hidrocele
hydrocephalus *The excessive accumulation of cerebral spinal fluid in the brain causing enlargement of the head.*	hidrocefalia
hydrochloric acid *A solution with a low pH formed by dissolving hydrogen chloride in water.*	ácido clorídrico
hydrochloride	cloridrato
hydrocortisone *A natural steroid hormone secreted by the adrenal cortex and used in a synthetic formulation for treatment of various medical conditions.*	hidrocortisona
hydrolysis *A reaction with water causing a compound to breakdown.*	hidrólise
hydronephrosis *Enlargement of a kidney due to interruption of outflow of urine from that kidney.*	hidronefrose
hydrophobia *Abnormal fear of water.*	hidrofobia
hydropneumothorax *Abnormal accumulation of fluid and air in the pleural space.*	hidropneumotórax
hydrops *The abnormal collection of fluid in a cavity.*	hidropsia
hydrops fetalis *The total body accumulation of fluid in a fetus; the result of a hemolytic reaction in a Rh neg mother.*	hidropsia fetal
hydrosalpinx *Collection of fluid in a fallopian tube.*	hidrossalpinge
hydrothorax *Accumulation of fluid within the thoracic cavity.*	hidrotórax
hygroma *A cyst or bursa filled with fluid.*	higroma
hygroscopic *The tendency to absorb moisture from the air.*	higroscópico
hymen *A membrane in the vagina.*	hímen
hymenotomy *Surgically creating an opening in the hymen.*	himenotomia
hyoid bone *A horseshoe shaped bone located between the chin and thyroid cartilage.*	osso hióde
hyperacidity *An abnormally high acid level.*	hiperácido
hyperactivity *Abnormal increase in activity.*	hiperatividade
hyperalgesia *Greater than normal sensitivity to pain.*	hiperalgesia
hyperbaric *Use of gas at a higher than normal pressure.*	hiperbárico
hyperbaric chamber *A device used to treat decompression illness.*	cámara hiperbárica
hyperbilirubinemia *Higher than normal level of bilirubin in the blood.*	hiperbilirrubinemia
hypercalcemia *Higher than normal level of calcium in the blood.*	hipercalcemia

English	Portuguese
hypercapnia *Higher than normal level of carbon dioxide in the blood stream.*	hipercapnia
hypercholesterolemia *Higher than normal level of cholesterol in the blood.*	hipercolesterolemia
hyperchromia *An excessive level of hemoglobin in erythrocytes.*	hipercromia
hyperemia *An increase in blood for the area of concern.*	hiperemia
hyperesthesia *Higher than normal skin sensitivity.*	hiperestesia
hyperextension *Extension of an articulation beyond the normal range.*	hiperextensão
hyperflexion *Flexion of an articulation beyond the normal range.*	hiperflexão
hyperglycemia *Higher than normal level of glucose in the blood.*	hiperglicemia
hypergonadism *A condition of excessive gonadal activity and subsequently precocious sexual development.*	hipergonadismo
hyperhidrosis *Excessive perspiration.*	hiperidrose
hyperkalemia *Higher than normal level of potassium in the blood stream.*	hipercalemia
hyperkeratosis *Excessive thickening of the outer layer of skin.*	hiperceratose
hyperkinesis *Excessive activity and inability to concentrate.*	hipercinese
hyperlipidemia *Higher than normal level of lipids in the blood stream.*	hiperlipemia
hypermetropia *Farsightedness.*	hipermetropia
hypermnesia *Unusually good memory.*	hipermnésia
hypermyotonia *Excessive muscle tone.*	hipermiotonia
hypernatremia *Elevated level of sodium in the blood.*	hipernatremia
hypernephroma *A renal tumor that mimic adrenal cortical tissue.*	hipernefroma
hyperonychia *Hypertrophic nails.*	hiperoníquia
hyperopia *Farsightedness.*	hiperopia
hyperosmia *Increased sense of smell.*	hiperosmia
hyperparathyroidism *Excessive level of parathyroid hormones in the blood stream causing weak bones and hypocalcemia.*	hiperparatireoidismo
hyperphagia *Excessive food ingestion.*	hiperfagia
hyperphoria *Upward deviation of the visual axis of the eye.*	hiperforia
hyperpituitarism *Excessive eosinophilic hormone resulting in acromegaly or excessive basophilic hormone resulting in pituitary compression and ultimately hypopituitarism.*	hiperpituitarismo
hyperplasia *Excessive growth of normal cells.*	hiperplasia
hyperpnea *Abnormal increase in rate and depth of respiration.*	hiperpnéia
hyperpyrexia *Fever.*	hiperpirexia
hyperreflexia *Abnormally brisk and vigorous reflex.*	hiper-reflexia
hypersensitivity *Abnormal increase in sensitivity.*	hipersensibilidade
hypersplenism *Excessive splenic activity resulting in decreased peripheral blood elements and sometimes splenomegaly.*	hiperesplenismo
hypertension *Higher than normal blood pressure.*	hipertensão
hyperthermia *Fever.*	hipertemia
hyperthyroidism *Increased thyroid activity resulting in exophthalmos and increased metabolic rate.*	hipertireoidismo
hypertonia *Excessive tone or tension.*	hipertonia
hypertonic *Increased osmotic pressure.*	hiperisotônico
hypertrichosis *Excessive hair growth.*	hipertricose
hypertrophy *Pathologic organ enlargement.*	hipertrofia

English	Portuguese
hyperuricemia *Elevated level of uric acid in the blood.*	hiperuricemia
hyperventilation *Rapid and deep respirations.*	hiperventilação
hypervolemia *Abnormally large amount of fluid in the blood stream.*	hipervolemia
hyphema *A blood collection in the front of the eye.*	hifema
hypnotic *Sleep inducing agent.*	hipnótico
hypocalcemia *Lower than normal level of calcium in the blood.*	hipocalcemia
hypocapnia *A decreased level of carbon dioxide in the blood.*	hipocapnia
hypochlorhydria *A state of decreased secretion of hydrochloric acid in the stomach.*	hipocloridria
hypochondriac *A person suffering from hypochondriasis.*	hipocondria
hypochondriasis *Abnormal increase in concern about one's own health.*	hipocondria
hypochondrium *The upper abdomen lateral to the epigastrium.*	hipocôndrio
hypochromic *Referring to the abnormal decrease in hemoglobin content of erythrocytes.*	hipocrômico
hypodermic injection *Subcutaneous injection.*	injeção hipodérmica
hypoesthesia *Abnormally decreased skin sensitivity.*	hipoestesia
hypofibrinogenemia *Diminished blood fibrinogen level.*	hipofibrinogenemia
hypogastric *Referring to the hypogastrium.*	hipogástrico
hypogastrium *The area of the central abdomen located below the stomach.*	hipogastro
hypoglossal nerve *Twelfth cranial nerve pair.*	nervo hipoglosso
hypoglycemia *Abnormally low blood sugar.*	hipoglicemia
hypogonadism *Abnormal decrease in gonadal function with associated diminished growth and sexual development.*	hipogonadismo
hypokalemia *Diminished level of potassium in the blood stream.*	hipocalemia
hypokalemic periodic paralysis *An inherited disorder that leads to muscle weakness related to a low serum potassium level.*	paralisia periódica hiperpotassêmica
hypomania *A moderate form of mania.*	hipomania
hyponatremia *Diminished level of sodium in the blood stream.*	hiponatremia
hypoparathyroidism *Abnormal decrease in parathyroid function.*	hipoparatireoidismo
hypophoria *Downward deviation of the visual axis of the eye.*	hipoforia
hypophosphatasia *A genetic defect of diminished alkaline phosphatase in the cells leading to bone demineralization.*	hipofosfatasia
hypophysectomy *Surgical removal of the pituitary gland.*	hipofisectomia
hypophysis *Pituitary gland.*	hipófise
hypopituitarism *Diminished pituitary activity exhibited by obesity and persistence of adolescent characteristics.*	hipopituitarismo
hypoplasia *Incomplete development.*	hipoplasia
hypopyon *The presence of purulent fluid in the anterior chamber of the eye.*	hipópio
hyposalivation *Secretion of saliva below the normal rate.*	hipossalivação
hypospadias *Congenital condition exhibited by development of the urethral meatus on the inferior aspect of the penis.*	hipospádia
hypostasis *The formation of a deposit.*	hipóstase
hypotension *Abnormally low blood pressure.*	hipotensão
hypothalamus *Located inferior to the thalamus it controls visceral activities, water balance, temperature and sleep.*	hipotálamo
hypothenar eminence *The prominence on the palm at the base of the fingers adjacent to the ulna.*	proeminência hipotenar

English	Portuguese
hypothermia *Lower than normal temperature.*	hipotermia
hypothyroidism *Reduced functioning of the thyroid.*	hipotireoidismo
hypotonia *Reduced tone or activity.*	hipotonia
hypoxia *Diminished oxygen content.*	hipoxia
hysterectomy *Surgical removal of the uterus.*	histerectomia
hysteria *A psychological condition exhibited by uncontrolled emotion or exaggerated manifestations.*	histeria
hysterography *1. Recording of uterine contractions. 2. Roentgenography of the uterus after administration of contrast media.*	histerografia
hysteromyomectomy *Surgical removal of a uterine myoma.*	histeromiomectomia
hysteropexy *Surgical fixation of the uterus by shortening of the round ligaments or by other means.*	histeropexia
hysterosalpingography *Roentgenography of the uterus and fallopian tubes after instillation of contrast media.*	histerossalpingografia
hysterotomy *Surgical opening of the uterus.*	histerotomia
i.e. *A latin derived abbreviation for "that is to say"(In latin: id est)*	id est
iatrogenic *A problem caused by medical treatment.*	iatrogênico
ichthyosis *A congenital anomaly exhibited by excessively dry, thick skin.*	ictiose
icterus *Yellowing of the skin and sclerae because of excess bilirubin.*	icterícia
identical twins *Twins from the same zygote.*	gêmeos idênticos
idiopathic *Relating to a disease with an unknown cause.*	idiopático
ileitis *Inflammation of the ileum.*	ileíte
ileocecal valve *The membranous folds between the ileum and cecum.*	válvula ileocecal
ileocolitis *Inflammation of the ileum and cecum.*	ileocolite
ileocolostomy *Creating a surgical opening between the ileum and colon.*	ileocolostomia
ileoproctostomy *Creating a surgical opening between the ileum and the rectum.*	ileoprotostomia
ileostomy *Surgical creation of an opening in the ileum that is placed at the skin surface.*	ileostomia
ileum *The portion of the small bowel from the jejunum to the cecum.*	ileo
ileus *A temporary obstruction in the intestine.*	íleo (obstrução mecânica)
iliac crest *The upper border of the ilium.*	crista ilíaca
iliococcygeal *Referring to the ilium and coccyx.*	iliococcígeo
ilium *The large bone at the superior aspect of the pelvis which is present bilaterally.*	osso ilíaco
illiterate *Unable to read or write.*	ileterado
immune *Being resistant to an infection.*	imune
immune response *The body's reaction to what is perceived as a foreign substance.*	resposta imune
immunization *A medication given to provide immunity.*	imunização
immunochemistry *The study of immune response and biochemistry.*	imunoquímica
immunodeficiency *An inadequate immune response.*	imunodeficiência
immunoelectrophoresis *A means of differentiating proteins and other compounds by comparing their mobility and antigenic specificities.*	imunoeletroforese

English	Portuguese
immunoglobulin *Serum and cellular proteins of the immune system.*	imunoglobulina
immunosuppression *The inhibition of the immune response.*	imunossupressão
impaction, tooth *A tooth that does not erupt because adjacent teeth prevent it.*	impactação dentária
impairment *A specific disability.*	enfraquecimento
imperforate *Lack of an opening. An infant with an imperforate anus has a congenital defect with no anal opening.*	imperfurado
impervious *Not affected by.*	impérvio
implant *A device or prosthesis implanted in a person.*	implante
implementation *The process of putting a plan into effect.*	implementação
impotence *Inability to act or inability to achieve a penile erection.*	impotência
inanition *Generalized weakness from lack of nutrition.*	inanição
inarticulate *Indistinct speech.*	inarticulado
incest *Sexual relations between related people.*	incesto
incipient *Starting to happen.*	incipiente
incision *An intentional surgical cut in the skin.*	incisão
incisor *Sharp-edged tooth; humans have four incisors.*	incisivo
incisura *A notch or indentation usually on the edge of a bone.*	incisura
incisure *A notch or incision.*	incisura
inclusion body *Variably shaped bodies in the nuclei of cells found in infections such as rabies and herpes.*	corpo inclusão
incoherent *Absence of intelligible speech.*	incoerente
incontinence *Inability to control urination.*	incontinência
incoordination *Absence of smooth, efficient body movement.*	incoordenação
increment *An increase on a fixed scale.*	incremento
incubator *A warming device for infants.*	incubador
incus *The middle ear bone between the stapes and malleus.*	bigorna
indeed *As a matter of fact.*	de fato
indigenous *Naturally occurring.*	indígeno
indigestion *Inadequate digestion for various reasons.*	indigestão
indolent *1. Causing little pain. 2. Slow healing ulcer.*	indolente
induce, to *Facilitated. When referring to labor, it means medication was given to assist in delivery of the fetus.*	induzir
induced abortion *Surgical or medical evacuation of the fetus.*	abortio induzido
induration *An area that is abnormally hard.*	endurecimento
indwelling catheter *Continuous use tube usually referring to a tube in the urinary bladder.*	cateter de demora
inebriation *Intoxication with drugs or alcohol.*	inebriação
ineffective *Unsuccessful or inefficient.*	ineficaz
inertia *The tendency to remain unchanged.*	inércia
inevitable *Not preventable.*	inevitável
infancy *Early childhood.*	infância
infant *Newborn.*	lactente; criança
infant, post-term *A neonate born after the normal gestation.*	lactente pósmaduro
infant, pre-term *A neonate born prior to normal gestation.*	lactente prematuro
infant, term *A neonate born at expected date.*	lactente termo
infantile *Referring to babies or young children.*	infantil
infarct *Referring to dead tissue.*	infarto
infarction *Dead tissue, for example, myocardial infarction.*	infartação
infectious *Contagious.*	infeccioso

English	Portuguese
inferior *The lower aspect.*	inferior
inferior pelvis strait *The pelvic outlet.*	abertura inferior da pelve
infestation *The presence of large numbers, as in lice infestation.*	infestação
inflammation *Localized redness, excessive warmth and swelling.*	inflamação
influenza *Viral infection causing fever, muscle aches and catarrh.*	influenza; gripe
infraspinous *Below the scapular spine.*	infra-espinhoso
infundibulum *The connection between the hypothalamus and the posterior pituitary gland.*	infundíbulo
infusion *The injection of fluid into tissue or a vein.*	infusão
ingestion *The intake of food or liquid orally.*	ingestão
ingrown nail *Also referred to as onychocryptosis.*	onicocriptose; unha encravada
inguinal *Referring to the groin.*	inguinal
inguinal ring (deep) *Indirect inguinal hernias exit the abdominal cavity via the deep inguinal ring.*	anel inguinal profundo
inhalation *The act of breathing in.*	inalação
injection *The act of a needle being inserted into a body.*	injecção
injure, to *To hurt or to wound.*	ferir
injury *A wound, abrasion or contusion.*	lesão
injury, closed head *Brain trauma not associated with damage to the dura or skull.*	lesão fechada da cabeça
injury, contrecoup of brain *An injury to the brain on the side opposite of that which was struck.*	lesão cerebral por contragolpe
injury, degloving *Trauma that involves the ripping of skin and subcutaneous tissue from the underlying tissue.*	lesão de desluvamento
injury, hyperextension-hyperflexion *An injury, usually to the cervical spine, that involves rapid deceleration, causing pronounced extension and flexion.*	lesão por hiperextensão e hiperflexão
inner ear *Made up of the cochlea and semicircular canals.*	ouvido interno
innervation *The presence of a nerve supply.*	inervação
innominate artery *The first branch off the aortic arch that branches into the right common carotid and right subclavian arteries.*	artéria inominada
innominate *Referring to the innominate artery.*	inominada
inoculation *Injection with a vaccine to provide immunity.*	inoculação
inorganic *Not coming from natural growth.*	inorgânico
insane *A term not used in formal medical evaluations that when used by a layperson means a serious mental illness.*	insano
insanity *Referring to a serious mental illness.*	insanidade
insensible *Unable to perceive a stimulus.*	insensível
insertion *The act of inserting something.*	inserção
inside *Inner part, center.*	interior
insidious *A slow, gradual and harmful advancement.*	insidioso
insomnia *Sleeplessness.*	insônia
inspiration *Drawing in a breath.*	inspiração
inspiratory reserve volume *The amount of air that can be inhaled after a normal inhalation.*	volume de reserva inspiratório
inspissate, to *To thicken or congeal.*	inspissado
instep *The medial aspect of the foot between the ankle and the ball of the foot.*	peito do pé
insulin *A hormone produced by the pancreas and synthetically to control blood glucose levels.*	insulina

English	Portuguese
insulinoma *An islet cell tumor that causes abnormally high insulin secretion and thus hypoglycemia.*	insulinoma
intake *An amount of food taken into the body.*	consumo
integument *Outer protective layer.*	integumento
intelligence quotient (IQ) *A number representing a person's ability to problem solve compared to a matched-control.*	quociente de inteligência
intensive *Very thorough or vigorous.*	intensivo
intensive care *Vigorous treatment of the acutely ill.*	cuidados intensiva
intention tremor *The tremulous movement noted when a person is beginning to perform a task but not seen at rest.*	tremor de intenção
interarticular *Between the articular surfaces of a joint.*	interarticular
intercellular *Between cells.*	intercelular
intermittent *Occurring at irregular intervals.*	intermitente
internal *Situated on the inside.*	interno
interosseous *Referring to something between bones, like the interosseous muscles of the hand.*	interósseo
interstitial *Referring to the interstices of tissue.*	intersticial
intertrigo *Irritation present because adjacent surfaces rub together.*	intertrigo
intertrochanteric *Referring to the space within the trochanter.*	intertrocantérica
interval *An intervening time.*	intervalo
interventricular *Between the ventricles.*	interventricular
intestinal obstruction *Blockage of the intestine by mass or volvulus.*	obstrução intestinal
intestinal *Referring to the intestines.*	intestinal
intestine *A general term used for the section of bowel from the stomach to the anus.*	intestino
intraabdominal abscess *A collection of pus in the abdomen.*	abscesso intra-abdominal
intraabdominal *Within the abdominal cavity.*	intra-abdominal
intraarticular *Within a joint space.*	intra-articular
intracellular *Within a cell.*	intracelular
intracerebral *Within the cerebrum.*	intracerebral
intracranial *Within the cranial vault.*	intracraniano
intradermal *Within the dermis.*	intradérmico
intradural *Within the dural space.*	intradural
intramedullary *1. Within the medulla oblongata. 2. Within the bone marrow.*	intramedular
intramuscular *Within a muscle.*	intramuscular
intraocular fluid *Fluid within the globe.*	fluido intra-ocular
intraosseous *Within a bone.*	intra-ósseo
intraperitoneal *Within the peritoneal cavity.*	intraperitoneal
intrathecal *Technically means within a sheath but this term is used when medication is instilled in the dura mater spinalis.*	intratecal
intrauterine contraceptive device (IUD) *A device used to physically prevent the implantation of a fertilized ovum.*	dispositivo contraceptivo intra-uterino (DIU)
intrauterine *Within the uterus.*	intra-uterino
intravenous infusion *Administration of fluid into a vein.*	infusão intravenoso
intravenous tubing *The tubing used to administer fluids.*	tubo intravenoso
intravenous *Within a vein.*	intravenoso
intubation *Placement of a tube; commonly used to refer to endotracheal intubation.*	intubação
intussusception *The inversion of one portion of the bowel into another.*	intossuscepção

English	Portuguese
inulin *A polysaccharide used in the testing of renal function.*	inulina
inunction *The application of lotion with friction.*	inunção
involucrum *A wrap or covering (referring to a sequestrum).*	invólucro
involutional *The shrinkage of an organ when it is not in use, as in the uterus after childbirth.*	involucional
involved *Difficult to comprehend.*	envolvido
iodine *A chemical used as an antiseptic and a deficiency of it can lead to goiter.*	iodo
iodism *A condition caused by excessive iodine intake resulting in diarrhea, weakness, and convulsions.*	intoxicação pelo iodo
ion channel *A selectively permeable cell membrane to certain ions.*	canal iônico
ionizing radiation *High energy radiation that produces ion pairs in matter.*	radiação ionizante
ipsilateral *On the same side.*	ipsolateral
iridectomy *Surgical removal of part of the iris.*	iridectomia
iridocyclitis *Inflammation of the ciliary body and the iris.*	iridociclite
iridoplegia *Paralysis of part of the iris with subsequent lack of contraction or dilation of the pupil.*	iridoplegia
iridotomy *A surgical opening of the iris.*	iridotomia
iris *The colored membrane posterior to the cornea.*	íris
iron *An element found in hemoglobin.*	ferro
iron-deficiency anemia *A microcytic anemia.*	anemia por deficiência de ferro
irradiation *The process of being irradiated.*	irradiação
irrelevant *Not pertinent.*	inaplicável
irritable bowel syndrome *A condition exhibited by chronic diarrhea or constipation and abdominal pain; it is sometimes associated with a labile emotional state.*	síndrome do intestino irritável
ischemia *Inadequate blood supply to a part of the body.*	isquemia
ischemic contracture *A muscle's resistance to passive stretch that is related to a decrease in arterial flow from any reason.*	contratura isquêmica
ischemic heart disease *Inadequate blood supply to the heart.*	doença isquémico cardíaco
ischemic optic neuropathy *A general category of a cause of blindness with several subcategories.*	neuropatia óptica isquêmica
ischium *The inferoposterior portion of the pelvis.*	ísquio
islet *Tissue that is structurally separate from adjacent tissues.*	ilhota
isoantibody *A situation in which an antibody of person A reacts with an antigen of person B.*	isoanticorpo
isolation *To be kept separate or apart.*	isolamento
isolation ward *A ward where patients with infectious disease are housed.*	enfermaria isolamento
isthmus *A narrow piece of tissue connecting two larger body parts.*	istmo
itch *A sensation that makes one want to scratch.*	prurido
jaundice *Yellowing of the sclerae and skin because of excessive bilirubin in the blood.*	icterícia
jaundice of the newborn *A form of jaundice seen in newborns in the first two weeks of life; also called icterus neonatorum.*	icterícia do recém-nascido
jaw *Mandible.*	mandíbula
jaw reflex *Contraction of the temporal muscles when a relaxed mandible is given a downward tap. Also, masseter reflex or jaw jerk.*	reflexo mandibular
jejunectomy *Surgical removal of the jejunum.*	jejunectomia
jejunostomy *Surgical creation of an opening in the jejunum.*	jejunostomia

English	Portuguese
Jendrassik's maneuver *A method of distracting a patient while checking the patellar reflex.*	manobra de Jendrassik
Job syndrome *Also known as hyperimmunoglobulin E syndrome, there are high levels if IgE, a leukocyte chemotactic defect, recurrent staph infections and cold abscess formation in the skin.*	síndrome de Job
jock itch *Pruritus caused by tinea cruris.*	tinha crural
joint *Articulation of two adjacent bones.*	articulação
jugular notch *The notch on the upper border of the sternum.*	incisura jugular
jugular *Referring to the neck, as in jugular vein.*	jugular
jugular vein (s) *Includes the internal, external and anterior jugular veins.*	veno jugular
juvenile angiofibroma *A noncancerous growth in the nose or pharyngeal region.*	angiofibroma juvenil
juxta-articular *Positioned near a joint.*	justarticular
juxtaglomerular apparatus *Cells located in the tunica media of the afferent glomerular arterioles.*	aparelho justaglomerular
kala-azar *A disease caused by Leishmania donovani that is exhibited by weight loss, fever, anemia and hepatosplenomegaly.*	calazar
Kaposi sarcoma *Typically seen in AIDS patients, it is characterized by cutaneous reddish-purple macules and plaques. Also called multiple idiopathic hemorrhagic sarcoma.*	sarcoma de Kaposi
karyokinesis *A part of mitosis involving the cell nucleus division.*	cariocinese
karyotype *The arrangement of chromosomes in a single cell.*	cariótipo
Kawasaki syndrome *Begins with fever for 5 days, skin rashes, strawberry tongue, lymphadenopathy and swollen hands and feet. It is known to cause coronary artery aneurysms. Also called mucocutaneous lymph node syndrome.*	síndrome do linfonodo cutaneomucoso; doença de Kawasaki
keloid *Hypertrophic scar tissue that forms after a minor cut or surgical procedure.*	quelóide
keratectasia *Obtrusion of the cornea.*	ceratoectasia
keratectomy *Excision of a portion of the cornea.*	ceratectomia
keratic *Referring to the cornea.*	cerático
keratin *A protein found in the skin, hair, nails and enamel of the teeth.*	ceratina
keratoma *A protuberance of horny tissue.*	ceratoma
keratomalacia *Softening of the cornea.*	ceratomalacia
keratosis *A growth of keratin such as a wart or callosity.*	ceratose
kernicterus *A condition associated with high bilirubin levels that causes yellow staining of cerebral tissues and subsequent neurologic dysfunction.*	icterícia nuclear
ketoacidosis *Usually referring to diabetic ketoacidosis in which ketones are broken down, causing a decrease in blood pH.*	cetoacidose
ketone body *One ketone with a decarboxylation product of acetone.*	corpo cetônico
ketonemia *Presence of ketone in the blood.*	cetonemia
ketonuria *Presence of ketone in the urine.*	cetonúria
ketosis *The presence of an abnormally high level of ketones in the blood and body tissues.*	cetose
kick, to *To strike an object with one's foot.*	espernear
kidney *One of two glandular organs that form urine.*	rim
kinase *An enzyme that facilitates movement of phosphate from ATP to another molecule.*	cinase

English	Portuguese
kineplasty *An amputation done in a fashion to facilitate ambulation.*	cineplastia
kinesis *Movement of a part in response to a stimulus.*	cinese
kinky-hair syndrome *Inborn error of copper metabolism, noted in the first few weeks of life. Exhibited by sparse kinky hair, failure to thrive and seizures. Also called Menke's syndrome or trichopoliodystrophy.*	síndrome de Menkes; doença do cabelo enroscado
Klinefelter's syndrome *Presence of an extra X chromosome, it is exhibited by longer legs, narrow shoulders, small testicles and gynecomastia.*	síndrome de Klinefelter
knee *The joint at the distal femur and proximal tibia.*	joelho
knee elbow position *Knees and elbows are on the table and the chest is in the air.*	posição genocubital
knee jerk reflex *Contraction of the quadriceps, yielding leg extension when the quadriceps tendon is tapped.*	reflexo patelar; reflexo de contração do joelho
kneecap *Common term for patella.*	patela
kneeling *Being on one's knees as in the prayer position.*	genuflexão
knock knees *Common term for genu valgum.*	genu valgum; joelho valgo
knot *A fastening made by tying a suture, for instance.*	nó
known *Recognized or familiar.*	sabido
knuckle *A metacarpophalagngeal joint or a finger joint when the fist is closed.*	junta; articulação
koilonychia *Thin and concave fingernails.*	quiloníquia
Koplik's spots *Red buccal macules with a blue center; seen in measles.*	manchas de Koplik
kopophobia *A morbid fear of fatigue.*	medo mórbido de fadiga
Köhler's disease *A genetic disease characterized by osteonecrosis and subsequent collapse of the tarsal navicular bone.*	doença de Köhler
kraurosis vulvae *Dryness and shrinkage of the vulva.*	craurose vulvar
Krebs cycle *The process of aerobic respiration by which living cells generate energy.*	ciclo de Krebs
kubisagari *Vestibular neuronitis.*	tontura epidêmica
Kussmaul respiration *The slow, deep breathing noted in patients with acidosis.*	respiração de Kussmaul
Kyasanur Forest disease *A viral fever noted in Mysore, India transmitted by Haemaphysalis spinigera. It is characterized by fever, headache, generalized pains, diarrhea, and intestinal bleeding.*	doença da Floresta de Kyasnur
kwashiorkor *A form of malnutrition from inadequate protein intake.*	pelagra infantil
kyphoscoliosis *An abnormal outward and lateral curvature of the spine.*	cifoescoliose
kyphosis *Abnormal outward curvature of the spine.*	cifose
lab result *The data obtained from a laboratory test.*	resultado laboratório
labial *Referring to the lip.*	labial
labile *Easily altered; emotionally unstable.*	lábil
labium majus (plural= labia majora) *The folds of skin forming the lateral borders of the pudendal cleft.*	grande lábio pudendo
labium minus (plural=labia minora) *The folds of skin posterior to the labia majora.*	lábio pudendo menor
labium *Referring to any lip shaped structure.*	lábio
labor onset *The time when a pregnant woman begins uterine contractions in the process of childbirth.*	começo do trabalho de parto

English	Portuguese
labor pains *The intermittent pain associated with uterine contractions.*	dores do parto
labor room *The hospital room used while a woman is in labor.*	sala de parto
laboratory *A room equipped to run blood, tissue and fluid samples.*	laboratório
labyrinthitis *Inflammation of the labyrinth.*	labirintite
labrum *An edge or lip. The labrum acetabular is the fibrocartilagous rim attached to the acetabulum.*	lábio
labyrinth *Inner ear structure concerned with balance.*	labirinto
laceration *An injury that produced a cut in the skin or tissue such as a tear during childbirth.*	laceração
lacrimal *Referring to the secretion of tears.*	lacrimal
lacrimal fluid *Fluid secreted by the lacrimal gland.*	fluido lacrimal
lacrimation *The secretion of tears.*	lacrimejamento
lactalbumin *Proteins found in milk.*	lactalbumina
lactase *An enzyme that facilitates the breakdown of lactose to glucose and galactose.*	lactase
lactation *The secretion of milk from mammary glands.*	lactação
lactic *Referring to milk.*	láctico
lactiferous duct *A canal that carries milk.*	ducto lactífero
lactose *A disaccharide present in milk.*	lactose
lactose intolerance *The inability of the small bowel to digest lactose.*	intolerância lactose
lacuna *A small cavity or depression.*	lacuna
lacunar infarction *Small non-cortical cerebral infarcts.*	infartação lacunar
lagophthalmos *Characterized by the inability to close the eyelid completely over the eye.*	lagoftalmia
laliophobia *Abnormal fear of speaking or stuttering.*	laliofobia
lalochezia *Relief of stress by uttering obscenities.*	laloquezia
lambdoid *The suture connecting the parietal bones with the occipital bone.*	lambdóide
lamella *A thin layer of bone.*	lamela
laminectomy *The surgical removal of part of a vertebrae.*	laminectomia
lancet *A small sharp instrument used to obtain a drop of blood for testing.*	lanceta
laparoscope *A fiber-optic instrument used to visualize the peritoneal contents.*	laparoscópio
laparoscopy *A procedure utilizing a laparoscope.*	laparoscopia
laparotomy *A surgical incision of the abdomen.*	laparotomia
laryngeal *Referring to the larynx.*	laríngeo
laryngectomy *Surgical removal of the larynx.*	laringectomia
laryngismus stridulus *Sudden, severe laryngeal spasm.*	laringismo estriduloso
laryngitis *Inflammation of the larynx.*	laringite
laryngology *The study of the larynx and related diseases.*	laringologia
laryngopharynx *The pharyngeal space between the superior aspect of the glottis and the opening of the larynx.*	laringofaringe
laryngospasm *Sudden, involuntary muscle contraction of the larynx.*	laringospasmo
laryngostenosis *Abnormal narrowing of the larynx.*	laringoestenose
laryngotomy *Surgical creation of an opening in the larynx.*	laringotomia
larynx *A hollow muscular structure that contains the vocal cords.*	laringe
last *Final.*	final

English	Portuguese
late *A time later than expected.*	tardio
lateral *Referring to the side of the body.*	lateral; de lado
laterodeviation *Pushed to the lateral aspect.*	látero-desvio
lathyrism *A disease characterized by tremors, spastic paralysis and paresthesias caused by Lathyrus sativus.*	latirismo
laugh, to	gargalhar
laxity *A description of a joint that is loose.*	frouxidão
layer *A stratum or thickness.*	camada
lead *An element with an atomic number of 82.*	chumbo
lead poisoning *The ingestion of lead, exhibited in severe cases by paralysis, encephalopathy, purple gingiva, and colic.*	intoxicação por chumbo
leaflet *Cusp.*	cúspide
leakage *Unintentional escape of gas or fluid.*	vazamento
learning *The intentional acquisition of knowledge.*	inclinação
lecithin *A compound widely used by tissues, derived from egg yolks and it consists of phospholipids linked to choline.*	lecitina
leech *An annelid used in some tropical regions for drawing out blood; they have an anticoagulant effect locally and have been attached to digits of persons with acute peripheral ischemia.*	sanguessuga
left	esquerdo
left-handed *The preference of using the left hand for common tasks.*	canhoto
leg *One of two lower extremities.*	perna
legionnaires' disease *The name was derived after an outbreak at a convention of the American Legion; it is manifested by fever, chills, dyspnea, and cough.*	doença dos legionários; legionelose
leishmaniasis *A condition caused by a flagellate protozoan parasite that is exhibited by visceral or dermatologic manifestations.*	leishmaniose
length *The end to end measurement.*	comprimento
lengthening *Becoming longer.*	alongamento
lens *The transparent chamber between the posterior chamber and the vitreous body.*	lente
lenticular *Referring to the lens of the eye.*	lenticular
lentigo *A benign condition exhibited by flat brown patches on the skin.*	lentigo
leontiasis ossea *Bilateral hypertrophy of the bones of the face and cranium.*	leontíase óssea; doença de Virchow
Leopold's maneuver *Used to determine fetal position.*	manobra de Leopold
leproma *A superficial granulatomous papule that is seen in leprosy.*	leproma
leprosy *A contagious disease caused by Mycobacterium leprae that causes insensate papules and disfiguration.*	lepra
leptomeningitis *A general term used to describe meningitis of the pia and arachnoid of the brain.*	leptomeningite
leptospirosis *A zoonosis caused by the spirochete Leptospira interrogans transmitted by rats and contaminated water.*	leptospirose
lesbian *A woman with same gender preference.*	lésbica
less *A smaller amount.*	menos
lethal *Deadly.*	letal
lethal dose *The amount of a drug required to cause death.*	dose letal
lethargy *Absence of energy.*	letargia

English	Portuguese
leucinosis; maple syrup urine disease *A condition characterized by an enzyme defect causing an increase in leucine in the urine.*	doença da urina em xarope de bordo; leucinose
leukemia *A malignant disease causing an increase in the number of abnormal and immature leukocytes.*	leucemia
leukine (or leucine) *An amino acid obtained from hydrolysis of some proteins.*	leucina
leukocyte *A white blood cell.*	leucócito
leukocythemia *Synonym of leukemia.*	leucocitemia
leukocytolysis *Destruction of white blood cells.*	leucocitólise
leukocytosis *An increase in the number of leukocytes.*	leucocitose
leukodermia *A localized loss of skin pigment.*	leucodermia
leukonychia *A whitish discoloration of the fingernails and toenails.*	leuconíquia
leukopenia *A decreased number of leukocytes in the blood.*	leucopenia
leukopoiesis *Production of white blood cells.*	leucopoiese
leukorrhea *Thick white vaginal discharge.*	leucorréia
levator *A muscle that raises part of the body; the levator labii superioris raised the upper lip.*	elevador
levulose *Synonym for fructose.*	levulose
libido *Sexual desire.*	libido
Libman-Sachs syndrome *A verrucous endocarditis associated with disseminated lupus erythematosus; also called nonbacterial verrucous endocarditis.*	síndrome de Libman-Sachs
library	biblioteca
lice *Plural for louse, a small parasite that lives on the skin. Pediculus humanus capitis is a head louse.*	piolhos
lichen *A term used to describe a variety of papular skin diseases. Lichen planus is a shiny, flat, violaceous eruption of the mucous membranes, skin and genitalia.*	líquen
life expectancy *The length of time a person is anticipated to live.*	expectativa vida
life-threatening *Potentially fatal.*	ameaçador vida
lifetime *Duration of a person's life.*	por toda a vida
lift, to *Raise to a higher level.*	erguer
ligament *A band of fibrous connective tissue that connects two bones or cartilage.*	ligamento
ligature *A thread used to tie a vessel.*	ligadura
light *Illumination, bright.*	luz
light *Not heavy.*	leve
light adaptation *The pupillary adjustment after going from a dark environment to one of bright light.*	adaptação à luz
likelihood *The probability or feasibility.*	probabilidade
limb *An extremity or branch.*	membro
limbus *The margin of a structure, for example, of the cornea and sclera.*	limbo
liminal stimulus *Referring to a stimulus of threshold strength.*	estímulo liminar
lincture *A medicine mixed with a sweet substance.*	linctura
linea alba *The tendinous portion of the anterior abdomen between the two rectus muscles.*	linha branca
lingua nigra *A condition characterized by a dark fur-like covering on the dorsum of the tongue.*	linha negra
lip, lower *Labium inferius oris.*	lábio inferior
lip, upper *Labium superius oris.*	lábio, superior

English	Portuguese
lipase *A pancreatic enzyme that facilitates the breakdown of fats.*	lipase
lipemia *Abnormally high fat content in the blood.*	lipemia
lipid *A compound that is a fatty acid which is insoluble in water but soluble in organic solvents.*	lipídeo
lipid-lowering agent *A medication used to treat hyperlipidemia.*	medicamento por hiperlipemia
lipoatrophy *Fatty tissue atrophy.*	lipoatrofia
lipochondrodystrophy *A congenital condition exhibited by short stature, kyphosis, mental deficiency and short fingers.*	dipocondrodistrofia
lipocyte *A fat cell.*	lipócito
lipodystrophy *Abnormal fat metabolism.*	lipodistrofia
lipoid *Referring to fat.*	lipóide
lipoidosis *Abnormal lipid metabolism.*	lipoidose
lipoma *A benign tumor consisting of fat cells.*	lipoma
lipoprotein *A soluble protein used to transport fat or lipids.*	lipoproteína
lipotrophic substance *A compound which causes an increase in body fat.*	substância lipotrófico
lisping *A speech problem in which "s" and "z" are pronounced "th".*	balbucio
listeriosis *A disease caused by Listeria monocytogenes that occurs in the pregnant and immunocompromised.*	listeriose
lithagogue *A treatment of a calculus.*	medicamento para cálculo
litholapaxy *The crushing and then removal of a calculus.*	litolapaxia
lithotomy *Surgical removal of a calculus.*	litotomia
lithotomy position *Buttocks positioned at the end of the OR table, the hips and knees flexed and the feet strapped in. Dorsosacral position.*	posição de litotomia
lithotriptor *An instrument used to crush a calculus.*	litotriptor
litmus *A dye that turns red with low pH and blue with high pH.*	litmo
liver *A large glandular organ in the right upper quadrant that functions in digestive processes, as well as, neutralizing toxins.*	fígado
liver abscess *A localized collection of pus in the liver.*	abscesso de fígado
lobar *Referring to a lobe.*	lobar
lobe *A body part divided by a fissure.*	lobo
lobectomy *Surgical removal of a lobe (generally lung or liver).*	lobectomia
lobotomy *Surgical incision into the prefrontal lobe; historically a treatment of mental illness.*	lobotomia
Lobo's disease *A condition exhibited by small, red, hard papules in the sacral region caused by Lacazia loboi.*	doença de Lobo; lobomycosis
lobule *A small lobe.*	lóbulo
localization *Establishment of a site of a disease process.*	localização
localized *Toward one point or area.*	localizado
lochia *Vaginal secretions noted within two weeks of childbirth.*	lóquios
locked-in syndrome *A neurologic condition characterized by a person being conscious of their surroundings but being unable to verbally communicate that understanding.*	síndrome pseudocoma
loculated *Divided into small cavities.*	loculação
loiasis *A disease caused by the filarial nematode Loa loa.*	loíasis
long-acting *Referring to a drug with long lasting effects.*	funcionamento prolongado
long-term care *Generally referring to nursing home care.*	cuidado de sanatório
long-standing *Having existed for a long time.*	antigo
longevity *Long life.*	longevidade
longsighted *Synonym of hyperopia.*	hiperopia

English	Portuguese
loose *Not tight.*	liberdade
looseness *Possessing a quality of not being tight.*	frouxidão
lordosis *An abnormal depth of the inward curvature of the spine.*	lordose
loss of consciousness *Unresponsive to verbal and tactile stimuli.*	consciência, perdir
loss of function *Inability to complete routine activities.*	função, perdir
lost to follow-up *This describes a situation in which a patient has a chronic medical problem but has not been seen regularly.*	sem responder a
lots of *An abundance of.*	muitos
low back pain *Pain in the lumbar region.*	dor em região lombar
low nasal bridge *A flattening of the top part of the nose.*	achatamento de eminência nasal
low-fat foods *Nutrients with lower than normal fat content.*	nutrição magro
lower extremity edema *Interstitial edema of the legs.*	edema de declive
lubricant *Emollient.*	lubrificante
lumbago *Pain in the region of the lumbar spine.*	dor em região lombar
lumbar puncture *Insertion of a needle into the spinal canal in the region of L3-4 to obtain a sample of CSF.*	poncionar lombar
lumbar *Referring to the spinal region inferior to the thoracic spine.*	lombar
lumen *A hollow cavity.*	espaço no interior de uma estrutura tubular
lump *A protuberance.*	pedaço
lunate bone; os lunatum *A carpal bone that articulates with the wrist.*	osso intermédio
lung *One of a pair of respiratory organs.*	pulmão
lung capacity, total *The amount of air in the lungs after a maximal inhalation.*	capacidade pulmonar total
lunula *The pale area at the base of a fingernail.*	lúnula
lupus erythematosous *An autoimmune inflammatory disease exhibited by a butterfly shaped rash on the face along with visceral and connective tissue abnormalities.*	lúpus eriematoso
luteinizing hormone (LH) *A pituitary hormone that stimulates ovulation in females and androgen in males.*	hormônio luteinizante
luteotropic *Synonym of prolactin.*	luteotrópico
Lyell's syndrome *Also called toxic epidermal necrolysis, there are large portions of the skin that become erythematous with epidermal necrosis as seen with 2nd degree burns. This reaction can be seen with use of nevirapine or Bactrim.*	síndrome de Lyell
lymph *A transparent and sometimes opalescent fluid that flows in the lymph channels.*	linfa
lymph node *An area of organized lymphatic tissue.*	linfonodo
lymphadenitis *Inflammation of a lymph node.*	linfadenite
lymphangiectasis *Distention of the lymph channels.*	linfangiectasia
lymphangioma *A mass composed of newly formed lymph tissue.*	linfangioma
lymphangitis *Inflammation of the lymph vessels.*	linfangite
lymphatic *Referring to the lymph system.*	linfático
lymphocyte *A white blood cell produced by the lymph tissue.*	linfócito
lymphocythemia *Abnormally high number of lymphocytes in the blood.*	linfocitemia
lymphocytic leukemia *Chronic accumulation of functionally incompetent lymphocytes.*	leucemia linfocítico
lymphocytopenia *Decrease in the usual number of lymphocytes in the blood.*	linfocitopenia
lymphocytosis *The organization of cysts containing lymph.*	linfocitose

English	Portuguese
lymphoid *Similar to lymph.*	linfóide
lymphoma *A malignant disease of the lymph system, Hodgkin's lymphoma for example.*	linfoma
lymphosarcoma *A malignant disease of the lymph system that does not include Hodgkin's lymphoma.*	linfossarcoma
lysine *An amino acid found in most proteins.*	lisina
lysis *The rupture of a cell wall or membrane.*	lise
lysosome *An organelle contained in the cytoplasm of eukaryotic cells.*	lisossoma
lysozyme *An enzyme in tears that facilitates destruction of certain bacterial cell walls.*	lisossoma; muramidase
lytic *Referring to lysis.*	lítico
macrocheilia *Abnormally large lips.*	macroquilia
macrocyte *A large red blood cell.*	macrócito
macrocytosis *Referring to the status of an increased number of large erythrocytes as seen in Vitamin B12 deficiency.*	macrocitose
macrodactyly *Abnormally large digits.*	macrodactilia
macroencephaly *Having an abnormally large head.*	macroencefalia
macroglobulinemia *A condition exhibited by an increase number of macroglobulins in the blood.*	macroglobulina
macroglossia *Abnormally large tongue.*	macroglossia
macromastia *Abnormally large breasts.*	macromastia
macromelia *Abnormally large head or extremity.*	macromelia
macrophage *A phagocytic cell that originates in the tissues.*	macrófago
macrostomia *Abnormal increase in the width of the mouth.*	macrostomia
macula *1. The area of the eye of greatest visual acuity that surrounds the fovea. 2. A small flat discoloration of the skin (synonym for macule).*	mácula
macula solaris *Formal medical term describing a freckle.*	máculas amareladas
maculopapule *A skin lesion that is similar to both a macule and a papule.*	maculopápula
mad cow disease *Bovine spongiform encephalopathy, a disease that cause cerebral degeneration exhibited by ataxia.*	encefalopatia espongiforme bovina
madness *Common term for insanity.*	loucura
magnet *A piece of iron with atoms ordered to make it magnetic.*	magneto
magnetic *Having the properties of a magnet.*	magnético
magnetic resonance imaging (MRI) *Images are produced by evaluating the response of body tissue. nuclei to radio waves in a magnetic field.*	imagem por ressonância magnética
maiden name *The surname a woman uses prior to being married.*	nome de solteira
maintenance therapy *Continuing a form of treatment long-term.*	terapia de manutenção
Malabar itch. *Pruritus associated with tinea imbricata which is characterized by overlapping rings of papulosquamous patches. It is also known as oriental ringworm.*	tinha imbricada
malacia *The abnormal softening of a body part or tissue.*	malacia
maladjustment *Having the trait of being unable to cope normally.*	inadaptação
malaise *A vague feeling of discomfort or unease.*	mal-estar
malalignment (dental) *Displacement of the teeth from their normal position.*	mal-alinhamento

English	Portuguese
malaria *A condition caused by a protozoan of the genus Plasmodium. It is transmitted by mosquitos and is exhibited by fever, chills, headache. In the severe form it can lead to convulsions, increased ICP and death.*	malária
malignant *Tendency of a tumor to invade normal tissue.*	maligno
malignant hypertension *Sudden, severe hypertension associated with neuroretinitis.*	hipertensão maligna
malingerer *A person who feigns illness.*	simulador
malleolus *A bony protrusion on medial and lateral aspect of each ankle.*	maléolo
malleolus, lateral *The lateral aspect of the distal fibula.*	maléolo lateral
malleolus, medial *The medial aspect of the distal portion of the tibia.*	maléolo medial
mallet finger *Flexion contracture of the distal phalanx.*	dedo em martelo; dedo de beisebol
malleus *Small bone in the inner ear that articulates with the incus.*	martelo
Mallory-Weiss syndrome *Upper GI bleeding related to a laceration at the gastroesophageal junction caused by vigorous vomiting.*	síndrome de Mallory-Weiss
malnutrition *Lack of appropriate nutrition.*	desnutrição
malpractice *Negligent professional activity.*	imperícia
maltose *A disaccharide hydrolyzed by amylase.*	maltose
malunion *The union of a fracture in a faulty position.*	má união
mammaplasty *Plastic surgery of the breast.*	mamoplastia
mammary *Referring to the breast.*	mamário
mammary gland *The mass of tissue posterior to the nipples which has the essential task of milk production.*	glande mamária
mammillary *Referring to a nipple.*	mamilar
mammography *Roentgenography of the breasts, used as a screening test for cancer.*	mamografia
man *Male human.*	homem
management *The process of dealing with things or people.*	administração
mandatory *Obligatory.*	madatário
mandible *The lower jaw.*	mandíbula
mania *A mental disorder exhibited by hyperexcitability, delusions and euphoria.*	mania
manic-depressive psychosis *A mental disorder exhibited by alternating periods of depression and mania.*	distúrbio maníco-depressivo
manometer *Device used for pressure monitoring.*	manômetro
manubrium sterni *The superior segment of the sternum which articulates with the clavicle and first rib.*	manúbrio esternal
maple syrup urine disease *A condition characterized by an enzyme defect causing an increase in leucine in the urine.*	doença da urina em xarope de bordo; leucinose
mapping *A collection of data points showing spatial distribution.*	mapeamento
marasmus *Progressive weight loss and emaciation.*	marasmo
Marfan syndrome *A connective tissue disease exhibited by long limbs, joint laxity and cardiovascular defects.*	síndrome de Marfan
marijuana *Cannabis.*	maconha
marital counseling *Therapy aimed at marriage reconciliation.*	conselheiro marital
marital status *Single versus married status.*	status marital
marsupialization *Creation of a surgical pouch.*	marsupialização
mass *Tumor.*	massa

English	Portuguese
mast cell *A cell containing basophilic granules that releases histamine and other substances during allergic reactions.*	célula mastócito
mastectomy *Surgical resection of one or both breasts.*	mastectomia
mastication *Chewing.*	mastigação
mastitis *Inflammation of the breast.*	mastite
mastodynia *Breast pain.*	mastalgia
mastoid *Referring to the mastoid process.*	mastóide
mastoid process *The posterior part of the temporal bone bordered by the parietal bone superiorly and the occipital bone posteriorly.*	processo mastóide
mastoidectomy *Surgical removal of the mastoid.*	mastoidectomia
mastoiditis *Inflammation of the mastoid process.*	mastoidite
matching *Corresponding in pattern or style.*	comparação
mattress *A fabric case filled with material, used for sleeping.*	colchão
mattress suture *A double stitch that forms a loop and there is eversion of the edges when tied.*	sutura de colchoeiro
maxilla *The upper jaw that also forms the inferior portion of the orbit and part of the nose.*	maxilar
maxillofacial *Referring to the maxilla and the face.*	maxilofacial
mazamorra *Dermatitis caused by hookworm larvae indigenous to Puerto Rico.*	mazamorra
Mcdonald's maneuver *A measurement of the uterus in centimeters that corresponds to gestational age in weeks.*	maneuver de Mcdonald
meaningless *Having no significance.*	insignificante
measles *A childhood viral, infectious disease exhibited by rash and fever.*	sarampo
meatus *Opening to the body, such as urethral meatus.*	meato
meconium *The first newborn feces which are green.*	mecônico
meconium aspiration *Presence of meconium on the newborn indicating there was fetal distress in-utero.*	aspiração mecônio
medial *Situated toward the midline.*	medial
medianstinoscopy *Visual inspection of the mediastinum with a scope.*	mediastinoscopia
mediastinum *The thoracic area between the lungs.*	mediastino
medical record *The electronic or paper report on a patient.*	registro médico
medication *A substance used for medical treatment.*	medicação; medicamento (P)
medicine *A substance used for medical treatment or the art and science of healing patients.*	medicamento; estudo de doenças
medicosurgical *Referring to medicine and surgery.*	medicocirúrgico
medulla oblongata *The inferior portion of the brainstem.*	medula oblonga
medullary *1. The inner part of an organ. 2. Referring to the medulla oblongata.*	medular
medulloblastoma *A malignant tumor of the cerebellum found mostly in children.*	meduloblastoma
megacephaly *Having a larger than normal cranial capacity.*	megacefalia
megacolon *Abnormal enlargement and dilatation of the colon.*	megacólon
megakaryocyte *A cell found in the bone marrow that is a source of platelet production.*	megacariócito
megaloblast *A large red blood cell noted primarily in pernicious anemia.*	megaloblasto
megalomania *A mental disorder characterized by abnormal feelings of self-importance.*	megalomania
meibomian cyst *An enclosed fluid collection along a sebaceous gland of the eyelid.*	cisto de Meibômio

English	Portuguese
meiosis *Cell division creating two daughter cells each with half the number of cells as the parent cell.*	meiose
melancholia *Profound sadness.*	melancolia
melanin *A dark pigment found on the skin, hair or iris.*	melanina
melanoma *Malignant cancer, typically found in the skin.*	melanoma
melena *The passage of black, tarry stools indicative of upper gastrointestinal bleeding.*	melena
melissophobia *Also called apiphobia, a fear of bees.*	melissofobia
melitis *Inflammation of the cheek.*	melite
member *Referring to an extremity (arm or leg).*	membro
memory *Ability to remember.*	memória
menarche *The time of the initial menstrual period.*	menarca
meningeal *Referring to the dura mater, arachnoid and the pia mater.*	meníngeo
meningioma *A tumor of the meningeal tissue; generally benign.*	meningioma
meningism *Signs and symptoms of meningitis without infection of the meninges.*	meningismo
meningitis *Inflammation of the meninges exhibited by fever, photophobia, nuchal rigidity and in severe cases coma and convulsions.*	meningite
meningocele *A congenital defect exhibited by protrusion of the meninges through a defect in the spinal column.*	meningocele
meningococcemia *Presence of N. meningitidis in the blood.*	meningococcemia
meniscectomy *Surgical excision of a meniscus.*	meniscectomia
meniscus *A thin cartilage between joint surfaces.*	menisco
menopause *The time when menstruation ceases.*	menopausa
menorrhagia *Abnormally large amount of menstrual blood.*	menorragia
menses *The blood and other material expelled from the uterus during menstruation.*	menstruação
menstruation *Synonym of menses.*	menstruação
mental *Cognitive or psychological.*	mentual
mention, to *Refer to or allude to.*	mencionar
mesarteritis *Inflammation of the middle layer of an artery.*	mesarterite
mesencephalon *Midbrain.*	mesencéfalo
mesenchyme *Organized mesodermal cells that produce connective tissue, lymphatics and bone.*	mesênquima
mesentery *The fold of peritoneum that connects the small bowel, pancreas and spleen to the posterior portion of the abdominal wall.*	mesentério
mesoappendix *The portion of the mesentery vermiform appendix.*	mesoapêndice
mesocolon *The mesentery connecting the colon to the posterior abdominal wall.*	mesocólon
mesoderm *The middle germ layer in an embryo that is the source of bone, muscle and skin.*	mesoderma
mesonephroma *Usually a tumor of the female genital tract that is thought to stem from the mesonephros.*	mesonefroma
mesosalpinx *A portion of the broad ligament supporting the fallopian tubes.*	mesossalpinge
mesothelioma *A tumor that stems from mesothelial tissue; a known cause is asbestos exposure.*	mesotelioma
mesovarium *The portion of the mesentery connecting the ovary with the abdominal wall.*	mesovário

English	Portuguese
metabolic *Referring to the physical and chemical reactions involved with keeping an organism functioning.*	metabólico
metacarpal *The name for any of the five hand bones.*	metacarpiano
metacarpophalangeal *Referring to the metacarpus and the phalanges.*	metacarpofalangiano
metaphysis *The region between the diaphysis and the epiphysis.*	metáfise
metaplasia *Abnormal change in the nature or character of tissue.*	metaplasia
metatarsal *Any of the bones of the foot.*	metatársico
metatarsalgia *Foot pain.*	metatarsalgia
meter *Unit if measurement. (instrument for measurement)*	metro
methemoglobin *A substance formed with the oxidation of hemoglobin.*	metemoblobina
methionine *A sulfur-containing amino acid used in the biosynthesis of cysteine.*	metionina
metric system	sistema métrico
metrorrhagia *Uterine bleeding in normal amounts but at irregular intervals.*	metrorragia
microbe *A microorganism.*	micróbio
microbiology *The study of microorganisms.*	microbiologia
microcephalic *A congenital deformity exhibited by an abnormally small head.*	microcefálico
microcyte *An unusually small erythrocyte associated with anemias, such as iron deficiency anemia.*	micrócito
micrognathia *Abnormally small maxilla or mandible.*	micrognatia
microgram *One millionth of one gram.*	micrograma
micrometer *One millionth of one meter.*	micrômetro
microorganism *An organism only seen with a microscope.*	microrganismo
microphthalmos *A congenital condition characterized by smallness of the eyes.*	microftalmia
microscope *A instrument used to magnify and view small objects.*	microscópio
micturition *Synonym of urination.*	micção
midbrain *The portion of the brainstem superior to the pons.*	cérebro médio
middle ear *The portion of the ear containing the stapes, incus and malleus.*	ouvido médio
midline *A median line of bilateral separation.*	linha do meio
midstream urine *A specimen of urine that is collected after the initial stream of urine is initiated and before one finishes urinating.*	urine meio do fluxo
midwife *A person trained to assist in childbirth.*	parteiro
midwifery *The occupation of assisting in childbirth.*	obstetrícia
migraine *An episodic, unilateral headache accompanied by nausea.*	hemicrânia; enxaqueca
mild *Slight, nominal.*	suave
milestone *An event indicative of a certain stage of development.*	aponta-caminho
miliary *Referring to a disease that is exhibited by small seed-like lesions (millet), such as miliary tuberculosis.*	miliária
Milkman syndrome *Osteomalacia with multiple pseudofractures.*	síndrome de Milkmann
milligram *A unit of weight, 1/1000 of a gram.*	miligrama
milliliter *A unit of volume, 1/1000 of a liter.*	mililitro
millimeter *A unit of measurement, 1/1000 of a meter.*	milímetro

English	Portuguese
Milroy's disease *Hereditary disease exhibited by leg edema.*	doença de Milroy; doença de Nonne-Milroy
minute *A unit of time.*	minuto
minute *Something very small.*	minúsculo
mirror *A device used for reflecting an image.*	espelho
miryachit *A disease of Siberia characterized by an exaggerated startle response; also referred to as jumping disease.*	miriachite
misanthropy *A severe dislike of homo sapiens.*	misantropia
miscarriage *Spontaneous abortion.*	abortamento
misspelling *Incorrect spelling of a word.*	ortografia errada
mite fever *Synonym of typhus fever.*	febre de tifo
mitochondria *Organelle found in cells responsible for energy production.*	mitocôndria
mitosis *Cell division in which two daughter cells are formed that have the same number of chromosomes as the parent cell.*	mitose
mitral *Referring to the mitral valve.*	mitral
mitral regurgitation *Backflow of blood from the left ventricle to the left atrium because of dysfunctional valve.*	regurgitação mitral
mitral stenosis *Narrowing of the left atrioventricular orifice.*	estenose mitral
mitral valve *The valve with two cusps between the left atrium and ventricle.*	valva mitral
modiolus *A column located in the cochlea.*	modíolo
moist *Damp or humid.*	chuvoso
molality *The number of moles of a solution per kilogram of pure solvent.*	molalidade
molar tooth *Any of the most posterior teeth bilaterally which includes 8 deciduous and usually 12 permanent teeth.*	dente molar
molecule *A combination of at least two atoms.*	molécula
monitor *A person that observes a process or a monitoring device.*	monitor
monkey-paw *An appearance due to median nerve palsy causing atrophy of the thenar eminence with adduction and elevation of the thumb, resembling that of a simian.*	gara de macaco
monkeypox *A viral disease that is similar to smallpox which occurs primarily in monkeys and rarely in humans.*	vírus da varíola do macaco
monoamine oxidase inhibitor (MAOI) *A drug used to treat depression that allows accumulation of serotonin and norepinephrine.*	inhibidor da monoamina oxidase
monoclonal *Asexual formation of a clone from a single cell.*	monoclonal
monocyte *A leukocyte with an oval nucleus and grey cytoplasm.*	monócito
monocytosis *An abnormal increase in the number of monocytes in the blood.*	monocitose
monodiplopia *Double vision in only one eye.*	diplopia monocular
monomania *A psychotic obsession about a single subject.*	monomania
mononeuritis *Inflammation of a single nerve.*	mononeurite
mononuclear *A cell having only one nucleus.*	mononuclear
mononucleosis *An infectious disease exhibited by malaise and lymphadenopathy.*	mononucleose
monoplegia *Paralysis of a single limb.*	monoplegia
mons pubis *The fleshy protuberance over the symphysis pubis.*	monte pubiano
mood *A temporary state of mind or feeling.*	modo
morbid *Indicative of disease.*	mórbido
morbidity *The state of disease.*	morbidade

English	Portuguese
Morgagni's syndrome *Also called metabolic craniopathy and Stewart-Morel syndrome, it is exhibited by hyperostosis frontalis interna, obesity and neuropsychiatric disorders.*	síndrome de Morgagni
morgue *A room where deceased patients are housed until sent to a funeral home.*	morgue; necrotério
moribund *Near death.*	moribundo
morning sickness *Nausea associated with pregnancy.*	doença matinal
morphea *A condition exhibited by an elevated or depressed patch of pink skin with a purple border.*	morféia
morphine *An opioid analgesic.*	morfina
morphology *The study of living organisms and the correlation between their structure.*	morfologia
morula *A solid mass created by the splitting of an ovum.*	mórula
mosquito net *A fine mesh fabric hung over a bed as a mosquito repellent.*	rede mosquito
mossy fiber *Nerve fibers that surround the nerve cells of the cerebellar cortex.*	fibras musgosas
motion sickness *Nausea associated with travel.*	doença do movimento
motor *Referring to muscles.*	motor
motor end plate *The expansions on a motor nerve where the branches terminate on muscle fiber.*	placa terminal
motor unit *The complex of one motor cell and its attached muscle fibers.*	unidade motora
mottled *An irregular arrangement of patches of color.*	mosqueamento
mourning *A period of grieving.*	luto
mouth *The orifice on the lower part of the face.*	boca
mouth to mouth resuscitation *A form of emergency management of respiratory failure.*	ressuscitação boca-a-boca
mouthful *A large quantity of something in one's mouth.*	bocado
mucilage *1. A viscous bodily fluid. 2. A polysaccharide used in medicines and glue.*	mucilagem
mucin *A glycoprotein that is the primary constituent in mucous.*	mucina
mucocele *An accumulation of mucous in a dilated cavity.*	mucocele
mucoid *Referring to mucous.*	mucóide
mucolytic *A substance that breaks down mucous.*	mucolítico
mucopolysaccharidosis type I *Also referred to as Hurler syndrome, persons cannot make lysosomal alpha-L-iduronidase which breaks down glycosaminoglycans.*	mucopolissacaridose do tipo I; síndrome de Hurler
mucopolysaccharidosis type II *Also referred to as Hunter syndrome, persons with this inherited condition cannot produce iduronate sulfatase. There are mild to severe forms but all forms have deafness, coarse facial features, hypertrichosis and macrocephaly.*	mucopolissacaridose do tipo II; síndrome de Hunter
mucopolysaccharidosis type III *Also referred to as Sanfilippo syndrome, persons cannot catabolize the heparan sulfate sugar chain. Symptoms include stiff joints, thick eyebrows, coarse facial features and developmental delays.*	mucopolissacaridose do tipo III; síndrome de Sanfilippo
mucopolysaccharidosis type Is *Also referred to as Scheie syndrome, persons cannot produce lysosomal alpha-L-iduronidase. Symptoms include cloudy cornea, hirsutism, prognathism and stiff joints.*	mucopolissacaridose do tipo IS; síndrome de Scheie
mucopolysaccharidosis type IV *Also referred to as Morquio syndrome, persons do not produce galactosamine-6-sulfatase or in some cases beta-galactosidase. Symptoms include hypermobile joints, macrocephaly, short stature and wide spaced teeth.*	mucopolissacaridose do tipo ; síndrome de Morquio

English	Portuguese
mucopolysaccharidosis type VI *Also referred to as Maroteaux-Lamy syndrome. It is characterized by hydrocephalus, macroglossia and coarse facial features but normal intelligence.*	mucopolissacaridose do tipo VI; síndrome de Marotaeux-Lamy
mucopurulent *That which contains both mucous and pus.*	mucopurulento
mucosa *A mucous membrane like the buccal mucosa.*	mucosa
Mucune-Albright syndrome *Polyostotic fibrous dysplasia with cutaneous brown patches, endocrine dysfunction that exhibits in females as precocious puberty.*	síndrome de Mucune-Albright
mucus *A substance secreted by mucous membranes.*	muco
multigravida *A woman who has been pregnant more than once.*	multigrávida
multilocular *The presence of more than one cell within a cavity.*	multilocular
multipara *A woman with more than one live births.*	multípara
multiple sclerosis *A chronic neurologic disease exhibited by numbness, vision and speech problems, and motor incoordination.*	esclerose múltipa
mumble, to *To speak quietly and indistinctly.*	resmungar
mumps *A contagious viral disease that is exhibited by parotid swelling and puts males at risk for sterility. Also called epidemic parotitis.*	caxumba
mural thrombus *A thrombus attached to a diseased portion of endocardium.*	trombo mural
murmur *An abnormal heart sound heard with a stethoscope.*	sopro
muscle *A band if fibrous tissue that can contract.*	músculo
muscle weakness *Decreased muscular function.*	debilidade muscular
muscular *Referring to muscles.*	muscular
muscular dystrophy *A hereditary condition exhibited by progressive muscular weakness and muscle atrophy.*	distrofia muscular
mutation *A gene alteration that can be passed to the next generation.*	mutação
mute *Refraining from or being speechless.*	mudo
mutism *Inability to speak.*	mutismo
myalgia *Muscle pain.*	mialgia
myasthenia gravis *An autoimmune disease characterized by fluctuating weakness of the ocular, limb and respiratory muscles.*	miastenia grave
mycetoma *Persistent inflammation of the tissues caused by an infection.*	micetoma
mycosis *A disease caused by a fungal infection.*	micose
mycotoxin *A substance toxic to fungus.*	micotoxina
mydriasis *Pupillary dilation.*	midríase
myelin *The substance that forms a sheath around some nerve fibers.*	mielina
myelitis *Inflammation of the spinal cord.*	mielite
myelocele *Protrusion of the spinal cord through a defect in the bony structure.*	mielocele
myelogram *CT scan or roentgenography of the spinal canal after injection of contrast media.*	mielograma
myeloid *Referring to the bone marrow or spinal cord.*	mielóide
myeloma *Malignant tumor of the bone marrow.*	mieloma
myelomatosis *A leukemic disease in which there is an abnormally high amount of myeloblasts in the blood.*	mielomatose
myelomeningocele *A protrusion of the spinal cord and its meninges through a defect in the vertebral canal.*	mielomeningocele
myelopathy *A condition of the spinal cord.*	mielopatia

English	Portuguese
myocardial *Referring to the muscular tissue of the heart.*	miocárdio
myocardial infarction *The death of myocardial tissue as a result of an interruption in flow to the region supplied by a coronary vessel.*	infartação miocárdico
myocarditis *An inflammation of the heart.*	miocardite
myocardium *The middle layer of the heart wall.*	miocárdio
myoclonus *Contraction or spasm of a group of muscles.*	mioclonia
myoglobin *A protein within muscle that carries and stores oxygen.*	mioglobina
myoma *A benign neoplasm of muscular tissue.*	mioma
myomectomy *Surgical resection of a myoma.*	miomectomia
myometrium *The smooth muscle layer of the uterus.*	miométrio
myopathy *Muscle disease.*	miopatia
myopia *Nearsightedness.*	miopia; visão curta
myosarcoma *A mass with myoma and sarcoma characteristics.*	miossarcoma
myosin *A protein that when coupled with actin form the contractile complex of a muscle cells.*	miosina
myositis *Inflammation of muscle tissue.*	miosite
myositis ossificans *Inflammation of muscle tissue with presence of bony deposits.*	miostie ossificante
myotomy *The surgical removal of muscle tissue.*	miotomia
myotonia dystrophica; Steinert's disease *A condition exhibited initially by hypertonic muscles followed by atrophy of the facial and neck muscles.*	doença de Steinert; distrofia miotônica
myringitis *Inflammation of the tympanic membrane.*	miringite
myringoplasty *Surgical repair of tympanic membrane defects.*	miringoplastia
myringotomy *Surgical opening of the tympanic membrane.*	miringotomia
mysophobia *Severe fear of dirt or contamination from common objects.*	misofobia
myxedema *Diffuse edema with a wax-like appearance of the skin; this condition is associated with hypothyroidism.*	mixedema
myxoma *A tumor composed of mucous tissue.*	mixoma
myxosarcoma *A sarcoma that also has mucous tissue.*	mixossarcoma
nail *The hard surface on the dorsal surface of the toes or fingers.*	unha
nail bed *The area just beneath a finger or toenail. Also called matrix unguis.*	leito de ungueal; matriz ungueal
nail biting *A habit of chewing on one's fingernails.*	tendência a roer as unhas; onicotilomania
nailing *Referring to placement of an intramedullary rod in a long bone in order to treat a fracture.*	encravamento
name *A word by which a person is known.*	nome
nap *A brief sleep or catnap.*	soneca
narcissism *Abnormally excessive self-interest.*	narcisismo
narcolepsy *A condition exhibited by a strong desire to sleep and by sudden onset of sleep at increased intervals.*	narcolepsia
narcosis *A reversible medication-induced condition of excessive drowsiness or unconsciousness.*	narcose
narcotic *A medication that produces narcosis.*	narcótico
nasal *Referring to the nose.*	nasal; rinal
nasogastric tube *A tube that is inserted into the nose with the distal tip in the stomach; it is used for irrigation or drainage of gastric contents.*	tubo nasogástrico

English	Portuguese
nasogastric tube placement *Insertion of a tube that is placed in the stomach via the nostril; it is used for administration of fluid or to suction gastric contents.*	inserção tubo nasogástrico
nasolacrimal *Referring to the nose and tear apparatus.*	nasolacrimal
nasopharyngeal *Referring to the nose and pharynx.*	nasofaríngeo
nasopharynx *The part of the pharynx which lies superior to the soft palate.*	nasofaringe
nausea *A feeling that one wants to vomit.*	náusea
navel *Umbilicus.*	umbigo
navicular *1. boat shaped 2. Referring to the navicular bone of the hand or foot.*	navicular
navicular bone *The most lateral bone in the proximal row of carpal bones.*	osso navicular de mão
near *In close proximity.*	próximo
nebula *An opaque spot on the cornea causing impaired vision.*	nébula
nebulizer *A device used for transforming a liquid into a fine mist for inhalation as in nebulized albuterol for an acute exacerbation of asthma.*	nebulizador
nebulizer treatment *Administration of medication such as albuterol via a fine mist using a nebulizer.*	tratamento nebulizador
neck *The part of the body that connects the body to the head.*	pescoço
neck of the femur *The portion of the femur between the shaft and head.*	colo do fêmur
necropsy *Synonym of autopsy.*	necroscopia
necrosis *The death of most of the cells of the affected part.*	necrose
necrotic *Referring to necrosis.*	necrótico
need *A want or obligation.*	carência
needle *The slender cylindrical device attached to a syringe.*	agulha
needle biopsy *Use of a needle to aspirate body contents for microscopic or pathologic examination.*	agulha de biopsia
needle for lumbar puncture	agulha de acupuntura
needle holder *A surgical instrument used to grasp a needle during suturing.*	porta-agulha
needle-stick injury *The inadvertent self-puncture with a needle that had been used previously to inject a patient.*	lesão de punção-agulha
negative *Contrary or opposing.*	negativo
nematode *An endoparasite belonging to the class of the Nemathelminthes including roundworms and threadworms.*	nematódeo
neonatal *Referring to the first four weeks after birth.*	neonatal
neonate *The term for a newborn infant for the first four weeks.*	neonado
neoplasm *A new and abnormal growth.*	neoplasma
nephrectomy *Surgical removal of a kidney.*	nefrectomia
nephritis *A general term meaning inflammation of a kidney that is further categorized depending on the associated pathology.*	nefrite
nephroblastoma *Congenital tumor of the kidney, also called Wilms' tumor.*	nefroblastoma
nephrocalcinosis *A condition exhibited by calcium phosphate deposition in the renal tubules; a cause of renal insufficiency.*	nefrocalcinose
nephrolithiasis *A calculus in the kidney.*	nefrolitíase
nephrolithotomy *Surgical removal of a renal calculus.*	nefrolitotomia
nephroma *A renal tumor.*	nefroma
nephron *A functional unit of the kidney that consists of the glomerulus, the proximal and distal convoluted tubules, the loop of Henle and the collecting tubule.*	néfron

English	Portuguese
nephropathy *Renal disease.*	nefropatia
nephropexy *The surgical fixation of a kidney that was previously floating.*	nefropexia
nephroptosis *Inferior displacement of the kidney.*	nefroptose
nephrosclerosis *Hardening of the kidney.*	nefrosclerose
nephrosis *A kidney disease exhibited by edema and proteinuria; also called nephrotic syndrome.*	nefrose
nephrostomy *Surgical creation of an opening between the renal pelvis and an opening in the skin.*	nefrostomia
nephrotic *Referring to nephrosis.*	nefrótico
nephrotomy *Surgical incision of the kidney.*	nefrotomia
nerve *A fibrous band made up of axons and dendrites that connects the nervous systems with other organs.*	nervo
nerve impulse *A signal transmitted along a nerve fiber.*	impulso nervo
nerve block anesthesia *Locally administered anesthesia.*	anestesia de bloqueio nervoso
neural *Referring to a nerve or nerve impulse.*	neural
neuralgia *Severe pain along the course of a nerve.*	neuralgia; neurodinia
neurapraxia *Paralysis from nerve injury but no degeneration of the nerve.*	neurapraxia
neurasthenia *A psychoneurosis exhibited by severe fatigue.*	neurastenia
neurectomy *Excision of a section of a nerve.*	neurectomia
neurilemma *The membrane covering a myelinated nerve fiber or the axon of an unmyelinated nerve fiber.*	neurolema
neuritis *Inflammation of a nerve.*	neurite
neuroblastoma *A nervous system malignant tumor composed of neuroblasts.*	neuroblastoma
neurodermatitis *A pruritic, thickened eruption in the axillary and inguinal thought to be exacerbated by emotions.*	neurodermatite
neuroepithelium *Cells specialized to serve as sensory cells such as cells of the cochlea and tongue.*	neuroepitélio
neurofibroma *A tumor formed by excessive growth of perineurium and endoneurium.*	neurofibroma
neurofibromatosis *A hereditary condition exhibited by formation of multiple soft tumors scattered throughout the skin surface. Also known as von Recklinghausen disease.*	neurofibromatose
neuroglia *A type of connective tissue of the nervous system.*	neuróglia
neuroleptic *A drug that causes neurologic symptoms.*	neuroléptico
neuroleptic malignant syndrome *A severe reaction to neuroleptic medications characterized by hyperthermia with autonomic and extrapyramidal symptoms.*	síndrome maligna meuroléptica
neurologist *A physician who specializes in the study of the nervous system.*	neurologista
neurology *The study of the nervous system.*	neurologia
neuroma *A mass composed of nerve cells and fibers.*	neuroma
neuron *A nerve cell.*	neurônio
neuropathic *Referring to neuropathy.*	neuropático
neuropathy *Structural of pathologic changes of the peripheral nervous system.*	neuropatia
neurosis *A mental disorder.*	neurose
neurosurgery *Surgery of the brain or spinal cord.*	neurocirurgia
neurosyphilis *Infection of the central nervous system with Treponema pallidum.*	neurossífilis
neurotmesis *The severing of a nerve.*	neurotmese
neurotomy *Surgical incision into a nerve.*	neurotomia

English	Portuguese
neurotransmitter *A substance released at the end of a nerve fiber that facilitates transmission of an impulse.*	neurotransmissor
neutropenia *Diminished number of neutrophils in the blood.*	neutropenia
neutrophil *A polymorphonuclear leukocyte.*	neutrófilo
nevus *A benign, well-circumscribed growth of tissue of congenital origin.*	nevo; espiloma
next *The following or upcoming.*	seguinte
nick *A small groove or notch.*	entalhe
nicotinic acid *A deficiency of this substance results in pellagra.*	ácido nicotínico
night blindness *Common term for nyctalopia, it refers to low vision with reduced illumination, often seen with Vitamin A deficiency.*	cegueira nocturna
night shift *The late shift, typically beginning at 19:00 or 23:00 hours.*	trabalho à noite; serviço noturno
night sweats *Profuse sweating at night occurring with tuberculosis among other conditions.*	suores noturnos
night terror *Sensation of profound fear upon wakening.*	terrores noturnos
nightmare *An unpleasant or frightening dream.*	pesadelo
nipple *The small projection on the breast thru which milk is secreted.*	mamilo
nitrogen *A colorless, odorless gas used as a coolant in the liquid form.*	nitrogênio
nitrous oxide *An inhalant gas used as an anesthetic agent.*	óxido nitroso
nocturia *Urination at night.*	noctúria
nocturnal emission *Involuntary emission of semen at night.*	emissão noturno
nocturnal *Referring to events that happen at night.*	noturno
node *A swelling or prominence.*	nodo
nodule *A small node in the skin of up to 1cm and in the lung up to 3cm.*	nódulo
nonpitting edema *Subcutaneous swelling that cannot be indented with compression.*	edema sólido
non-rebreather mask *A type of oxygen mask used to deliver a higher oxygen concentration.*	máscara de não-reinalação
non-resorbable suture (nylon) *Suture used to be permanent as it is not removed by normal body processes.*	sutura cirúrgica inabsorvível
noon *The 12 o'clock mid-day hour.*	meio-dia
norepinephrine *A hormone secreted by the adrenal medulla and a synthetic drug used as a pressor agent.*	norepinefrina
normoblast *A precursor cell for erythrocytes.*	normoblasto
normocyte *A normal erythrocyte.*	normócito
Norway itch *A severe pruritus caused by scabies and is associated with immune disorders such as AIDS.*	escabiose norueguesa
nose *The midface protuberance used for smelling and breathing.*	nariz
nosebleed *Common term for epistaxis.*	nariz sangrante
nosocomial infection *An infection occurring after admission to a hospital.*	infecção nosocomial
nosology *The medical science of disease classification.*	nosologia
nosophobia *Unwarranted, excessive fear of any disease.*	nosofobia
nostril *One of two openings in the nose used for air passage.*	narinas
noxious *Harmful or poisonous.*	nocivo
nuclear magnetic resonance (NMR) *A type a diagnostic body imaging utilizing electromagnetic radiation in a magnetic field.*	ressonância magnética nuclear (RMN)

English	Portuguese
nuclear medicine *The branch of medicine associated with the use of radioactive material in the evaluation and treatment of disease.*	medicina nuclear
nuclear *Referring to a nucleus.*	nuclear
nucleic acid *An organic compound found in living cells; its molecules contain nucleotides linked in long chains.*	ácido nuclear
nucleoprotein *A substance composed of a nucleic acid and a protein.*	nucleoproteína
nulligravida *A woman who has never been pregnant.*	nuligrávida
nullipara *A woman who has never given birth.*	nulípara
numb chin syndrome. *Generally associated with metastatic breast or prostate cancer, it is characterized by unilateral sensory loss of the chin and lower lip.*	síndrome de mento entorpecimento
numbness *Decreased sensation to tactile stimuli.*	entorpecimento
nummulation *Formed as round, flat discs.*	numulação
nurse *A person trained to care for the sick.*	enfermeira
nurse practitioner *A person with advanced training capable of acting as a patient's primary care provider.*	enfermeira especializada
nursing care *The assessment and treatment provided by nurses.*	cuidados enfermagem
nutation *Referring to nodding of the head.*	nutação
nutrient *A substance that provides essential nourishment.*	nutriente
nutrient foramen *A conduit for passage of nutrient vessels in the marrow of bone.*	forame nutriente
nutrition *The process of supplying food needed for growth.*	nutrição
nutritional status *The relative state of one's nutrition.*	estado nutricional
nystagmus *Rapid involuntary movement of the eyes; it can be horizontal, vertical or rotary.*	nistagmo
nyxis *Paracentesis or a puncture.*	paracentese
obesity *Having a body mass index over 30kilograms/meters squared.*	obesidade
obsession *A pathologic preoccupation.*	obsessão
obsolete *No longer in use; antiquated.*	obsoleto
obstetric *Referring to The management of pregnancy, labor and the peuperium.*	obstétrico
obstetrician *A physician who specializes in the management of pregnancy, labor and the peuperium.*	obstetra
obstructed *To be blocked or halted.*	obstrução
obturator *A device used to close an artificial or natural opening.*	obturador
obtuse *Rather insensitive or hard to understand.*	obtuso
occipital *Referring to the back part of the head.*	occipital
occipitofrontal muscle *Raises the eyebrows.*	músculo occipitofrontal
occlusion *A pathway that is blocked or obstructed.*	oclusão
occlusive dressing *A synthetic covering for a wound that has a semipermeable membrane.*	curativo oclusivo
occult blood *Presence of blood from an unknown source.*	sangue oculto
occupational therapy *Rehabilitation focusing on activities of daily living.*	terapia ocupacional
ocular paralysis. *Paralysis of intraocular and extraocular muscles.*	paralisia ocular
ocular *Referring to the eye.*	ocular
oculogyric *Referring to movement of the eye around the anteroposterior axis.*	oculogírico

English	Portuguese
oculomotor nerve *Referring to cranial nerve III which is one of the nerves responsible for extraocular movements.*	nervo oculomotor
odiferous *Having an unpleasant or distinctive smell.*	odorífero
odontalgia *Tooth pain.*	odontalgia
odontoid *A prominence on the second cervical vertebra on which the first cervical vertebra pivots.*	odontóide
odontology *Synonym of dentistry.*	odontologia
odor *A smell that is given off someone or something.*	odor; cheiro
odynophagia *Pain associated with swallowing.*	odinofagia
odynophonia *Pain associated with speaking.*	odinofonia
offspring *One's children.*	descendência
ointment *A petroleum jelly based topical medication.*	ungüento; pomada
old age *A relative term for the period of advanced years.*	velhice
older *Being around more than compared with another.*	mais velho
olecranon *The bony protrusion at the proximal ulna at the elbow.*	olecrânio; olécrano
olfactory *Referring to the sense of smell.*	olfatório
oligodactyly *Presence of fewer than 5 digits on a hand or foot.*	oligodactilia
oligodendroglia *The ectodermal cells forming part of the central nervous system.*	oligodendria
oligohydramnios *Inadequate amount of amniotic fluid.*	oligoidrâmnios
oligomenorrhea *Infrequent menstruation or low volume menstrual flow.*	oligomenorréia
oligoptyalism *Insufficient secretion of saliva; also oligosialia.*	oligoptialismo
oligospermia *Abnormally low sperm count.*	oligospermia
oligotrophia or hypotrichosis *Less than normal amount of head/body hair.*	oligotrofia
oliguria *Abnormally low urine output.*	oligúria
ombrophobia *An abnormal fear of rain.*	ombrofobia
omentocele *A herniated protrusion of omentum.*	omentocele
omentopexy *Surgically fastening the omentum to an adjacent tissue it was not previously attached to.*	omentopexia
omentum *A fold of peritoneum fastening the stomach to other organs in the viscera.*	omento
omphalitis *Inflammation of the umbilicus.*	onfalite
omphalocele *A large congenital, umbilical hernia with only a thin membranous covering.*	onfalocele
on going *Continuing,*	acontecimento
oncologist *A physician specializing in the treatment of cancer.*	oncologista
oncology *The study of cancer.*	oncologia
onion bulb neuropathy *Also known as hypertrophic interstitial neuropathy which is a sensorimotor polyneuropathy.*	neuropatia em bulbo de cebola; neuropatia intersticial hipertrófica
onset *The beginning of an event.*	começo
onychia *Inflammation of the toenail or fingernail matrix.*	oniquia
onychia sicca *Brittle fingernails or toenails.*	oniquia seca
onychocryptosis *Ingrown toenail.*	onicocriptose
onychogryphosis *A deformed nail that is incurved or hooked.*	onicogrifose
onychomycosis *Fungal disease of the toenails or fingernails.*	onicomicose
onychophagia *Habitually chewing on one's fingernails.*	onicofagia
oocyte *An ovarian cell that needs to undergo meiotic division to become an ovum.*	oócito
oogenesis *The initiation and development of an ovum.*	oogênese

English	Portuguese
oophorectomy *Surgical removal of an ovary.*	ooforectomia
oophoritis *Inflammation of an ovary.*	ooforite
oophoron *Synonym for ovary.*	oóforo
oophorosalpingectomy *Surgical removal of an ovary and fallopian tube.*	ooforossalpingectomia
ooze, to *To slowly leak.*	escoar lentamente
open reduction (of fractures) *The realignment of a fractured bone using a surgical approach.*	redução aberta (de fraturas)
operation *A surgical procedure.*	operação
operative note *A detailed description of a surgical procedure performed on a specific patient.*	registro operatório
ophthalmia *Profound inflammation of the eye or its structures.*	oftalmia
ophthalmic *Referring to the eye.*	oftálmico
ophthalmologist *A physician specializing in diseases of the eye.*	oftalmologista
ophthalmology *The study of diseases of the eye.*	oftalmologia
ophthalmoplegia *Paralysis of the eye muscles.*	oftalmoplegia
ophthalmoscope *A device used to visually inspect the interior eye.*	oftalmoscópio
opiate *Referring to opium.*	opiáceo
opioid *A substance similar to opium that binds to at least one of the opium receptors in the body.*	opióide
opisthotonos *A profound spasm in which the head/neck is hyperextended, the feet are touching the bed and with the patient supine the body arched upward.*	opistótono
opium *An addictive drug derived from opium poppy; synthetic versions are used as analgesics.*	ópio
Oppenheim reflex *Extension of the toes elicited by scratching of the medial leg; present when the patient has cerebral irritation.*	reflexo de Oppenheim
opponens *Synonym for opponent muscle.*	oponente
opsonin *An antibody used to facilitate phagocytosis of a bacterium.*	opsonina
optic *Referring to the eye.*	óptico
optic disk *The area of the retina where the optic nerve enters.*	disco óptico
optician *A person who makes eyeglasses.*	óptico
optometrist *A person who practices optometry.*	optometrista
optometry *The profession of examination of the eyes for disease (not a medical doctor).*	optometria
oral *Relating to the mouth.*	oral
oral contraceptive *Tablet taken by mouth to prevent pregnancy.*	anticoncepcional oral
oral hygiene *Cleansing of the mouth and associated structures.*	higiene oral
orally *By mouth.*	oralmente
orbicular *Rounded or circular.*	orbicular
orbit *The bony structure enclosing the eyeball.*	órbita
orbital *Referring to the orbit.*	orbitário
orchialgia *Testicular pain.*	orquialgia
orchidectomy *Synonym of orchiectomy; removal of one or both testes.*	orquidectomia
orchidopexy *Surgical repair of an undescended testis.*	orquiopexia
orchiepididymitis *Inflammation of the testis and epididymis.*	orquiepididimite
orchitis *Inflammation of one or both testes.*	orquite
organ *A part of the body that is self contained and serves a vital function.*	órgão

English	Portuguese
organomegaly *Enlargement of an organ, typically referring to an intraabdominal organ.*	organomegalia
oriental sore *A stigmata of cutaneous leishmaniasis caused by a bite from a sand fly.*	úlcera oriental
orifice *Synonym of foramen.*	orifício
ornithosis *A viral infection transmitted by birds that is manifested by chills, headache, photophobia, fever, nausea and vomiting.*	ornitose
oropharynx *The portion of the pharynx between the soft palate and the superior aspect of the epiglottis.*	orofaringe
orthodontics *A subspecialty of dentistry concerned with treatment of dental irregularities and malocclusion, including the use of braces.*	ortodôntica
orthopedics *A surgical specialty concerned with treatment of skeletal problems.*	ortopedia
orthopnea *The inability to breath comfortably except in the upright position.*	ortopnéia
orthosis *Straightening of a malaligned part with the use of braces and other supportive devices.*	ortose
orthostatic *Referring to the standing position. Orthostatic hypotension is low blood pressure in the standing position.*	ortostático
oscillating nystagmus *Abnormal movement of the eyes in a wave-like pattern.*	nistagmo pendular
osmolality *The concentration expressed in total number of solute particles per kilogram.*	osmolalidade
osmole *The recognized unit of osmotic pressure.*	osmol
osmosis *The movement of a solvent from a solution of greater concentration to one of lower concentration through a semi-permeable membrane until the two solutions have equal concentration.*	osmose
osmotic *Referring to osmosis.*	osmótico
osseous *Possessing the quality of bone.*	ósseo
ossicle *A small bone. (auditory ossicle)*	ossículo
ossification *The formation of bone.*	ossificação
osteitis *Inflammation of the bone.*	osteíte
ostensibly *Synonym of apparently and seemingly.*	ostensivamente
osteoarthritis *A long term, progressive degenerative joint disease.*	osteoartrite
osteoarthrosis *Arthritis without inflammation.*	osteoartrose
osteoblast *A cell that matures from a fibroblast and produces bone.*	osteoblasto
osteochondral *Referring to bone and cartilage.*	osteocondroso
osteochondritis *Inflammation of bone and cartilage.*	osteocondrite
osteochondroma *A tumor with bony and cartilaginous characteristics.*	osteocondroma
osteoclasis *The surgical fracture of a bone usually in order to restore proper alignment.*	osteoclasia
osteoclast *A large bone cell that is associated with bone reabsorption and removal.*	osteoclasto
osteoclastoma *A tumor composed of giant cells or osteoclasts.*	osteoclastoma
osteocyte *An osteoblast within the bone matrix.*	osteócito
osteodystrophy *Abnormal bone formation.*	osteodistrofia
osteogenesis *Development of new bones.*	osteogênese
osteolytic *Referring to the removal or loss of calcium from the bone.*	osteolítico

English	Portuguese
osteomalacia Softening of the bones because of a deficiency of vitamin D, calcium or phosphorus.	osteomalacia
osteomyelitis Inflammation of the bone or bone marrow because of a microorganism.	osteomielite
osteopathy 1. Any disease of the bone. 2. Medical practice concerning treatment of disease by manipulation and massage of bones, joints, and muscles.	osteopatia
osteopetrosis Increased bone density with no change in modeling.	osteopetrose; doença de Albers-Sc
osteophony The sound conduction of bone.	osteofonia
osteophyte Abnormal growth of a bone protuberance.	osteófito
osteoporosis Loss of bone substance because the osteoblasts fail to produce bone matrix.	osteoporose
osteosarcoma A tumor composed of a sarcoma and osseous material.	osteossarcoma
osteosclerosis Abnormal hardening of bone.	osteosclerose
osteotomy Creation of a surgical opening in bone.	osteotomia
ostium A vessel or body cavity opening.	óstio
ostogenesis imperfecta A connective tissue disorder characterized by bone fragility, skeletal deformity, blue sclerae, ligament laxity, and hearing loss.	osteogênese imperfeita
otalgia Ear pain.	otalgia
otitis Inflammation of the ear. (otitis media or otitis externa)	otitie
otolaryngologist Surgical specialist concerned with organs of the ears, nose and throat.	otolaringologista
otolith A calcium based calculus in the inner ear.	otólito
otology Study of conditions and anatomy of the ear.	otologia
otomycosis Fungal infection of the ear.	otomicose
otosclerosis A hereditary condition exhibited by progressive hearing loss because of bone overgrowth in the inner ear.	otosclerose
otoscope A device used for inspection of the tympanic membrane.	otoscópio
ototoxic A substance harmful to the ear or its nerve supply.	ototóxico
outbreak (of a disease) A sudden start of a disease in a population.	erupção
ouch-ouch disease Common term for Itai-Itai disease that is derived from "it hurts, it hurts" said by patients suffering from cadmium poisoning.	doença de Itai-Itai
outdated Something that has passed the expiration date.	antiquado
ovarian cysts Generally used to describe benign tumors.	cisto ovariano
ovaritis Synonym for oophoritis.	ovarite
overdose An above normal dose of a medication.	dose excessiva
overriding suture The overlapping of cranial sutures noted on vaginal exam when the head is descended.	acavalgamento
overt Not hidden.	visível
overweight Defined as BMI over 25kilograms per meters squared.	excesso de peso
oviduct The channel which an ovum passes from the ovary.	oviduto
ovulation The release of an ova from the ovary.	ovulação
ovule An immature ovum.	óvulo
owing to On account of.	devido à
oxaluria Existence of oxalates in the urine.	oxalúria
oxidation The process of a chemical combining with oxygen.	oxidação

English	Portuguese
oximeter *A medical device used to measure the percent of oxygen that is saturated in the blood (oxygen saturation).*	oxímetro
oxycephaly *The deformation of the skull so that it appears pointed.*	oxicefalia
oxygen *A colorless, odorless gas with atomic number 8.*	oxigênio
oxygen consumption *The body's utilization of oxygen per unit of time.*	consumo oxigênio
oxygen tent *A manner of giving supplement oxygen to a neonate.*	tenda de oxigênio
oxygen therapy *Utilization of supplemental oxygen.*	oxigenoterapia
oxygenation *Saturated with oxygen.*	oxigenação
oxyhemoglobin *The combination of oxygen and hemoglobin using a covalent bond.*	oxyemoglobina
oxytocic *Referring to rapid parturition.*	oxitócico
oxytocin *A natural hormone released by the pituitary or a synthetic hormone that facilitates uterine contraction.*	oxitocina
ozena *Various nasal conditions, all of which include fetid discharge.*	ozena
ozone *A toxic chemical that has profound oxidizing properties. It has three atoms in its molecule compared with oxygen which has two.*	ozônio
pace *Consistent and continuous movement.*	passo
pacemaker *An electrical device used to stimulate the heart used for bradyarrhythmias.*	marca-passo cardíaco
pachydermia *An abnormally thick skin.*	paquidermia
pachymeningitis *Inflammation of the dura mater.*	paquileptomeningite
pad *A thick piece of soft clothing.*	almofada
pagophagia *Compulsive need to eat ice which is usually associated with iron deficiency anemia.*	pagofagia
pain *Physical suffering or discomfort.*	dor
painful *Affected with pain.*	doloroso
palatal myoclonus *An involuntary, persistent, rapid regular tremor of the soft palate and face.*	mioclonia palatal
palate *The roof of the mouth.*	palato
palatoplegia *Paralysis of the palate.*	palatoplegia; estafiloplegia
palliative *A treatment used to reduce pain when cure is not possible.*	paliativo
pallidectomy *Surgical resection of all or part of the palate.*	palidectomia
pallor *Unusually pale appearance.*	palidez
palm *The anterior aspect of the hand.*	palma da mão
palmar *Referring to the palm.*	palmar
palpation *The assessment of the body with the use of one's hands.*	palpação
palpebra, palpebrae *Eyelid, eyelids.*	pálpebra
palpitation *Sensation of a forceful, rapid, irregular heartbeat present after exercise or with anxiety.*	palpitação
palsy *Paralysis that is usually associated with tremors.*	paralisia
paludism *Synonym of malaria.*	paludismo
pamper, to *Indulge with comfort and kindness.*	acariciar
panarthritis *Inflammation of the joints.*	pan-artrite
pancarditis *Inflammation of pericardium, myocardium and endocardium.*	pan-cardite
pancreas *A gland that secretes digestive enzymes into the duodenum and insulin and glucagon into the blood.*	pâncreas

English	Portuguese
pancreatectomy *Surgical excision of part or all of the pancreas.*	pancreatectomia
pancreatitis *Inflammation of the pancreas.*	pancreatite
pancreozymin *A duodenal mucosal enzyme that facilitates the secretion of amylase and other enzymes from the pancreas.*	pancreozimina
pandemic *When a disease is present over an entire region.*	pandêmico
panhypopituitarism *Insufficiency of the anterior pituitary.*	pan-hipopituitarismo
panic attack *Sudden, profound anxiety.*	ataque de pânico
panniculitis *Inflammation of a section of subcutaneous tissue containing large amounts of fat.*	paniculite
panophthalmia *Inflammation of the eye and all its structures.*	pan-oftalmite
panotitis *Inflammation of each part of a bone.*	pan-otite
papilledema *Swelling of the optic disc.*	papiledema
papillitits *Swelling of a papilla.*	papilite
papilloma *A benign, lobulated tumor coming from epithelium.*	papiloma
papule *A small, well-circumscribed elevation of the skin.*	pápula
para-aminobenzoic acid *A natural product (not FDA approved) reportedly beneficial for Peyronie's disease and scleroderma. It is a component of folic acid.*	ácido para-aminobenzóico
para-aminohippuric acid (PAH) *A chemical used for calculation of renal plasma flow.*	ácido para-aminohipúrico
paracentesis *A procedure involving aspiration of fluid from the abdominal cavity.*	paracentese
paracusia *Any abnormality in the sense of hearing.*	paracusia
paradoxical pupil *Constriction of the pupil when exposed to darkness.*	pupila paradoxal
paralysis agitans *Synonym of Parkinson's disease.*	paralisia com agitação
paralytic *1. Referring to paralysis. 2. A person who is paralyzed.*	paralítico
paramedian *Situated toward the middle of the body.*	paramediano
paramedical *Hospital support staff excluding physicians.*	paramédico
parametritis *Inflammation of the parametrium.*	parametrite
parametrium *The connective tissue and smooth muscle between the broad ligament serous layers.*	paramétrio
paramnesia *A condition exhibited by a person's belief they have memory for an event that never happened.*	paramimia
paranasal sinuses *Any of the sinuses (ethmoidal, frontal, maxillary or sphenoidal) that communicate with the nasal cavity.*	seios paranasais
paranasal *Situated adjacent to the nose.*	paranasal
paranoia *A mental condition exhibited by delusions of persecution.*	paranóia
paranoid *Having the symptom of paranoia.*	paranóide
paraphimosis *A condition in which the foreskin is retracted but cannot be replace because of a restricted foreskin.*	parafimose
paraplegia *Paralysis of the lower extremities.*	parapleglia
parapraxis *1. Unable to perform purposeful movements. 1. Irrational behavior.*	parapraxia
pararectal *Adjacent to the rectum.*	pararretal
parasite *An organism that lives on or within another organism without benefit to the latter.*	parasita
parasympathetic *Part of the autonomic nervous system that opposes sympathetic stimulation.*	parassimpático
parathormone *Synonym for parathyroid hormone.*	paratormônio

English	Portuguese
parathyroid *Positioned adjacent to the thyroid.*	paratireóide
paravertebral *Positioned adjacent to the vertebra.*	paravertebral
parenchyma *The functional elements of an organ.*	parênquima
parenteral *Other than the alimentary canal.*	parenteral
paresis *Incomplete paralysis.*	paresia
paresthesia *An abnormal sensation usually described as pins and needles.*	parestesia
parietal *Referring to the wall of a part or cavity.*	parietal
parietal cell *Acid secreting cells of the stomach.*	célula parietal
Parkinson's disease *A progressive neuromuscular disease exhibited by masklike facial expression, resting tremor, cogwheel rigidity and abnormal gait.*	doença de Parkinson
paronychia *Inflammation of the tissue bordering a fingernail*	paroníquia
parosmia *An alteration in the sense of smell.*	parosmia
parotid *A gland near the ear.*	parótida
parotiditis *Inflammation of the parotid gland.*	parotidite
paroxysmal *Occurring in sudden attacks.*	paroxístico
parrot-beak nail *A curved fingernail.*	unha em bico de papagaio
parthenogenesis *Reproduction that occurs without an egg being fertilized by sperm.*	partenogênese
parting *Separating.*	partida
parturition *The process of giving birth.*	parturição
passive *Not achieved through active effort.*	passivo
past history *Prior medical problems experienced by a patient.*	doença antecedentes
paste *A thick, soft moist substance usually with medicine mixed in.*	grude
patch test *A test used to determine which substances provoke an allergic response in a patient.*	teste de emplastro
patella *The bone situated in the anterior portion of the knee.*	rótula; patela
patellectomy *Surgical excision of the patella.*	patelectomia
patellofemoral stress syndrome *Overuse syndrome causing anterior knee pain from excessive lateral motion.*	síndrome de patelofemoral
patent ductus arteriosus *A condition exhibited by failure of the ductus arteriosus (communication between the aorta the the pulmonary artery normally noted in a fetus) to close.*	ducto arterioso permeável
patent foramen ovale *A congenital anomaly in which there is a defect in the wall between the right and left atria; this can be a benign condition or result in cryptogenic strokes.*	forame oval permeável
pathogenesis *The course of a disease.*	patogênese
pathogenic *Referring to an organism that can cause disease.*	patogênico
pathognomonic *Characteristic of something.*	patognomônico
pathological *Referring to pathology.*	patológico
pathology *1. The branch of medicine dealing with the study of tissues and the forensic application. 2. Referring to a condition that is abnormal.*	patologia
patient *The client being treated for a medical or surgical condition.*	paciente
patient chart *The file containing the client's medical record.*	registro médico
peak flow *A measurement of lung function used in asthma.*	fluxo máximo
pectineal ligament *A continuation of the lacunar ligament along the pectineal line in the pubis.*	ligamento pectíneo
pectoral *Referring to the pectoral muscle.*	peitoral

English	Portuguese
pectoriloquy *The examiner's voice is clearly audible when the patient speaks as when the examiner listens to an area of consolidation in the lungs of the speaker.*	pectorilóquia
pediatrician *Physician who is a specialist in pediatrics.*	pediatra
pediatrics *Medical specialty concerned with the treatment and prevention of childhood disease.*	pediatria
pedicle *Part of a skin/tissue graft temporarily left connected to the original site.*	pedículo
pediculate *Referring to pedicle.*	pediculado
pediculosis *Lice infestation.*	pediculose
peduncle *1. A stalk-like protrusion. 2. A bundle of nerve fibers connecting two parts of the brain.*	pedúnculo
pellagra *A deficiency in nicotinic acid exhibited by diarrhea and dermatitis.*	pelagra; coceira de Santo Inácio
pelvic inflammatory disease *Generally a bacterial infection affecting a woman with potential involvement of the uterus, fallopian tubes, ovaries and cervix.*	doença inflamatória pélvica
pelvic *Referring to the pelvis.*	pélvico
pelvimetry *Measurement of the dimensions of the pelvis to determine whether a patient is capable of natural childbirth.*	pelvimetria
pelvis *The bony structure at the base of the spine.*	pelve
pemphigus *A skin disorder with large bullous lesions.*	pênfigo
penetration *The process of making a way through something.*	penetração
penicillin *A synthetic antibiotic originally produced from blue mold.*	penicilina
penis *Male genital organ used for the transfer of sperm and elimination of urine.*	pênis
pentosuria *The presence of pentose in the urine (a monosaccharide with five carbon atoms in the molecule).*	pentosúria
pepsin *A proteolytic gastric enzyme.*	pepsina
peptic *Referring to pepsin or concerning digestion.*	péptico
peptide *A compound with low molecular weight and containing two or more amino acids.*	peptído
percussion *A manual procedure involving tapping a body part to determine the size or density (liquid or air) of a part.*	percussão
perforation *Presence of a hole.*	perfuração
periaqueductal gray matter *Refers to the brain gray matter adjacent to the periaqueductal.*	substância cinzenta periaqueduto do cérebro
periarthritis *Inflammation of the tissues around a joint.*	periartrite
pericardial *Referring to around the heart.*	pericardíaco
pericarditis *Inflammation of the pericardium.*	pericardite
pericardium *The structure enclosing the heart which contains a fibrous outer layer and serous inner layer.*	pericárdio
perichondritis *Inflammation of the perichondrium.*	pericondrite
perichondrium *The membrane that encloses a cartilage.*	pericôndrio
pericolitis *Inflammation of the membrane covering the colon.*	pericolite
pericorneal ring *Also known as Kayser-Fleischer rings exhibited by presence of brown or grey-green rings on the cornea. This is from the deposition of copper and seen in Wilson's disease.*	anel de Kayser-Fleischer
perilymph *The fluid separating the membranous and osseous labyrinth.*	perilinfa
perinatology *The study of disease in the period just before and right after birth.*	perinatologia
perineal *Referring to the perineum.*	períneal

English	Portuguese
perineal laceration *Tearing of the tissue adjacent to the vaginal that can occur during childbirth.*	colporrexe
perineorrhaphy *Surgical repair of the perineum.*	perineorrafia
perinephric *Around the kidney.*	perinéfrico
perineum *The area between the anus and scrotum or anus and vulva.*	períneo
periodic paralysis *A familial muscle disorder exhibited by recurrent episodes flaccid paralysis without change in level of consciousness.*	paralisia periódica
periodontal disease *Present around to a tooth.*	doença periodontal
periosteal *Referring to the periosteum.*	perióstico
periosteum *A layer of connective tissue covering the bones.*	periósteo
periostitis *Inflammation of the periosteum.*	periostite
peripheral *Referring to an outward part or surface.*	periférico
periproctitis *Inflammation of the tissue encircling the anus and rectum.*	periproctite
peristalsis *The contraction of the longitudinal and circular muscle fibers of the alimentary canal so food is propelled.*	peristaltismo
peritomy *Surgically creating an opening of the periosteum.*	peritomia
peritoneal *Referring to the peritoneum.*	peritoneal
peritoneum *The serous membrane covering the abdominal organs and lining the abdominal walls.*	peritônio
peritonitis *Inflammation of the peritoneum.*	peritonite
peritonsillar abscess	abscesso peritonsilar
peritonsillar *Surrounding the tonsils.*	peritonsilar
periurethral *Surrounding the urethra.*	periuretral
permanent teeth *Dentition that comes in after the primary teeth.*	dentes permanente
pernicious *1. Having a detrimental effect. 2. Pernicious anemia is a reduced red blood cell count due to Vitamin B12 deficiency.*	perniciose
peroneal *Referring to the fibula or the outer part of the leg.*	peroneiro
peroneal atrophy *Progressive muscle atrophy in the peroneal region.*	atrofia peroneiro
personality *Qualities that form a person's unique character.*	personalidade
perspiration *The process of sweating.*	perspiração
pertussis *Synonym for whooping cough.*	coqueluche
pes cavus *Excessive height of the longitudinal arch of the foot.*	pé cavo
pes planus *Medical term for flat foot.*	pé plano
pes valgus *Abnormal longitudinal arch- it is flat.*	pé valgo
pessary *A supportive device placed in the rectum or vagina.*	pessário
pet *An animal kept for companionship.*	animal de estimação
PET scan Positron emission tomography. *Production of tomographic images revealing biochemical tissue properties by analyzing positrons emitted when radioactively tagged substances are taken in tissues.*	tomografia com emissão de pósitrons (PET)
petechia *A small red or purple macule on the skin caused by bleeding.*	petéquias
petrissage *Massage using a kneading action.*	malaxação
petrous *Possessing a density of a stone.*	petroso
Peyronie's disease *Curvature of the penis during an erection to to plaque.*	doença de Peyronie; doença de van Buren; fibromatose peniana
phagocyte *A cell capable of surrounding and digesting microorganisms.*	fagócito
phagocytosis *The action of a phagocyte.*	fagocitose

English	Portuguese
phalanx *One of the long bones of the fingers or toes.*	falange
phantom limb pain *Pain sensed in an area where one has had an amputation as though the limb is still present.*	dor do membro-fantasma
pharmacist *A professional who prepares and sells medicine through various systems, including governmental organizations like the Veterans Administration.*	farmacêutico
pharmacokinetics *The study of the distribution, absorption and excretion of drugs within the body.*	farmacocinética
pharmacology *The study of all aspects of medicines.*	farmacologia
pharmacy *A business that sells prescription medication.*	farmácia
pharyngeal pouch *A lateral diverticulum of the pharynx.*	bolsas faríngeas
pharyngeal *Referring to the pharynx.*	faríngeo
pharyngectomy *Surgical excision of part of the pharynx.*	faringectomia
pharyngitis *Inflammation of the pharynx.*	faringite
pharyngolaryngectomy *Surgical removal of part of the pharynx and larynx.*	faringolaríngectomia
pharyngotympanic tube *Synonym for eustachian tube.*	tubo faringotimpânico
pharynx *The membranous cavity from the mouth to esophagus.*	faringe
phenotype *The visual expression exhibited by a person from the association of the genotype with the environment.*	fenótipo
phenylketonuria *A hereditary condition in which a person cannot excrete phenylalanine; untreated it causes brain and spinal cord dysfunction.*	fenilcetonúria
phimosis *Stricture of the prepuce preventing it from being pulled back over the glans penis.*	fimose
phlebectomy *Surgical excision of a vein.*	flebectomia
phlebitis *Inflammation of a vein.*	flebite
phlebothrombosis *Presence of a clot in a vein, without associated inflammation.*	flebotrombose
phlegmasia alba dolens *Phlebitis of the femoral vein that can occur after pregnancy or typhoid fever.*	perna de leite ou branca; flegmasia trombótica
phlegmasia *Inflammation or fever.*	flegmasia
phlyctenular *Related to the formation of small vesicles on the cornea or conjunctiva.*	flictenular
phobia *An profound fear of something.*	fobia
phonation *The vocalization of sounds.*	fonação
phoniatrics *The treatment of speech abnormalities.*	foniatria
phosphaturia *Presence of phosphates in the urine.*	fosfatúria
phospholipid *A substance, such as lecithin, that when hydrolyzed produces fatty acids, glycerin, and a nitrogen compound.*	fosfolipídeo
phosphonecrosis *The breakdown of the mandible caused by excessive exposure to phosphorus.*	fosfonecrose
photophobia *Abnormal sensitivity to light.*	fotofobia
photosensitization *The process of reacting to sunlight by developing edema and dermatitis.*	fotossensibilização
phrenic *Referring to the diaphragm.*	frênico
phrenicectomy *Surgical excision of the phrenic nerve.*	frenicectomia
phrenoplegia *Paralysis of the diaphragm.*	frenoplegia
physical exam *Examination of a client to assess their medical status.*	exame físico
physical therapy *Treatment of disease by heat, massage and exercise as opposed to medications.*	terapia físico
physician *Medical practitioner.*	médico

English	Portuguese
physiologic dead space *The combination of anatomic and alveolar dead space.*	espaço morto fisiológico
physiological saline *0.9% normal saline.*	solução salina fisiológica
physiology *A subspecialty of biology that studies the normal functioning of the body.*	fisiologia
physiotherapy *Physical therapy.*	fisioterapia
pia mater *The first layer of three covering the brain and spinal cord.*	pia-máter
pica *A desire for unusual substances as occurs in pregnancy and some psychological conditions.*	pica
pill *A medicated tablet or capsule.*	pílula
pillow *An encased fabric covering soft material used for a cushion.*	traseiro
pilonidal cyst *A small cone-shaped cluster of tissue situated posterior to the third ventricle of the brain.*	ciclo pilonidal
pin *Hardware used in surgery.*	cravo; pino
pin, intramedullary *Hardware used for fracture management or during joint replacement.*	pino intramedular
pineal gland *A small body posterior to the third ventricle of the brain.*	glande pineal
pinguecula *The yellow tissue on the bulbar conjunctiva adjacent to the sclerocorneal junction.*	pinguécula
pink eye *Common term for acute contagious conjunctivitis.*	conjuntivite
pinocytosis *The absorption of fluid into a cell by the formation of vesicles on the cell membrane.*	pinocitose
pinworm *Common term for Enterobius vermincularis; a nematode worm that is a parasite.*	oxiúro
pipet *A slender tube with a bulb used for transferring liquids.*	pipeta
pitting edema *Edema of the lower extremities characterized by an indentation being left when the examiner applies pressure with their thumb.*	edema depressível
pituitary gland *A gland at the base of the hypothalamus.*	glande pituitário
pityriasis rosea *A skin disease characterized by dry pink oval papulosquamous eruptions.*	pitiríase rósea
placebo controlled study *When a study is placebo controlled it means part of the group received an inactive treatment while the other group received active therapy.*	estudo de controle de placebo
placenta *The vascular tissue that nourishes a fetus through an umbilical cord.*	placenta
placenta praevia *A condition in which the placenta covers the cervical os.*	placenta prévia
placental *Referring to the placenta.*	placentário
plagiocephaly *A condition characterized by an asymmetric skull because the cranial sutures do not close normally.*	plagiocefalia
plantar *Referring to the bottom of the foot.*	plantar
plantar fibromatosis *Deep fascia nodules on the plantar aspect of the feet.*	fibromatose plantar
plantar wart *A viral epidermal growth on the bottom of the foot.*	verruga plantar
plasma cell *A cell that produces only one type of antibody.*	célula plasma
plasmacytosis *The existence of plasma cells in the blood.*	plasmacitose
plasmapheresis *A method of removing blood and reinfusing it after the elimination of antibodies.*	plasmaferese
plaster cast *Use of gypsum impregnated gauze to immobilize fractured extremities.*	molde gessado

English	Portuguese
plaster *Dehydrated gypsum that has water added to it in order to immobilize fractured extremities.*	emplastro; gesso
platelet *An oval cell without a nucleus used in coagulation; also called a thrombocyte.*	plaqueta
pledget *A small plug of cotton or other synthetic material inserted into a wound.*	chumaço
pleomorphism *The ability of an organism or substance to attain distinct forms.*	plesiomorfismo
plethora *An excess of something.*	pletora
plethysmograph *A device used to measure the amount of blood flowing through a body part; impedance plethysmography is used to check for deep venous thrombosis.*	pletismógrafo
pleura *The serous membrane lining each lung.*	pleura
pleural effusion *An abnormal collection of fluid between the internal chest wall and the pleura.*	efusão pleural; pleurisia com derrame
pleurisy *Inflammation of the pleura.*	pleurisia
plica *A fold, as in a fold in the peritoneum.*	prega
Plummer-Vinson syndrome *Also called sideropenic dysphagia. Exhibited by iron deficiency anemia, dysphagia, esophageal stenosis and atrophic glossitis. The cause is not known.*	síndrome de Plummer-Vinson; disfagia sideropênica
pneumatocele *1. A hernia-like protrusion of lung tissue. 2. A collection of gas in a sac such as the scrotum.*	pneumatocele
pneumaturia *Presence of air or gas in the urine.*	pneumatúria
pneumococcus *A bacterium causing pneumonia and meningitis. A common type is Streptococcus pneumoniae.*	pneumococos
pneumoconiosis *Fibrosis of the lung due to dust inhalation.*	pneumoconiose
pneumocystis jiroveci pneumonia. *A pulmonary infection associated with AIDS. Formerly called pneumocystis carinii pneumonia*	pneumonia pneumocística jiroveci
pneumonectomy *Surgical excision of all or part of a lung.*	pneumonectomia
pneumonia *Inflammation of the lung due to an infection caused by a virus or bacterium.*	pneumonia
pneumoperitoneum *Abnormal or induced presence of air or gas in the peritoneum.*	presença de ar na cavidade peritoneal
pneumothorax *Abnormal presence of air between the lung and chest wall.*	pneumotórax
poikilocytosis *The presence of abnormally shaped erythrocytes.*	pecilocitose
poikilothermy *A condition of cold-blooded animals in which their temperature varies based on the ambient temperature.*	pecilotermia
poison *A substance that causes illness or death.*	veneno
polioencephalitis *Polio infection of the brain.*	polioencefalite
poliomyelitis *An infectious viral disease exhibited by constitutional symptoms that can lead to quadriplegia.*	poliomielite
polyarteritis nodosa *A systemic necrotizing vasculitis that effects medium sized arteries.*	poliarterite nodosa
polychondritis *Inflammation of the cartilage at more than one site.*	policondrite
polycystic *Possessing more than one cyst.*	policístico
polycythemia *Excess in the number of erythrocytes in the blood.*	policitemia
polycythemia vera *Condition characterized by increase in erythrocytes, thrombocytes and leukocytes, as well as, splenomegaly.*	policitemia rubra
polydactyly *Congenital anomaly exhibited by more than 5 digits on the hands and/or feet.*	polidactilia

English	Portuguese
polydipsia *Profound thirst.*	polidipsia
polymenorrhea *Increase in the frequency of menstruation.*	polimenorréia
polymyositis *Inflammation of several muscle groups at once.*	polimiosite
polyneuritis *Inflammation of more than one nerve.*	polineurite
polyneuropathy *A condition involving more than one nerve.*	polineuropatia
polyopia *A condition in which one object is seen abnormally as two or more.*	poliopia
polyposis *The formation of multiple polyps.*	polipose
polypus *Synonym of polyp (a prominent growth from a mucous membrane).*	polipo
polysaccharide *A carbohydrate that upon hydrolysis forms more than ten monosaccharides.*	polissacarídeo
polysialia *Abnormal increase in saliva.*	poliptialismo
polytrauma *A condition exhibited by multiple injuries from blunt or penetrating trauma.*	politraumatiso
polyuria *Abnormal increase in volume of urine excreted.*	poliúria
pompholyx *A condition exhibited by interdigital vesicles of the hands and feet.*	ponfólige
pons *The part of the brainstem that connects the medulla oblongata with the thalamus.*	ponte
pontine *Referring to the pons.*	pontino
popliteal *Referring to the posterior aspect of the knee.*	poplíteo
popliteal fossa *The hollow in the posterior aspect of the knee joint.*	fossa popliteo
porphyria *A hereditary condition currently classified based on the specific enzyme deficiency. The most common form is porphyria cutanea tarda that causes blistering lesions.*	porfiria
porphyrin *A class of pigments that contain a flat ring of four heterocyclic groups.*	porfirina
port-wine mark *Also called nevus flammeus, it is a vascular anomaly characterized by purplish skin discoloration.*	marca de vinho do Porto; nevo flâmeo
portal *Referring to an entrance such as porta hepatis.*	portal
portal hypertension *Hypertension in the portal system of the liver as seen in conditions causing obstruction to the portal vein.*	hipertensão porta
positive *Indicating the presence of something.*	positivo
post-mortem lividity *The purplish discoloration occurring 30-120 minutes after death in dependent body parts.*	lividez pós-morte
post-nasal drip *The descent of sinus drainage.*	gotejamento pós-nasal
post-term birth *An infant born after the normal length of pregnancy.*	parto pósmaduro
posterior *Further back in position; opposite of anterior.*	posterior
posterior chamber of the eye *An aqueous filled space between the cornea and the lens.*	câmara posterior do olho
posterior columns *The dorsal portion of the gray matter of the spinal cord.*	coluna posterior
postictal *The period of time after a seizure.*	pós-íctico
postmaturity *Generally referring to a pregnancy that goes beyond the due date.*	pós-maduro
postpartum psychosis *A episode of abnormal thought or hallucinations following delivery.*	psicose pós-parto
postpone, to *To delay.*	pospor
postural hypotension *A significant drop in blood pressure when going from the supine or sitting position to standing.*	hipotensão postural; hipotensão ortostática
postural *Referring to position or posture.*	postural

English	Portuguese
potassium *A chemical of the alkali metal group.*	potássio
potency *Strength or power.*	potência
Pott's disease *Also referred to as tuberculous spondylitis it is caused by a spinal deformity caused by a tuberculosis infection of the spine.*	doença de Pott; espondilite tuberculosa
Potter's syndrome *A group of findings associated with oligohydramnios. Renal failure is the primary problem but the infant has abnormal limbs, broad nasal bridge, low set ears and receding chin. Death usually ensues due to renal and respiratory failure.*	síndrome de Potter
poultryman's itch *Pruritus associated with the mite Dermanyssus gallinae.*	erupção devida à infestação com o ácaro
powder *Fine dry particles.*	polvilho
pox *A general term for fluid filled papules that upon rupturing leave pockmarks.*	pústula
preauricular *Anterior to the ear.*	pré-auricular
precancerous *Referring to an early stage in cancer development.*	pré-canceroso
precipitin *An antibody-antigen reaction producing a precipitate.*	precipitina
precordialgia *Pain in the precordium.*	precordialgia
precordium *The area occupying the epigastrium and lower sternum.*	precórdio
preeclampsia *Hypertension with proteinuria and/or edema in the setting of pregnancy.*	pré-eclâmpsia
pregnancy *The period of being pregnant.*	gravidez
premature *Occurring earlier than expected.*	prematuro; pré-madura
premenstrual *Occurring prior to the onset of menstruation.*	pré-menstrual
premenstrual syndrome *A cluster of emotional, behavioral, and physical symptoms that occur in the premenstrual phase of the menstrual cycle and resolve with the onset of menstruation.*	síndrome pré-menstrual
premolar *The teeth anterior to the molars.*	dentes pré-molar
prenatal care *Medical care received while one is pregnant.*	cuidados pré-natal
prenatal *Referring to the time prior to birth.*	pré-natal
presbyacusia *An age related, progressive hearing loss.*	presbiacusia
presbyopia *Farsightedness associated with aging.*	presbiopia
prescription *The action of prescribing a medication or treatment.*	prescrição; receita (P)
presenting symptom *The initial subjective complaint that initiated a visit.*	sintoma apresentado
pressure dressing *A dressing used for compression to reduce bleeding.*	curativo compressivo
pressure ulcer *Loss in skin integrity due to a portion of the body being in the same position for too long and possibly other factors.*	úlcera compressivo
presystolic *The time just before systole.*	pré-systólico
prevent, to *To stave off or hinder.*	prevenir
priapism *A painful and abnormally prolonged erection.*	priapismo
prickly heat *A rash with small vesicles that is pruritic and associated with a warm moist environment.*	calor pruriginoso
primipara *A woman giving birth for the first time.*	primípara
prior status *Referring to a person's previous state of health.*	estado prévio
probe *A device used for exploration.*	sonda
problem *Difficulty or complaint.*	problema

English	Portuguese
proctalgia *A chronic high, dull rectal pain worse with sitting position.*	proctalgia
proctectomy *Surgical excision of the rectum.*	proctectomia
proctitis *Inflammation of the rectum.*	proctite
proctocele *A hernia-type protrusion of the rectum into the vagina.*	proctocele
proctoscopy *Inspection of the rectum with a scope.*	proctoscopia
progeria *A childhood disorder exhibited by signs of aging including gray hair, wrinkled skin and short height.*	progeria
progesterone *A steroid hormone that prepares the uterus for pregnancy.*	progestogênio
proglottis *Any segment of a tapeworm.*	proglote
prognathism *Protrusion of the mandible which can cause malocclusion.*	prognatismo
prognosis *The likely course of a disease.*	prognóstico
progressive *Developing gradually.*	progressivo
prolactin *A pituitary hormone that facilitates milk production.*	prolactina
prolapse of the uterus *Eversion of the uterus through the vagina.*	prolapso uterino
prolapse of the umbilical cord *Refers to the umbilical cord protruding from the cervix during active labor.*	prolapso do cordão umbilical
prolapse *The slipping downward of a body part, such as rectal prolapse.*	prolapso
prolonged rupture of the membranes *Rupture of the membranes more than 24 hours before delivery.*	ruptura prolongamento de membrano placentário
promonocyte *An intermediate cell stage between monocyte and monoblast.*	promonócito
promontory *A protruding eminence.*	promontório
pronation *Turning posteriorly. When the hand is pronated, it is turned medially until the palm is facing posteriorly (when the body was initially in the anatomic position).*	pronação
prone *Lying with the abdomen and face downward.*	prono
prophylaxis *That which is done to prevent disease.*	profilaxia
proprioceptor *A receptor that responds to sensory input including position sense.*	proprioceptor
proptosis oculi *Synonym of exophthalmos; bulging of the eye.*	proptose do olho
prostacyclin *A prostaglandin that functions as an anticoagulant and vasodilator.*	prostaciclina
prostaglandin *A compound first found in semen (thus "prosta" in the name from prostate) with many effects including uterine contraction.*	prostaglandina
prostate *A gland found in men that surrounds the neck of the urethra and bladder.*	próstata
prostatectomy *Surgical excision of the prostate.*	prostatectomia
prosthesis *An artificial body part. (above the knee) [below the knee]*	prótese
prostration *Profound exhaustion.*	prostração
protein *A class of nitrogenous organic compound.*	proteína
proteinuria *The presence of protein in the urine.*	proteinúria
proteolysis *Enzyme action on proteins to form amino acids.*	proteólise
prothrombin *A compound converted to thrombin during coagulation of blood.*	protrombina
protoplasm *The cytoplasm, organelles and nucleus of a living cell.*	protoplasma

English	Portuguese
Protozoa *A single celled microscopic organism including amoebas among others.*	Protozoa
provoke, to *To evoke or elicit.*	provocar
proximal *Situated closer to the center of the body (opposed to that which is farther away, as in distal).*	proximal
prurigo *A chronic, pruritic papular skin eruption.*	prurigo
pruritus *A general term for conditions exhibited by itching.*	prurido
pseudarthrosis *Deossification of weight bearing long bones.*	pseudartrose
pseudobulbar palsy *Sudden outbursts of laughter or tearfulness sometimes seen in amyotrophic lateral sclerosis.*	paralisia pseudobulbar
pseudomnesia *Sensing the memory of an event that has never happened.*	pseudomnésia
psittacosis *A chlamydial pneumonia that is transmitted by birds.*	psitacose
psoriasis *A chronic papulosquamous dermatosis characterized by silver plaques.*	psoríase
psychasthenia *Essentially any non-hysterical neuroses.*	psicoastenia
psychiatry *A branch of medicine specializing in the treatment of mental disorders.*	psiquiatria
psychologist *A professional specializing in psychology.*	psicólogo
psychology *The study of the human mind and emotions.*	psicologia
psychoneurosis *A mental disorder that could include depression or anxiety but does not include hallucinations.*	psiconeurose
psychopathology *Scientific examination of mental disease.*	psicopatologia
psychosis *A profound mental disorder that can include delusions and hallucinations.*	psicose
psychosomatic *Physical ailments arising from mental disease.*	psicossomático
psychotherapy *Treatment of mental disease with cognitive-behavioral approaches.*	psicoterapia
pterygium *A membrane in the interpalpebral fissure present from the conjunctiva to the cornea.*	pterígo
ptosis *Drooping of the upper eyelid usually due to paralysis of the third cranial nerve.*	ptose
ptyalin *An enzyme found in saliva.*	ptialina
puberty *The time when adolescents become capable of sexual reproduction.*	puberdade
pubic hair *Hair present in the perineal area.*	cabelo pubiano
pubis *The anterior inferior part of the hip bone on each side that articulates at the pubic symphysis.*	púbis
pudendal *Referring to the female genitalia*	pudendo
pudendum *The mons, pubis, labia majora, labia minora and the vagina.*	pudendo; os genitais externos
puerpera *A woman who just gave birth.*	puérpera
puerperium *The six week period after childbirth.*	puerpério
puffiness *Having a soft, swollen area.*	inchação
pull, to *To exert force on something.*	puxar
pulmonary edema *Characterized by abnormal fluid buildup in the lungs.*	edema pulmonar
pulmonary embolism *A sudden blockage of a lung artery frequently emanating from a blood clot in one's leg.*	embolismo pulmonar
pulmonary *Referring to the lungs.*	pulmonar
pulmonary stenosis *A stricture between the pulmonary artery and the right ventricle.*	estenose pulmonar
pulp *The tissue filling the root canals of a tooth.*	polpa
pulpitis *Dental pulp inflammation.*	pulite

English	Portuguese
pulsatile *Relating to pulsation.*	pulsátil
pulsation *The action of expanding and contracting.*	pulsação
pulse *The rhythmic throbbing of arteries felt at major vessels.*	pulso
pulsus alternans *A regular alternation of weak and strong beats of the pulse.*	pulso alternante
pupil *The opening at the center of the iris.*	pupila
purpura *The presence of patches of ecchymosis or petechiae.*	púrpura
purulent *Referring to pus.*	purulento
pus *Thick yellow or green opaque liquid as seen with infection.*	pus
putrefaction *The rotting or decaying of organic matter.*	putrefação
pyelitis *Renal pelvis inflammation.*	pielite
pyelography *Use of a contrast agent to radiologically study the kidney, ureters and bladder.*	pielografia
pyelolithotomy *Surgical excision of a calculus from the renal pelvis.*	pielolitotomia
pyelonephritis *Inflammation of the renal parenchyma usually due to bacterial infection.*	pielonefrite
pyelonephrosis *Term, rarely used anymore,used to describe disease of the renal pelvis.*	pielonefrose
pyemia *Sepsis characterized by the presence of secondary abscesses.*	piemia
pyknic *Possessing a short, stocky physique.*	pícnico
pyknosis *The degeneration of a cell with the nucleus shrinking.*	picnose
pyloric *Referring to the pylorus.*	pilórico
pyloroplasty *Surgical enlargement of a pylorus that previously was stenotic.*	piloroplastia
pylorus *The opening at the distal stomach that opens into the duodenum.*	piloro
pyoderma *A purulent skin infection.*	piodermatite
pyogenic liver abscess *A pus filled fluid collection in the liver.*	abscesso piogênico de fígado
pyogenic *Referring to the formation of pus.*	piogênico
pyonephrosis *Injury to the renal parenchyma due to pus.*	pionefrose
pyorrhea *Emission of pus.*	piorréia
pyosalpinx *Purulent material in the oviduct.*	piossalpinge
pyramidal *A term that is used to describe various spinal tracts that originate in the cerebral cortex.*	piramidal
pyrexia *Fever.*	pirexia
pyridoxine *Synonym for vitamin B6.*	piridixina
pyrogen *A fever producing substance released by bacteria.*	pirogênio
pyrosis *Synonym for heartburn.*	pirose
pyuria *Presence of purulent material in the urine.*	piúria
Q fever *A disease caused by rickettsiae from the ingestion of unpasteurized milk.*	febre de query
quadranic hemianopia *Loss of a quarter of the visual field in one or both eyes. If bilateral, it may be further described as homonymous, heteronymous, binasal, bitemporal, or crossed.*	hemianopsia quadrântica
quadriceps jerk (reflex) *Also referred to as the patellar reflex.*	reflexo do quadríceps
quadriceps *The anterior thigh muscle composed of four muscles.*	quadríceps
quadrigeminal bodies *The cranial and caudal colliculi.*	corpos quadrigêmeos
quadriplegia *Paralysis of all four extremities.*	quadriplegia
qualify *To become eligible by fulfilling a necessary standard.*	qualificar

English	Portuguese
quarantine *A place of isolation for infectious persons until it can be certain it is safe to let them mingle.*	quarentena
quickening *Signs of life noted by a mother as the fetus moves.*	sinais de vida
querulousness *Whining or complaining.*	lamentação
quiescent *A time of inactivity.*	quiescente
quiet *Making little or no noise.*	veloz
quinsy *Peritonsillar inflammation or abscess.*	esquimência
quintan fever *Also known as trench fever as it was first noted during trench warfare in WW I. It is a rickettsial fever caused by Bartonella quintana and transmitted by a louse; signs and symptoms are myalgia, headache, malaise, fever and chills.*	febre quintã; febre das treincheiras
rabies *An infectious viral disease transmitted through the bite of a mammal. Symptoms include hydrophobia, pharyngeal spasms and hyperactivity.*	rábico
racemose *A gland having the form of a cluster.*	racemoso
radial *Referring to the radius.*	radial
radiation *1. The emission of energy in the form of electromagnetic waves. 2. Divergence from a common point.*	radiação
radiculitis *Inflammation of a spinal nerve root.*	radiculite
radioactive *Referring to the emission of ionizing particles or radiation.*	radioativo
radioactive isotope *An isotope with an unstable nucleus that is used in diagnostic imaging.*	isótopo radioativo
radiobiology *The study of the effects of radiation on organisms.*	radiobiologia
radioepithelitis *The injury to epithelial cells due to effects of radiation.*	radioepitelite
radiography *The department where images are produced on sensitive film by x-rays.*	radiografia
radiologist *A physician specializing in radiology.*	radiologista
radiology *The branch of medicine concerned with roentgenography and other high-energy radiation.*	radiologia
radionuclide *A radioactive nuclide.*	radionuclídeo
radiosensitivity *The susceptibility of the skin to radiation.*	radiossensibilidade
radiotherapy *Treatment of cancer with radiation.*	radioterapia
rage *Uncontrollable anger.*	raiva
raise, to *To lift or bring up.*	levantar
rale *An abnormal lung sound noted during auscultation.*	estertor
ramus *A branch; a term used to describe a smaller vessel branching off from a larger one.*	ramo
ranula *A retention cyst formed because of obstruction of a salivary gland in the floor of the mouth.*	rânula
rape *Forced sexual relations.*	estupro
Rapid Eye Movement *The movement of a person's eyes during this period of sleep.*	movimentos oculares rápidos (MOR)
rash *Exanthema or urticaria.*	exantema; erupção cutânea
rat bite fever *As the name implies, it is a condition exhibited by fever, nausea and skin erythema after one is bitten by a rat.*	febre da mordida de rato
reaction *A response to an action.*	reação
reactive *A response to a stimulus.*	reactivo
rebound *A term used to describe a type of tenderness found with peritonitis.*	ressalto
receptor *A cell or organ that accepts stimuli and transmits data to a sensory nerve.*	receptor

English	Portuguese
recessive This refers to genetic controlled traits that are only inherited when code from both parents is the same.	recessivo
recollection Memory.	recordação
recovery room The immediate post-operative room where patients are stabilized prior to going to a general ward.	sala de recuperação
rectal digital examination Use of a gloved finger to assess the rectal vault.	exame retal digital
rectal Referring to the rectum.	retal
rectocele A herniation of the wall between the rectum and vagina.	retocele
rectoscopy Visualization of the rectum with a scope.	retoscopia
rectosigmoidectomy Surgical resection of the rectum and sigmoid colon.	retossigmóidectomia
rectovesical septum The wall between the rectum and the urinary bladder.	septo retovesical
rectus abdominis muscle The pair of long, flat muscles that connect the sternum with the pubis.	músculo reto abdominal
recumbent Lying down.	recúbito
red nucleus A collection of gray matter near the subthalamus that receives data from the superior cerebellar peduncle.	núcleo vermelho
reduction Return of a dislocated joint or fractured bone to its proper position.	redução
referred pain Pain felt in an area distinct from the original source.	dor referida
regardless of Without consideration of.	apesar de
regurgitation 1. Backflow of blood in the heart. 2. Movement of gastric contents into the mouth.	regurgitação
relapse The return to a prior state of ill health.	recorrência
relapsing fever A recurrent bacterial infection, with fever, caused by Spirochetes.	febre recorrente; febre da foma
related to Causally connected.	ligado a
relation 1. A person who has a blood or marriage connection.	parentesco
relaxant Term generally used to refer to a muscle relaxant.	relaxante
relaxin A hormone secreted by the placenta which dilates the cervix.	relaxina
releasing hormone Hormones that come from one gland such as the thalamus that cause release of hormones from another gland such as the pituitary.	hormônio liberador
reliable Trustworthy.	confiança, de
relief Alleviation from pain or discomfort.	alívio
relieve, to (pain) To make less severe.	aliviar
REM (rapid eye movement) sleep This period of sleep is associated with irregular respirations and heart rate, involuntary movements and dreaming.	movimento rápido dos olhos
remission A decrease in severity or a temporary resolution.	remissão
removal The act of removing something.	remoção
renal Referring to the kidney.	renal; néfrico
renal colic Pain caused by passage of a calculus through the ureter.	cólico renal
renal failure Diminution of kidney function.	insuficiência renal
renal pelvis The kidney collecting system.	pelve renal
renin A renal enzyme that facilitates the production of angiotensin.	renina
resection The removal of tissue.	ressecção

English	Portuguese
residual urine *The amount of urine remaining in the bladder after a person voids.*	urina residual
residual volume (RV) *The amount of air left in the lung after a maximal exhalation.*	volume residual
resin *An organic substance that is insoluble in water. There are many types. Cholestyramine resin is used for hypercholesterolemia.*	resina
resorbable suture (chromic) *Suture that is not intended to be permanent as it is dissolved by normal body processes.*	sutura absorvível
respirator *A device used to artificially ventilate a patient.*	respirador
respiratory *Referring to respiration or the organs of respiration.*	respiratório
respiratory distress syndrome *A disease in infants that is caused by a surfactant deficiency.*	síndrome da angústia respiratório
respiratory rate *The number of breaths per minute.*	freqüência respiratória
rest *Relaxation or respite.*	repouso
restless legs *Associated with a syndrome exhibited by continuous movement of the legs from uncertain etiology.*	síndrome das pernas inquietas
retching *Spasm of the stomach without presence of gastric material.*	vômito seco
reticular *Referring to a matrix of membranous tubules inside the cytoplasm of a eukaryotic cells.*	reticular
reticulo-endothelial *Referring to the system of phagocytes involved in the immune system.*	reticuloendotelial
reticulocyte *A red blood cell without a nucleus.*	reticulócito
reticulocytosis *An abnormal increase in circulating reticulocytes.*	reticulócite
retina *The innermost of three layers of the eyeball; it surrounds the vitreous body and is continuous with the optic nerve.*	retina
retinal detachment *A tear or hole in the retina caused by vitreous traction.*	retina descolada
retinitis *Inflammation of the retina.*	retinite
retinoblastoma *A tumor consisting of retinal germ cells.*	retinoblastoma
retinopathy *Any one of a number of retinal inflammatory conditions.*	retinopatia
retraction *Being drawn back.*	retração
retractor *A device for pulling back tissue during surgery.*	retrator
retrobulbar optic neuritis *An inflammatory, demyelinating condition in the retrobulbar region.*	neurite retrobulbar
retroflexed uterus *Bending back of the uterus so that the top portion pushes against the rectum.*	útero retroflexão
retrograde *Referring to backward movement.*	retrógrado
retroperitoneal *Situated or referring to the area posterior to the peritoneum.*	retroperitônio
retropharyngeal abscess *A collection of purulent material posterior to the pharynx.*	abscesso retrofaríngeo
retropharyngeal *Referring to the area posterior to the pharynx.*	retrofaríngeo
Rett syndrome. *A rare inherited disorder causing developmental delays and is seen mostly in girls.*	síndrome de Rett
rhabdomyolysis *A acute destruction of muscle documented by myoglobinemia and myoglobinuria.*	rabdomiólose
rhagade *Fissures in the skin, particularly adjacent to body orifices.*	rágades
rheumatic *Referring to rheumatism.*	reumático

English	Portuguese
rheumatic fever *A febrile streptococcal disease causing pain and joint swelling.*	febre reumática
rheumatic heart disease *A manifestation of rheumatic fever, frequently causing valvular dysfunction.*	doença reumática do coração
rheumatism *Any condition exhibited by inflammation and pain in the joints and muscles.*	reumatismo
rheumatoid arthritis *A symmetric peripheral polyarthritis.*	artrite reumatóide
rhinitis *A viral infection or allergic reaction exhibited by nasal mucosal inflammation.*	rinite
rhinoplasty *Plastic surgery performed on the nose.*	rinoplastia
rhinorrhea *Abundant nasal mucosal drainage.*	rinorréia
rhinoscopy *Examination of the nasal passages.*	rinoscopia
rhizotomy *Interruption of the spinal nerve roots within the spinal canal.*	rizotomia
rhodopsin *A reddish purple light sensitive pigment in the human retina.*	rodopsina
rhomboid *A back muscle that elevates, retracts and adducts the scapula.*	rombóide
rhonchus *A coarse, dry sound heard on auscultation of the lungs.*	ronco
rhythm *The pattern or cadence.*	ritmo
rib *A series of curved paired boney articulations protecting the thorax.*	costela
riboflavin *Also called vitamin B2, this essential vitamin is present in food such as eggs and is synthesized in the small bowel.*	riboflavina
ribonucleic acid *An acid present in all living cells, it is a messenger for DNA.*	ácido ribonucléico
ribosomal RNA *Four chains designated by their appropriate coefficients.*	ARN ribossômico
rice-field fever *An infection cause by a species of Leptospira, affecting rice workers in Italy and Sumatra.*	febre dos arrozais
rickets *A condition exhibited by softening and bowing of the long bones; caused by Vitamin D deficiency.*	raquitismo
rickettsia *A genus of bacteria transmitted by ticks or fleas; Rocky Mountain Spotted fever is one of many diseases caused by this bacterium.*	rickettsia
Rift valley fever *A human febrile illness that is an endemic disease in sheep, transmitted by mosquitos and direct contact and caused by a virus of the family Bunyaviridae.*	febre do Vale Rift
right *Opposite of left.*	direito
right-handed *Having a preference to use the right hand.*	destro
rigor mortis *The normal stiffening of the muscles and joints that occurs a few hours after death.*	rigidez cadavérica
ring *A small circular band.*	anel
ringing in the ears *Common term for tinnitus.*	zumbido; tinido
ringworm *A fungal skin infection exhibited by pruritic well circumscribed patches on the scalp or feet.*	tinha ; tinea
risus sardonicus *A spasm of the facial muscles causing what appears to be a smile on one's face.*	riso sardônico
Ritgen's maneuver *A procedure that controls the rate of delivery of the infant's head during childbirth.*	manobra de Ritgen
rodent *A gnawing mammal that includes rats and mice.*	roedor
Roentgen *One unit of ionizing radiation named after the German physicist Wilhelm Conrad Röntgen.*	roentgen

English	Portuguese
room *A division in a building surrounded by walls.*	sala
root *An embedded part of an organ or structure.*	raiz
rosacea *Erythema of the cheeks and nose caused by chronic vascular and follicular dilation.*	rosácea
Rossolimo reflex *Flexion of the toes when the tips of the toes are flicked. This abnormal response is present in pyramidal tract lesions.*	reflexo de Rossolimo
rotation *Movement around an axis.*	rotação
rotator cuff *The structure around the capsule of the shoulder joint formed by the infraspinatus, supraspinatus, teres minor and subscapularis muscles.*	manguito rotador do ombro; manguito musculotendinoso
round ligament of the uterus *The supporting structure of the uterus.*	ligamento redondo do útero
rub *A sound heard at times with pericarditis called more specifically a pericardial friction sound.*	atrito
rubefacient *A substance that reddens the skin.*	rubefaciente
rubella *Also called German measles, it is characterized by a rash, fever, headache.*	rubéola; sarampo alemão
Rubeola *Another term for measles, an acute exanthematous disease.*	sarampo; rubéola
rude *Ill-mannered.*	rude
rugine *A surgical instrument that resembles a rasp.*	rugina
rule out, to *To perform a test or exam to exclude an illness or disease.*	excluir
running suture *A method of sewing a wound in which there is a knot at each end and continuous otherwise.*	sutura contínua
rupia *A sign of tertiary syphilis in which there are bullae or vesicles formed on the skin that erupt and form crusts.*	rúpia
rupture *An instance of bursting suddenly.*	ruptura
sacral *Referring to the sacrum.*	sacral
sacral canal *The portion of the vertebral canal that progresses into the sacrum.*	canal sacro
sacralization *The fusion of the fifth lumbar vertebra to the sacrum.*	sacralização
sacrum *The bone formed by five fused vertebrae that is situated between the two hip bones.*	sacro
saddle joint *A joint that exhibits two saddle type surfaces at a 90 degree angle to each other, such as the carpometacarpal joint.*	articulação em sela
sadness *The state of being sad.*	tristeza
sagittal suture *The line where the two parietal bones meet.*	sutura sagital
Saint Ignatius' itch *Pruritus noted with a cluster of symptoms related to niacin deficiency. Generally referred to as pellagra.*	prurido de Santo Inácio; pelagra
Saint Vitus' dance *Historic name for chorea minor characterized by hypotonia and emotional lability months after a streptococcal infection.*	coréia de Sydenham; coréia menor
saline *A solution of sodium chloride.*	salino
saliva *The watery liquid secreted by the salivary glands.*	saliva
salivary gland *The parotid, submandibular and sublingual glands that secrete saliva.*	glande salivar
salivation *The process of secreting saliva.*	salivação
salpingectomy *Surgical resection of the fallopian tubes.*	salpingectomia
salpingitis *Inflammation of the fallopian tubes.*	salpingite
salpingography *Roentgenography of the fallopian tubes after administration of contrast media.*	salpingografia

English	Portuguese
salpingostomy *A surgical procedure involving cutting the fallopian tube.*	salpingostomia
salt *Typically referring to sodium chloride.*	sal
saluretic *An agent that promotes excretion of sodium and chloride in the urine.*	salurético
sampling *The taking of samples.*	amostragem
sandfly fever *A febrile illness transmitted by a sandfly, from the genus Phlebotomus, and found in the Mediterranean.*	febre do mosquito-palha
sanitary napkin *Cloth or synthetic material used to absorb menstrual blood.*	tampão
saphena *Referring to either of the two superficial saphenous veins.*	safena
saponify,to *The creation of soap from oil using an alkali.*	saponificar
saprophyte *Any organism living on dead organic material.*	saprófita
sarcoid *Referring to sarcoidosis.*	sarcóide
sarcoidosis *A chronic disease characterized by lymphadenopathy and widespread granulomas.*	sarcoidose
sarcolemme *The sheath that covers skeletal muscle fibers.*	sarcolema
sarcoma *A non-epithelial malignant tumor.*	sarcoma
sartorius muscle *The thigh muscle that runs from the pelvis to the proximal, medial aspect of the tibia.*	músculo sartório
saturation *An amount, expressed in a percentage, that expresses the degree something is absorbed versus the maximal absorption possible.*	saturação
saw *A hand or power-driven tool used for cutting.*	serra
scabies *A skin condition exhibited by intense pruritus and a macular rash commonly in the perineal and interdigital spaces.*	escabiose
scald *A burn injury from extremely hot water.*	escaldadura
scale *A device to check a person's weight.*	escala
scalp *The skin covering the head except for the face.*	escalpo
scalp avulsion *An injury causing the skin along with some subcutaneous tissue to be pulled from the skull.*	avulsão escalpo
scalpel *A knife used during surgery for incision of skin and tissue.*	escalpelo
scaphocephaly *A condition exhibited by a long narrow skull because of early closure of the sagittal sutures.*	escafocefalia
scaphoid bone *The most lateral of the carpal bones; it articulates with the radius.*	osso escafóide
scapula *Medical term for the shoulder blade.*	escápula
scarification *Multiple small scratches of the skin, as is sometimes used for vaccine administration.*	escarificação
scarlet fever *A condition caused by streptococci that is exhibited by fever and a bright red (scarlet) rash.*	febre escaraltina
scatter *The degree to which repeated measurements differ.*	despersão
scheme *A program or plan.*	esquema
schistocyte *Part of a red blood cell seen in hemolytic anemia.*	esquistócito
schistosomiasis *A condition, sometimes known as bilharzia, which involves infestation with flukes of the genus Schistosoma.*	esquistossomíase
schizophrenia *A chronic mental condition exhibited by delusions, hallucinations, and faulty perception.*	esquizofrenia
Schmorl's nodule *Protrusion of the nucleus pulposus through the vertebral body endplate into the adjacent vertebra.*	nódulo de Schmorl
sciatica *Pain radiating from the buttock down the back of the leg; it is caused by a compressed spinal nerve root.*	ciática

English	Portuguese
scimitar sign *An abnormal radiologic finding associated with anomalous pulmonary venous drainage.*	sinal da cimitarra
scirrhus *A cancer that is hard to palpation.*	cirro
scissors *A cutting instrument with two blades, joined at the middle.*	tesoura
sclera *The white outer covering of the eyeball.*	esclera
scleritis *Inflammation of the eyeball.*	esclerite
sclerodactylia *Scleroderma of the digits.*	esclerodactilia
scleroderma *A systemic disease of the connective tissues.*	esclerodermia
sclerotomy *Surgical incision of the sclera.*	esclerotomia
scolex *The front end of a tapeworm.*	escólex
scoliosis *A lateral curvature of the spine.*	escoliose
scopophilia *Sexual please attained by viewing sexual organs.*	escopofilia
scotoma *A blind spot within an otherwise normal visual field.*	escotoma
scrape *An injury caused by having a body part rubbed against a rough surface.*	raspado
scratch *A long, narrow superficial wound.*	arranhadura
screening *An evaluation as part of a methodical study.*	triagem
scrofula *Cervical tuberculous lymphadenitis.*	escrófula
scrotal *Referring to the scrotum.*	escrotal
scrotal hydrocele *A benign collection of fluid in the scrotum.*	hidrocele funicular
scrotum *The sac which contains the testes.*	escroto
scurvy *A disease of vitamin C deficiency exhibited by bleeding gums.*	escorbuto
scutulum *A crust of tinea capitis.*	escútulo
scybalum *A hard, dry formation of stool in the bowel.*	cíbalo
seal *A device or substance used to bind two things together.*	selo
sebaceous *Referring to a sebaceous gland or what it secretes.*	sebáceo
sebaceous gland *A gland in the skin that secretes sebum.*	glande sebáceo
seborrhea *Abnormal amount of sebum production.*	seborréia
secretin *A hormone that increases secretion from the pancreas and liver.*	secretina
secretion *The discharge of substances from cells or glands.*	secreção
sedative *A medication used to facilitate sleep or calm a person.*	sedativo
seizure *An episode of tonic/clonic movement noted in epilepsy.*	ataque; convulsão
semen analysis *Evaluation of semen used as part of a fertility workup.*	análise sêmen
semicircular canal *The anterior, posterior and lateral canals in the inner ear that assist in balance control.*	canal semicircular
seminiferous tubules *Used for transport of semen.*	túbulos seminífero
seminoma *A malignant tumor of the testis.*	seminoma
senescence *The normal process of deterioration with age.*	senescência
senile *Generally referring to mental deterioration associated with aging.*	senil
senility *The process of being senile.*	senilidade
sensation *A perception when one is touched.*	sensação
sensibility *Ability to feel or perceive.*	sensibilidade
sensible *When referring to a choice, chosen with wisdom.*	sensível
sensitization *The change in an organ by a hormone so it will respond to another stimulus.*	sensibilização
sensitized *Being abnormally sensitive to a substance.*	sensibilizar

English	Portuguese
sensory nerve *A nerve that receives input from various receptors.*	nervo sensitivo
sepsis *A condition exhibited by overwhelming inflammation due to infection.*	sépsis
septic *Referring to a state of sepsis.*	séptico
septicemia *A systemic disease in which microorganisms or their toxins are in the blood stream.*	septicopiemia
septum *A wall separating two chambers, the nasal septum for example.*	septo
sequela *A medical problem related to an initial injury or disease.(late sequelae)*	seqüela
sequestrum *Necrotic bone present in an injured or diseased bone.*	seqüestro
serial *In a series.*	em série
serotonin *A neurotransmitter that constricts blood vessels.*	serotonina
serous *Referring to serum or similar to serum.*	seroso
serpiginous *A skin lesion having wavy margin.*	serpiginoso
serum *The fluid that isolates out when blood coagulates.*	soro
sessile *Having a broad base with no stalk.*	séssil
severe *Intense or very great.*	severo
sex *Gender.*	sexo
sexual intercourse *The act of copulation.*	relações sexuais
sexually transmitted disease (STD) *A condition one obtains from another during sexual relations.*	doença transmitida sexualmente
Sézary syndrome *Symptoms are exfoliative dermatitis with intense itching caused by cutaneous infiltration by mononuclear cells,*	síndrome de Sézary
shake, to *To tremble uncontrollably.*	sacudir
sharp (pain) *When describing pain, a piercing sensation.*	aguçado
sheath *A covering.*	bainha
sheet (bed) *A rectangular fabric covering a bed.*	roupa de cama
shellfish *An aquatic shelled crustacean or mollusk.*	marisco
shield *A protective device, as in face shield.*	escudo
shin *Refers to the anterior tibial region.*	canela
shingles *A reactivation of herpes zoster.*	herpes zóster
shiver *A trembling.*	tremor; calafrio
shock *A condition characterized by systemic hypoperfusion.*	choque
shoe *Article of clothing worn on each foot.*	sapato
shortening *Notable for having a shorter length.*	encurtamento
shoulder *The joint were the scapula joins the clavicle and humerus. (right shoulder, left shoulder)*	ombro (ombro direito, ombro esquerdo)
shunt *An alternate path for blood or fluid.*	derivação
sialadenitis *Inflammation of a salivary gland.*	sialoadenite
sialogogue *A substance that increase salivary flow.*	sialogogo
sialolith *A calculus in a salivary duct.*	sialólito
sibling *A brother or sister.*	irmão
sickle-cell anemia *A hereditary type of anemia characterized by crescent shaped red blood cells.*	anemia de células falciformes
sickness *Illness or a state of disease.*	doença
side *A position medial or lateral to center.*	lado
side effect *An expected but unwanted effect of a medication.*	efeito colateral
siderosis *Discoloration of a part due to iron deposition.*	siderose

English	Portuguese
sigh *A long deep exhalation that expresses an emotion, as in relief.*	suspiro
sigmoid flexure *The S shaped curve located between the descending colon and rectum.*	flexura sigmóide
sigmoid *Referring to the portion of the colon that leads into the rectum.*	sigmóide
sigmoidoscopy *Visualization of the sigmoid colon with a scope.*	sigmoidectomia
sigmoidostomy *Formation of an opening in the sigmoid colon that communicates with the outside of the body.*	sigmoidoscopia
silent *Absence of noise or no indication of something.*	silencioso
silicosis *Grinders's disease; fibrotic lung disease caused by inhalation of silica.*	silicose
silver *A precious metal with atomic number 47.*	prata
silver nitrate stick *A medical device used to treat hypergranulation tissue.*	nitrato de prata
simultaneous *Occurring at the same time.*	simultâneo
single *Only one.*	solitário
single *Not married.*	solteiro
sinistrocardia *Location of the heart toward the left (more than normally seen).*	sinistrocardia
sinistrotorsion *Distorsion toward the left; in reference to the eye generally.*	sinstrotorção
sinoatrial *Referring to the cardiac node of the same name.*	sinoatrial
sinoatrial node *A mass of cardiac tissue that acts as the pacemaker.*	nodo sinoatrial
sinus arrhythmia *Cardiac dysrhythmias related to sinoatrial nodal dysfunction.*	disritmia atrial
sinusitis *Inflammation of the sinuses.*	sinusite
sinusoid *An irregular vessel having almost no adventitia that is found in the liver, heart, parathyroid, spleen and pancreas.*	sinusóide
sip, to *To slowly take small drinks of a fluid.*	bebericar
Sister Mary Joseph nodule *A nodule at the umbilicus associated with metastatic abdominal cancer.*	nódulo da Irmã Joseph
site *Location.*	sítio
size *The dimensions of something.*	tamanho
Sjogren's syndrome. *Characterized by dryness of the mouth and eyes, it is sometimes linked to rheumatoid arthritis.*	síndrome de Sjogren
skeletal traction *Use of a pulley system to reduce a fracture.*	tração óssea
skeleton *Internal bony framework.*	esqueleto
skin *Flesh.*	pele
skin fold *An overlapping of skin formed by subcutaneous tissue.*	dobra do pele
skin lesion *An abnormal but not necessarily cancerous lesion.*	lesão de pele
skin rash *Dermal exanthema.*	exantema
sleep *A nap or a snooze.*	sono
sleep apnea *Episodic apnea during sleep that is exhibited by daytime symptoms of fatigue, difficulty concentrating and sleepiness.*	apnéia do sono
sleeping sickness *Also called Trypanosomiasis, this disease is caused by a parasitic protozoa and transmitted by the tsetse fly.*	doença do sono; tripanossomíase gambiense
slice *A sliver or shaving.*	fatia
slide *A thin, rectangular piece of glass used for viewing specimen under a microscope.*	lâmina
slight *Minor or small.*	desprezo
sling *A device used to give support to an injured extremity.*	tipóia

English	Portuguese
slow *Unhurried.*	lento
sludge *A viscous fluid.*	lodo
slurring *Indistinct yet comprehensible speech.*	pronunciar indistintamente
smallpox *Variola.*	varíola
smear *Used to refer to a specimen smeared on a slide.*	esfregaço
smegma *A thick curdled secretion found around the clitoris and the prepuce.*	esmegma
smoke, to *To inhale on a cigarette.*	fumar
sneeze, to *To suddenly expel air from the nose and mouth because of nasal irritation.*	espirrar
sniffing *Short, rapid nasal inhalation.*	fungada
snore, to *To snore or grunt while breathing during sleep.*	roncar
soap *A compound made with fats/oils and an alkali; it is used for washing.*	sabão
sob, to *To cry uncontrollably.*	soluçar
socket *An anatomical hollow that is part of an articulation. (eyeball socket)*	concavidade
socks *Worn on the feet before one puts on shoes.*	meias
sodium chloride *A colorless, crystalline compound; also table salt.*	cloreto de sódio
soft *Easy to mold or compress.*	pessoa
solar plexus *A cluster of ganglia and nerves, located at the base of the sternum, that surround the celiac trunk.*	plexo solar
sole of foot *Common term for plantar aspect of the foot.*	sola de pé
soleus muscle *Assists with ankle plantar flexion.*	músculo solear
solvent *Able to dissolve with other chemicals.*	solvente
somatic *Referring to the body.*	somático
somnambulism *Sleepwalking.*	sonambulismo
somnolence *Drowsiness.*	sonolência
soporific *Promoting drowsiness or sleep.*	soporífico
sore throat *Common term for pharyngitis.*	faringite
sorrow *A feeling of deep despair.*	tristeza
sound *Vibrations that travel through air and are heard when reaching the ears.*	som
sour *An acid or bitter taste.*	coisa
span *A distance between two objects.*	palmo
sparing *Economical.*	escasso
spasm *An involuntary contraction of muscles.*	espasmo
spasmolytic *A substance that diminishes spasms.*	espasmolítico
spastic *Stiff, awkward movement of the muscles.*	espático
spasticity *Refers to continuous spastic movement.*	espasticidade
specific *Clearly defined.*	específico
specimen *A sample for medical testing.*	espécime
spectrometry *The use of a device to measure spectra.*	espectrometria
spectroscope *A device for producing and recording spectra.*	espectroscópio
speculum *A device used to open a canal for inspection. (vaginal speculum)*	espéculo
speech *Oral articulation.*	fala
speech therapist *A person trained to assist people with speech and language disorders.*	terapeuta de fala
sperm *Short term for spermatozoon.*	esperma

English	Portuguese
spermatic cord *The structure containing the ductus deferens, testicular artery, and nerves that goes from the inguinal ring to the testis.*	cordão espermático
spermatocele *A cyst in the epididymis containing spermatozoa.*	espermatocele
spermatogenesis *The production of spermatozoa.*	espermatogênese
spermatozoon *A mature male germ cell that is capable of fertilizing an ovum.*	espermatozóide
spermicide *A substance capable of killing sperm.*	espermicida
sphenoidal sinus *Part of the sphenoid bone; it communicates with the most superior aspect of the nasal meatus.*	seio esfenoidal
spherocyte *An erythrocyte without the usual central pallor; it is noted in spherocytosis and some hemolytic anemias.*	esferócito
spherocytosis *The presence of spherocytes in the blood.*	esferocitose
sphincter *A muscle the surrounds an orifice or duct so it closes when the muscle contracts.*	esfíncter
sphincterotomy *Surgical incision of the anal sphincter.*	esfincterotomia
sphygmomanometer *Device for measuring blood pressure.*	esfigmomanômetro
spica *A figure of eight bandage.*	espiga
spicule *A sharp, slender part.*	espícula
spider nevus *A papule with telangiectases radiating from the center.*	nevo arâneo
spinal *Referring to the spine.*	espinhal
spinal cord abscess *A localized collection of purulent material in or adjacent to the spinal cord.*	abscesso de cordão espinhal
spinal cord *The bundle of nerves that with the brain comprise the central nervous system.*	cordão espinhal
spinal ganglion *The ganglion located on the dorsal root of each spinal nerve.*	gânglio espinhal
spinal nerve *The term for each of the thirty pairs of nerves that originate in the spine and traverse between the vertebrae. There are eight cervical, twelve thoracic, five lumbar, five sacral and one coccygeal nerve pairs.*	nervo espinhal
spinal reflex *A reflex that has an arc passing through the spine.*	reflexo espinhal
spinal shock *Hypotension related to injury or intervention of the spine.*	choque medular
spine *The spinal column or a thorny protrusion.*	espinha
spirograph *A device used to record respiratory movements.*	espirógrafo
spirometer *A device used to measure pulmonary capacity.*	espirômetro
spit *A term used to describe saliva that is ejected from the mouth.*	saliva
splanchnic nerves *The nerves supplying the abdominal viscera and blood vessels.*	nervo esplâncnico
spleen *The visceral organ that is involved with production and removal of blood cells.*	baço
splenectomy *Surgical excision of the spleen.*	esplenectomia
splenic flexure of the colon *The portion of the colon that turns from the transverse to the descending colon.*	flexura esplênica
splenic *Referring to the spleen.*	esplênico
splenomegaly *An abnormally enlarged spleen.*	esplenomegalia
splint *A rigid support used to immobilize and extremity.*	aparelho
splinter *A small, thin object; usually refers to the object being imbedded in the body.*	lasca
spondylitis *Inflammation of the vertebrae.*	espondilite
spondylolisthesis *The overlapping of one vertebra over another.*	espondilolistese

English	Portuguese
spondylolysis *Dissolution of the vertebra.*	espondilólise
sponge *Sterile fabric used to soak up fluid during surgery.*	esponja
spongiosis *Edema of the spongy layer of the skin.*	espongiose
spontaneous *Occurring without provocation.*	espontâneo
spoon nail *Also referred to as koilonychia, the nail is concave and is generally associated with anemia.*	unha em colher
spoonful *A measurement that does not specify teaspoon or tablespoon.*	colherada
sporotrichosis *A Sporotrichum schenckii infection manifested by formation of lymphatic and subcutaneous nodules.*	esporotricose
sprain *A joint injury without fracture.*	entorse
spray *Liquid blown through the air in the form of fine droplets.*	aerossol
sputum *A mixture of respiratory tract secretions and saliva.*	esputo
squama *A scale or platelike body.*	escama
squamous *Scaly.*	escamoso
square root *The result noted when a number is multiplied by itself.*	raiz quadrada
squeeze, to *To apply pressure.*	comprimir
squint, to *To look at something with the eyes partially closed.*	sofrer de estrabismo
squirt, to *To eject a liquid from a small opening.*	esguichar
stab wound *An injury occurring with a sharp object.*	ferida puntiforme
stabbing pain *A sharp piercing quality to pain.*	dor do afiado
stagger, to *To walk in an unsteady fashion.*	cambalear
staging *Refers to a stratification of cancer for example.*	estadiamento
stamina *Ability to maintain physical or mental exertion for a long period.*	sobrevivência
stammering *The impulse to repeat the first letter of words and involuntary pauses while speaking.*	gagueira
standing *Position or status.*	estagnado
stapedectomy *Surgical excision of the stapes.*	estapedectomia
stapedius muscle *Located in the tympanic interior, it reduces stapedial movement.*	músculo estapédio
stapes *This auditory ossicle is the innermost of three ossicles and is shaped like a stirrup.*	estribo
staphyloma *Protrusion of the cornea due to inflammation.*	estafiloma
staphylorrhaphy *Surgical repair of a defect between the soft palate and uvula.*	estafilorrafia
starvation *Death related to starvation.*	inanição
stasis *Lack of movement.*	estase
state *Status.*	estado
statement *A written or oral commentary.*	declaração
static *Not changing.*	estático
status *Position or condition*	estado
steady state *In equilibrium.*	estado de equilíbrio
steatoma *A sebaceous cyst or lipoma.*	esteatoma
steatorrhea *Excrement with an abnormally high fat content.*	esteatorréia
steatosis *Fatty degeneration; when referring to the liver it involves invasion of fat into hepatocytes.*	esteatose
stellate ganglion *Formed by the seventh cervical, eighth cervical and first thoracic ganglia.*	gânglio estrelado
stenosis *Narrowing of an orifice.*	estenose
stercobilin *A substance created by the reduction of bilirubin and gives excrement the brown hue.*	estercobilina

English	Portuguese
stereognosis *The ability to identify an object by touch.*	esterognose
sterile *1. Infertile 2. Refers to equipment that is free of contamination.*	estéril
sterilization *A procedure done to prevent production of offspring.*	esterilização
sternal *Referring to the sternum.*	esternal
sternocleidomastoid *The pair of muscles that connect the sternum, clavicle and mastoid process.*	esternocleidomastóide
sternum *Commonly called the breast bone, it consists of the corpus, manubrium and xiphoid process.*	esterno
sterol *Unsaturated steroid alcohols such as cholesterol.*	esterol
stethoscope *Device used to auscultate the heart, lungs and over arteries to assess for abnormalities.*	estetoscópio
stiff *Not easily bent.*	rijo
stiff-neck *Cervical sprain with reduced range of motion.*	colo rígido
stillborn *Refers to a newborn that died in utero.*	narimorto
sting *A small puncture as in a bee sting.*	picada
stippling *Having numerous small specks or spots.*	pontilhado
stirrup *An attachment to an exam table where a woman puts her legs to assist examination of the genitalia.*	estribo
stomach *Organ of digestion between the esophagus and small bowel.*	estômago
stomach cramps *Sensation of muscle contraction in the epigastric area.*	cãibras por estômago
strabismus *An anomaly of ocular movement.*	estrabismo
strain *As in a muscle strain.*	cepa
strait-jacket *A device used to temporarily restrain the arms of patients who are psychotic and violent.*	camisa-de-força
strange *Unusual in an unsettling way.*	estranho
straw itch *Pruritus associated with exposure to straw that is infested with the mite Pyemotes ventricosus. Also referred to as dermatitis pediculoides ventricosus.*	prurido da palha
strawberry tongue *A characteristic discoloration of the tongue seen in an early phase of scarlet fever.*	língua de framboesa
stream *The flow of a liquid.*	corrente
strength *Force, might or vigor.*	força
stress *Strain or pressure.*	tensão
stress fracture *A long bone fracture caused by repetitive mechanical stress.*	fratura por tensão
stretcher *A device used to carry a patient in the supine position.*	uma maca
stria *A narrow bandlike body.*	estria
stricture *A narrowing of a canal or duct.*	estreitamento
stride *Walk with long definitive steps.*	passo
stridor *An abnormal, high-pitched, musical sound caused by an obstruction in the larynx or stenosis of the vocal cords.*	estridor
stroke *Common term for cerebrovascular accident.*	acidente vascular cerebral
stroke volume *The amount of blood ejected from the ventricle with each contraction.*	volume sistólico
stroma *A term used to describe the framework of an organ.*	estroma
strong *Having the power to move heavy objects.*	forte
stump *Term used to designate what remains of an amputated extremity.*	coto

English	Portuguese
Strümpell's disease *Also known as spondylitis deformans, it is characterized by arthritis and osteitis deformans of the spinal cord with a rounded kyphosis and rigidity.*	doença de Strümpell; espondilite deformante
Strümpell reflex *Flexion of the leg and adduction of the foot elicited by stroking of the thigh or abdomen.*	reflexo de Strümpell
stupor *A reduced level of consciousness.*	estupor
stuttering *Involuntary repetition of the first consonant.*	tartamudez
sty *Also called hordeolum externum, it is inflammation of the sebaceous gland of an eyelash.*	terçol
stylet *A thin wire within a catheter that is removed after the catheter is in place.*	estilete
subacute *A stage between acute and chronic.*	subagudo
subarachnoid *The layer of the brain covering between the arachnoid and pia mater.*	subaracnóide
subareolar abscess *A purulent fluid collection in the areolar gland.*	abscesso subareolar
subclavian *Refers to the area under the clavicle; the subclavian vein runs below the clavicle.*	subclávio
subclavian steal syndrome *Retrograde vertebral artery flow due to ipsilateral subclavian artery stenosis.*	síndrome do roubo subclávio
subdural *The area between the dura mater and the arachnoid membrane.*	subdural
subdural hematoma *Formation of a blood clot between the dura mater and the arachnoid membrane.*	hematoma subdural
suberosis *A type of hypersensitivity pneumonitis related to inhalation of moldy cork dust.*	suberose
sublingual *Situated under the tongue.*	sublingual
submaxillary *Situated below the maxilla.*	submaxilar
subphrenic *Referring to below the diaphragm.*	subfrênico
succussion *The presence of a splashing sound when a body cavity is moved indicating presence of both air and fluid.*	sucussão
suck, to *As in, to suction fluid.*	sugar
suckle, to *An infant taking to his mother's nipple.*	amamentar
sudamina *White vesicles noted because of retained sweat in the layers of the epidermis.*	sudames
sudden infant death syndrome *A leading cause of death of infants from one month to one year; the etiology is unknown.*	síndrome da morte súbita do lactente
suffer, to *To be affected by an illness or sickness.*	sofrer
suffocation *To die from a lack of air or inability to breathe.*	sufocação
sugar *A sweet crystalline substance made from a plant such as sugar cane.*	açúcar
suicide *To kill oneself intentionally.*	suicídio
sulcus *A groove, like in the brain.*	sulco
sulfonamide *A class of drugs derived from sulfanilamide that are antibacterial.*	sulfonamidas
sulfur *A chemical element with atomic number of 16.*	enxofre
summer itch *Pruritus noted upon exposure to hot weather, also known as pruritus aestivalis.*	prurido do verão;
superciliary arch *The area superior to the upper border of each orbit.*	arco superciliar
superfecundation *The fertilization of two different ova by spermatozoa of two different males.*	superfecundação
superficial inguinal ring *The opening of the aponeurosis of the external oblique muscle for the round ligament or spermatic cord.*	anel inguinal superficial

English	Portuguese
superior *In a position above something else.*	superficial
supination *Turning the sole of the foot or the palm of the hand upward..*	supinação
supine *Flat on one's back.*	supino
supplies *Stock or reserves.*	suprimento
suppository *A delivery system for medication placed in an orifice.*	supositório
suppuration *Formation of purulent material.*	supuração
supranuclear ophthalmoplegia *A disorder that effects the extraocular movements especially limiting the upward movement of the eyes.*	oftalmoplegia supranuclear
supraorbital *Situated above the orbit.*	supra-orbitário
suprapubic *Situated above the pubis.*	suprapúbico
sural *Referring to the calf of the leg.*	sural
surfactant *A substance that reduces surface tension in the lungs.*	surfactante
surgeon *A physician who performs surgery.*	cirurgião (P)
surgery *The incision of a body part using sterile technique in order to treat disease or injury.*	cirurgia
surgical *Referring to surgery.*	cirúrgico
surname *One's given "last" name that generally changes for women upon marriage to that of the man's surname.*	sobrenome
sustain, to *To keep or maintain.*	sustentar
sustained release tablet *Describes a medicine that is slowly dispersed so it has a lasting effect.*	comprimido de ação prolongada
suture *Thread used for sewing together a wound.*	sutura
swab *An absorbent material used for cleaning wounds or applying ointment.*	chumaço de algodão
swallow, to *To cause something to pass down the esophagus.*	deglutir
sweat *Moisture exuded through the pores of the skin.*	suor
sweat, to *The action of releasing moisture through pores of the skin.*	suar
swelling *An abnormal enlarged from fluid collection.*	tumefação
swimmer's itch *Pruritus caused by exposure to schistosomes.*	prurido do nadador
swollen (distended) abdomen	tumefação abdominal
sycosis *A bacterial infection affecting the hair follicles on a person's face.*	sicose
Sydenham chorea *Historically known as Saint Vitus' dance, it is a childhood chorea associated with rheumatic fever.*	coréia de Sydenham; coréia menor
symbiosis *The living together of two organisms.*	simbiose
symmetry *Being equally bilaterally.*	simetria
sympathectomy *The surgical resection of a sympathetic nerve to reduce undesired effects.*	simpatectomia
sympathetic nervous system *The nerves responsible for the flight or fight response.*	sistema nervoso simpático
symptom *A physical feature that is characteristic of disease.*	sintoma
synapse *The intersection of two nerve cells.*	sinapse
synarthrosis *Adjacent bones connected by a joint but the joint is fixed.*	sinartrose
synchondrosis *A joint with little motion that uses cartilage such as the vertebral bodies.*	sincondrose
syncope *Sudden loss of consciousness.*	síncope
syncytial knot *Aggregation of syncytiotrophoblastic nuclei in the villi of the placenta during early pregnancy.*	nó sincicial

English	Portuguese
synechia *The adhesion of two body parts, such as synechia vulvae in which the labia minora are congenitally adherent.*	sinéquia
synovectomy *Surgical resection of a synovial membrane.*	sinovectomia
synovial fluid *The fluid that surrounds, for example, the knee within a capsule.*	fluido sinovial
synovitis *Inflammation of the synovium.*	sinovite
syphilis *A infectious disease caused by Treponema pallidum that causes a painless penile ulcer in the primary stage but can lead to irreversible brain damage in the untreated tertiary stage.*	sífilis
syringe *A device used for administering medication through various routes.*	seringa
syringomelia *A condition exhibited by fluid-filled cavities in the spinal cord.*	siringomielia
syrup *A thick sweet liquid.*	xarope
systole *The phase of the cardiac cycle in which the ventricles contract.*	sístole
systolic *Referring to systole or that which occurs during systole.*	sistólico
tablespoon *An eating utensil that holds 15milliliters of fluid.*	colher de sopa
tablet *A small disk of a compressed solid substance.*	comprimido; tablete
tachycardia *Heart rate higher than physiologic normal.*	taquicardia
tachypnea *Breathing faster than normal.*	taquipnéia
tactile *Able to be felt.*	tátil
talipes calcaneus *A foot deformity exhibited by abnormal dorsiflexion.*	talipe calcaneus
talipes equinovaro *Medical term for what is commonly known as club foot.*	talipe eqüinovaro
talipes equinus *A foot deformity exhibited by abnormal plantar flexion.*	talipe eqüino
talon *The ball of the ankle joint.*	tálon
talus *The most superior tarsal bone that articulates with the tibia.*	talo
tampon *Disposable intravaginal product used to collect blood from menstruation.*	tampão
tamponade *1. Stopping bleeding during surgery with a cotton pledget. 2. When referring to cardiac tamponade, it is the limitation of cardiac contraction because of blood or fluid accumulation in the pericardial sac.*	tamponamento
tap *A puncture with the intent of draining fluid as in spinal tap.*	puncionar
tape measure *A long length of tape, marked at intervals for measuring.*	fita métrica
tapeworm *A parasitic, intestinal flatworm.*	tênia
tarantula *A large hairy spider found mainly in the tropics.*	tarântula
target *An objective towards which efforts are directed.*	alvo
target cell *An abnormal cell that is present in liver disease and certain hemoglobinopathies.*	célula alvo
tarsal *Referring to any bone in the tarsus.*	társico
tarsal tunnel syndrome *Characterized by impingement of various nerves of the ankle.*	síndrome do túnel do tarso
tarsalgia *Pain in any of the tarsal bones.*	tarsalgia
tarsectomy *Surgical excision of all or part of the tarsus.*	tarsectomia
tarsorrhaphy *Suturing the eyelids in order to tighten the palpebral fissure.*	tarsorrafia
tarsus *The group of seven bones of the ankle or foot (three cuneiform bones, talus, calcaneus, navicular, cuboid bones).*	tarso

English	Portuguese
taste *Sensation of flavor perceived in one's mouth.*	sabor; gosto
tattoo *A design made by inserting indelible ink into the skin.*	tatuagem
taurocholic acid *A bile acid composed of cholic acid and taurine.*	ácido taurocólico
tear *As in, to shed a tear.*	lágrima
tear *Referring to a vaginal tear after childbirth.*	laceração
teaspoon *A measure instrument that holds 5 milliliters of fluid.*	colher de chá
tectum *A roof-like body.*	teto
tectum mesencephali *The posterior portion of the mesencephalon including the sup. and inf. colliculi and tectal lamina.*	teto do mesencéfalo
telangiectasis *A condition exhibited by red, dilated capillaries on the skin.*	telangiectasia
telemetry *Use of radio signals to transmit patient data. The most common form is for electrocardiography in a patient who is ambulatory.*	telemetria
temperature *The degree of internal heat in a person's body.*	temperatura
temporomandibular joint *The hinged joint of the temporal bone and mandible.*	articulação temporomandibular
tendinitis *Inflammation of a tendon.*	tendinite
tendon *Fibrous tissue that connects muscle to bone.*	tendão
tendon reflex *A deep reflex elicited by gently tapping the tendon.*	reflexo do tendão
tenesmus *The attempt to defecate but attempts elicit pain and are ineffective.*	tenesmo
tennis elbow *Inflammation at the lateral aspect of the epicondyle where the muscle and tendon join; lateral epicondylitis.*	cotovelo do tenista; epicondilite umeral lateral
tenoplasty *Surgical repair of a tendon.*	tenoplastia
tenorrhaphy *The surgical repair with suture of a separated tendon.*	tenorrafia
tenosynovitis *Inflammation and swelling of an articulation.*	tenossinovite
tenotomy *Incision of a tendon as is done for strabismus.*	tenotomia
tepid *Lukewarm.*	tépido
teratogen *A substance that induces fetal anomalies.*	teratógeno
teratoma *A tumor made up of tissue not usually at the location (a mass of hair, teeth and gingival tissue in a leg tumor for instance).*	teratoma
terebrant *Having a piercing quality.*	terebrante
terminal illness *A disease with no viable treatment with death being inevitable.*	enfermidade terminal
tertian fever *A febrile syndrome caused by Plasmodium vivax which produces a fever spike every 48 hours.*	febre terçã
tertiary *Third in order or designating medical care at a specialized hospital.*	terciário
test tube *A glass or plastic tube used to hold a medical specimen.*	tubo de teste; tubo de ensaio
testicle *One of a pair of organs in the male scrotum that produces sperm.*	testículo
testicular torsion *Rotation of the spermatic cord resulting in testicular ischemia.*	torção do testículo
testosterone *This steroid hormone produces secondary male sexual characteristics.*	testosterona
tetanus *A condition caused by Clostridium tetani which produces spasm and rigidity of voluntary muscles.*	tétano

English	Portuguese
tetany *A condition caused by the hypocalcemic effect of hypoparathyroidism, exhibited by periodic muscle spasms, convulsions, and peri-oral numbness.*	tetania
tetracycline *An antibiotic used for gram positive and gram negative infections.*	tetraciclina
tetradactylous *Referring to a condition of having only four digits on a hand or foot.*	tetradáctilo
thalamic syndrome *Caused by an infarct of the posteroinferior thalamus, there is transient hemiparesis, severe sensory loss with preserved crude pain in the hypalgic limbs.*	síndrome talâmica
thalamus *A paired structure located adjacent to the third ventricle.*	tálamo
thalassemia *A hereditary hemolytic anemia first observed in people from the Mediterranean area.*	talassemia
thalidomide *A drug used originally as a sedative, after it was found to cause congenital anomalies, its use was restricted. Now it is used for a few conditions such as multiple myeloma.*	talidomida
theca *A tendon or ovarian follicle sheath.*	teca
thecoma *A tumor composed of theca cells.*	tecoma
thenar eminence *Formed by the bellies of the abductor pollicis brevis, flexor pollicis brevis and opponens pollicis.*	eminência tenar
therapeutic range *The highest to lowest value that will produce a desired effect.*	variação terapêutica
thermometer *A device used to measure temperature.*	termômetro
thiamine *Also called vitamin B1; a deficiency causes beriberi.*	tiamina
thigh *The body region between the inguinal crease and knee.*	coxa
thin *Lean or slender.*	fino
thirst *The desire to drink.*	sede
thoracentesis *Insertion of a needle into the pleural space to drain and or obtain a specimen for analysis.*	toracocentese
thoracic *Referring to the thorax.*	torácico
thoracoplasty *Surgical removal of ribs.*	toracoplastia
thoracoscopy *Visualization of the thoracic cavity with a scope.*	taracoscopia
thoracotomy *Surgical incision of the thorax.*	taracotomia
thorax *The part of the body between the neck and abdomen.*	tórax
three way foley *A urinary tube used for irrigation of the bladder.*	sonda de canal triplo
threonine *An amino acid needed for the growth in infants.*	treonina
throat *The anterior aspect of the neck.*	garganta
throb, to *The beat with strong regular rhythm.*	pulsar
thrombectomy *Excision of a thrombus from a vein or artery.*	trombectomia
thrombin *An enzyme that is a catalyst for the conversion of fibrinogen to fibrin in the formation of a clot.*	trombina
thromboangiitis *Inflammation and thrombosis in a blood vessel.*	tromboangeíte
thromboarteritis *Thrombosis of an inflamed artery.*	tromboarterite
thrombocytopenia *Abnormal decrease in the number of blood platelets.*	trombocitopenia
thrombophlebitis *Inflammation of a venous wall associated with a thrombus.*	tromboflebite
thrombosis *Formation of a clot in a vein or artery.*	trombose
thrush *Candida albicans*	afta; sapinho
thumb *The first digit of each hand.*	polegar
thymectomy *Surgical excision of the thymus.*	timectomia

English	Portuguese
thymine *A chemical with a pyrimidine base found in DNA.*	timina
thymocyte *A lymphocyte located in the thymus.*	timócito
thymoma *A tumor composed of thymic tissue and is sometimes associated with myasthenia gravis.*	timoma
thymus *A body organ located in the neck and it produces T cells to improve immune function.*	timo
thyroglossal cyst *A common congenital growth in the thyroglossal duct.*	cisto de tireoglosso
thyroid *A gland in the neck that secretes hormones regulating metabolism.*	tireóide
thyroid stimulating hormone (TSH) *A thyroid secreted by the pituitary that regulates the thyroid.*	hormônio estimulante da tireóide
thyroidectomy *Surgical resection of all or part of the thyroid.*	tireoidectomia
thyrotoxicosis *Abnormal increase in thyroid activity exhibited by thinning hair, hypertension, tachycardia and at times atrial fibrillation.*	tireotoxicose
thyroxine *An iodine containing hormone, referred to T4.*	tireoxina
tibia *The larger of two long bones in the lower leg.*	tíbia
tic *Periodic spasmodic facial muscle contractions.*	tique
tic douloureux *Also referred to as trigeminal neuralgia.*	tique doloroso
tick bite	mordedura por carrapato
tick-borne fever *A relapsing fever caused by a spirochete of the genus Borrelia.*	febre transmitida por carrapato
tickle, to *To lightly touch a person to cause one to laugh.*	fazer cócegas
tidal volume *The amount of air inspired with each breath. One can set a ventilator to deliver a preset number of milliliters of oxygenated air with each breath.*	volume corrente
tight junction *An intercellular junction with an impermeable membrane.*	junção estreita
tincture *1. A very small amount of something. 2. A medicine dissolved in alcohol.*	tintura
tinea barbae *Ringworm on the face in the region a man shaves.*	tinha da barba
tinea capitis *Ringworm of the scalp, a fungal infection.*	tinha da cabeça
tinea corporis *Ringworm of the body, a fungal infection.*	tinha do corpo
tinea cruris *Ringworm in the inguinal region, a fungal infection.*	tinha crural
tinea *Medical term for ringworm.*	tinha
tinea pedis *Ringworm of the feet, a fungal infection.*	tinha do pé
tingling *Prickling or stinging sensation.*	formigamento
tinnitus *Medical term for ringing in the ears. It is associated with Meniere's syndrome among other conditions.*	tinido
tired *Fatigued.*	cansado
tissue *Any of the distinct materials people are made of.*	tecido
tocopherol *Vitamin E.*	tocoferol
toe *Any of the digits of of the feet.*	dedo (do pé)
toenail *The nail at the tip/dorsal aspect of each toe.*	unha do dedo do pé
tongs *A medical device used for holding or grasping.*	tenazes
tongue *The fleshy muscular organ of the mouth.*	língua
tongue depressor; tongue blade *As the name implies, the stick pushes the tongue down so the posterior aspect of the mouth can be viewed more readily.*	abaixa-lingua
tonometer *A device used to measure ocular pressure in glaucoma.*	tonômetro

English	Portuguese
tonsil *A rounded mass of lymphoid tissue, most commonly referring to the pharyngeal tonsil.*	tonsila
tonsillectomy *Excision of the tonsils.*	tonsilectomia
tonsillitis *Inflammation of the tonsils.*	tonsilite
tooth *One of a set of hard, bony enamel coated structure in the jaw.*	dente
toothache *Dental pain.*	odontalgia
toothless *Edentulous.*	sem dentes
torpor *Unresponsiveness to normal stimuli.*	torpor
torsade de pointe *Ventricular cardiac rhythm disturbance.*	paroxismos de taquicardia ventricular
torsion *Refers to twisting. Testicular torsion is the twisting of the spermatic cord that can lead to ischemia and gangrene of the testicle.*	torção
torsion spasm *Also called dystonia musculorum deformans, a genetic condition exhibited by twisting contortions sideways and forward while walking.*	espasmo de torção
torso *The trunk of the body.*	torso
torticollis *A condition exhibited by the head being turned to one side continuously.*	torcicolo
touch *Tactile stimulation.*	toque
tourniquet *A device tied tightly around an extremity to diminish blood flow or blood loss.*	garrote
toxemia *The release of toxic substances into the blood stream from a local infection. Toxemia of pregnancy is a synonym for preeclampsia.*	toxemia
toxic *Relating to or caused by poison.*	tóxico
toxicology *The study of the nature, effects and detection of poisons.*	toxicologia
toxin *A poison of plant or animal origin.*	toxina
toxoid *A chemically modified toxin that can be used as a vaccine.*	toxóide
toxoplasmosis *A disease caused by an organism from the genus Toxoplasma. One can have simple malaise to central nervous system involvement.*	toxoplasmose
trabecule *A connective tissue strand that goes from a capsule to the enclosed organ.*	trabécula
trabeculotomy *A surgery for open angle glaucoma.*	trabeculectomia
trachea *The ringed canal between the pharynx and bronchi.*	traquéia
tracheitis *Inflammation of the trachea.*	traqueíte
trachelorrhaphy *Surgical repair of a lacerated cervix.*	traquelorrafia
tracheobronchitis *Inflammation of the trachea and bronchi.*	traqueobronquite
tracheostomy *Creation of a surgical opening in the trachea so a tube could be placed in the trachea.*	traqueostomia
tracheotomy *Surgical incision of the trachea.*	traqueotomia
trachoma *An infection of the cornea and conjunctiva caused by Chlamydia.*	tracoma
tract *A large bundle of fibers or a major passage in the body.*	tracti; tracto
traction *Sustained pull on a muscle or bone to correct alignment.*	tração
tragus *The fleshy prominence anterior to the opening of the ear.*	trago
tranquilizer *A medication used to diminish anxiety.*	tranqüilizante
transabdominal *Through the abdominal wall.*	transabdominal

English	Portuguese
transaminase *An enzyme that facilitates the transfer of an amino group to an amino acid.*	transaminases
transdermal *Through the skin.*	transdermico
transfusion *Administration of blood products intravenously.*	transfusão
transient ischemic attack *Cerebral ischemic changes resulting from transitory hypoperfusion.*	ataque isquêmico transitório
transpire, to *To release vapor from the skin or respiratory mucosa.*	transpirar
transplant, to *To move a body part from one location to another.*	transplante
transplantation *The grafting of tissues.*	transplante
transrectal ultrasound *Insertion of an ultrasound probe into the rectum to view adjacent structures.*	ultra-som transretal
transudation *The movement of body tissue through a membrane that is usually the result of inflammation.*	transudação
transvaginal ultrasound *Insertion of an ultrasound probe in the vagina to view adjacent structures.*	ultra-som transvaginal
trapezium *The lateral bone in the distal row of carpal bones.*	trapézio
trapezius muscle *The muscle with an origin of occipital bone and seventh cervical vertebra, insertion of clavicle and scapula, and it draws the scapula backward.*	músculo trapézio
trapezoid bone *A bone that articulates with the second metacarpal, trapezium, capitate and scaphoid.*	osso trapezóide
trauma *A physical injury or emotional shock.*	trauma; traumatismo
treadmill *An exercise machine on a continuous belt used for walking.*	trabalho monótono
treatment *Medical care one receives for illness or injury.*	tratamento (P)
trematoda *A parasitic fluke such as Schistosoma.*	trematódeo
tremor *Involuntary contraction and relaxation of small muscle groups.*	tremor
trench mouth *Inflammation and ulceration of the gingivae.*	boca de trincheira
trephination *Cutting away a circular disc of bone or the cornea.*	trepanação
triceps *Referring to something having three heads like the triceps muscle.*	tríceps
triceps reflex *A tendon reflex causing extension of the arm when the triceps tendon is gently tapped.*	reflexo do tríceps
trichiasis *Inversion of the eyelashes.*	triquíase
trichinosis *A disease caused by meat infected by Trichinella spiralis causing fever and gastrointestinal effects.*	triquinose
trichomoniasis vaginitis *Infection related to a species of Trichomonas.*	vaginite tricomoníase
trichophytosis *A skin or nail fungal infection caused by Trichophyton.*	tricofitose
tricuspid valve *The cardiac valve located between the right atrium and right ventricle.*	valva tricúspide
trigeminal *Generally refers to the fifth cranial nerve.*	trigeminal
trigeminal nerve *The fifth cranial nerve which supplies the motor function of mastication and has three sensory branches, the ophthalmic, maxillary and mandibular.*	nervo trigêmeo
trigeminal neuralgia *Pain in the region of one or more branches of the fifth cranial nerve sensory branches.*	neuralgia trigêmeo
trigger finger *A condition in which one's finger gets stuck in the flexed position and when extended it snaps like a trigger. Also called stenosing tenosynovitis.*	dedo em gatilho

English	Portuguese
trigone of bladder *Refers to the area at the base of the bladder between the openings of the ureters and the urethra.*	trígono da bexiga
triplegia *Paralysis of three extremities.*	triplegia
triplets *Three infants born during one birth.*	tripleto
triploid *Referring to a cell with three homologous sets of chromosomes.*	triplóide
trismus *Commonly called lockjaw, it is a spasm of the muscles supplied by the trigeminal nerve and is an early symptom of tetanus.*	trismo
trisomy 21 *A congenital anomaly in which chromosome 21 is effected and results in Down's syndrome.*	trissomia 21
trisomy *A general category of congenital anomalies in which there is an extra set of chromosomes in the cell nucleus.*	trissomia
trivial *Of little importance or value.*	comum
trocar *A device enclosed in a catheter that is used to withdraw fluid from a body cavity.*	trocarte
trochanter *Refers to the greater or lesser trochanter; the prominences on the femoral neck.*	trocânter
trochlea *A pulley-shaped structure such as the groove at the distal humerus.*	tróclea
trochlear *Referring to a trochlea.*	troclear
trochlear nerve *The fourth cranial nerve that supplies the superior oblique muscle of the eyeball.*	nervo troclear
trophoblast *A layer of endodermal tissue that helps attach an ovum to the uterine wall.*	trofoblasto
truncal *Referring to the trunk of a body or a nerve.*	tronco
truss *A synthetic device for containing a hernia within the abdomen.*	funda
trypanosomiasis *A disease caused by a protozoa of the genus Trypanosoma that can cause sleeping sickness and Chagas' disease.*	tripanossomíase
trypsin *An enzyme whose precursor is secreted by the pancreas that breaks down proteins in the intestine.*	tripsina
trypsinogen *The precursor to trypsin that is secreted by the pancreas.*	tripsinogênio
tryptophan *An amino acid that is a precursor of serotonin. If present in the body in appropriate levels it can prevent pellagra even if niacin levels are low.*	triptofano
tsetse fly *An insect that transmits the protozoa trypanosoma and can cause sleeping sickness.*	glossina; moscas tsé-tsé
tsutsugamushi disease *An acute febrile infectious disease caused by Rickettsia tsutsugamushi. It is characterized by fever, pain lymphadenopathy, small black lesions on the genitals, neck or axilla.*	doença de tsutsugamushi
tubal *Referring to a tube, as in fallopian tube.*	tubárino
tubercle *1. A granulomatous nodule produced by Mycobacterium tuberculosis. 2. A small prominence on a bone.*	tubérculo
tuberculin *A solution containing M. tuberculosis or M. bovis that is used to test for tuberculosis by injecting the solution intradermally and looking for a reaction.*	tuberculina
tuberculoma *1. A tuberculous growth in the brain. 2. A mass that is produced from enlargement of a caseous tubercle.*	tuberculoma
tuberculosis *Any infectious disease caused by Mycobacterium.*	tuberculose
tuberculous *Referring to tuberculosis.*	tuberculoso
tuberosity *A protuberance. For instance the iliac tuberosity is a prominence on the surface of the ilium.*	tuberosidade

English	Portuguese
tuberous sclerosis *An inherited neurocutaneous disorder exhibited by benign hamartomas of the brain, lung, kidney, skin and other organs.*	esclerose tuberosa
tubo-ovarian *Referring to the fallopian tube or ovary.*	tubovariano
tubular *Referring to a hollow, round-shaped organ.*	tubular
tularemia *An infectious disease caused by Francisella tularensis. The symptoms range from mild constitutional complaints to septic shock.*	tularemia
tumefaction *An area of swelling.*	tumefação
tumor *A benign or malignant overgrowth of tissue.*	tumor; neoplasia
tunica *Generally a covering of a body part or organ. The tunica mucosa nasi is the mucous membrane lining the nasal cavity.*	túnica
tuning fork *A device used to distinguish between perceptive and conductive hearing loss.*	diapasão
tunnel vision *Constriction in the visual field as though looking through a tube or hollow cylinder. Also called tubular vision.*	visão em túnel
turbinate bones *The three curved shelves in the nasal cavity.*	ossos turbinadso
turbinectomy *Surgical excision of a turbinate bone.*	turbinectomia
turgid *Congested and swollen.*	túrgido
turgor *Referring to the elasticity of skin. If one pinches skin and it remains in place the patient is dehydrated.*	turgor
twins *Two infants born at the same birthing.*	gêmeos
twitch *A sudden jerking movement.*	contrair espasmodicamente
two times *One action being done on two occasions.*	duas vezes
tympanic *Referring to the tympanic membrane or having a resonant quality to percussion.*	timpânico
tympanic cavity *The air chamber medial to the tympanic membrane in the temporal bone, between the external acoustic meatus and the inner ear.*	cavidade timpânico
tympanic membrane *The membrane between the external and middle ear.*	membrana timpânico
tympanoplasty *Restoration of the tympanic membrane's continuity.*	timpanoplastia
typhoid fever *A condition caused by ingestion of food or water containing salmonella typhi that is exhibited by fever and abdominal signs and symptoms.*	febre tifóide
typhus fever *A rickettsiae infection exhibited by rash, fever, headache and myalgia.*	febre do navio; tifo epidêmico
tyrosine *An amino acid important in the synthesis of hormones.*	tirosina
ulcer *A concave wound caused by a break in the integrity of skin or mucous membrane. (duodenal ulcer)*	úlcera
ulcerative *Referring to ulceration.*	ulcerativo
ulcerative colitis *Recurrent episode of inflammation of the membranous layer of the colon.*	colite ulcerativa
ulnar nerve *Arises from the C8-T1 nerves and supplies the hand. (Injury to the ulnar nerve causes loss of flexion of the metacarpophalangeal joints and extension at the interphalangeal joints, thus the common term, claw hand.)*	nervo ulnar; nervo cubital
ultrasonography *Visualization of body structures with the echoes of ultrasound pulses.*	ultra-sonografia
ultrasound *A sound or vibration of ultrasonic frequency.*	ultra-som
ultraviolet rays *Electromagnetic radiation with wavelength longer than x rays.*	raios ultravioleta
umbilical cord *The stalk between the placenta and the unborn infant.*	cordão umbilical

English	Portuguese
umbilicated *Referring to depressed areas that resemble the umbilicus.*	umbilicado
umbilicus *The scar that denotes the end of the umbilical cord.*	umbigo; ônfalo
unciform *Another term for hamate bone in the wrist.*	unciforme; osso hamato
uncinariasis *Hookworm infestation of genus Uncinaria.*	uncinaríase
unciforme bone *Hamate bone. The bone on the ulnar side of the distal row of the carpus. It articulates withe the 4th and 5th metacarpal, triquetral, lunate and capitate.*	osso hamato; unciforme
unconsciousness *Unable to respond to sensory stimuli.*	inconsciência
under; infra *Sometimes used when indicating a patient is "under treatment" for a condition (active treatment).*	debaixo
underlying *Causative, unexposed, or fundamental.*	subjacente
undulant fever *Wave-like variations in the fever, going from very high to normal and back again, as seen in Brucellosis.*	febre ondulante; febre de Malta
unexpected *Unforeseen.*	inesperado
unicellular *A term describing organisms like protozoans that only have cell.*	unicelular
unilateral *One side only.*	unilateral
uniovolar *Referring to one fertilized ovum.*	uniovular; unioval
unknown *Uncertain or undisclosed.*	desconhecido
unstable knee *A condition with giving way of the knee due to ligamentous or cartilaginous dysfunction.*	joelho travado
unsteady *Unstable or wobbly.*	oscilante
upper limb *Referring to either arm.*	membro superior
upper respiratory tract *Generally considered the part of the respiratory tract superior to the vocal cords.*	trato respiratório superior
upright *Vertical or standing.*	vertical; em pé
urachus *A connection between the bladder and the allantois in the fetus.*	úraco
urate *The salt of uric acid.*	urato
urea *A nitrogenous product of protein metabolism; excreted in urine.*	uréia
uremia *An excess of urea and creatinine in the blood.*	uremia
ureter *The conduit between each kidney and the urinary bladder.*	ureter
ureteral *Referring to one of two tubes from the kidneys to the bladder that carry urine.*	ureteral; uretérico
ureterectomy *Surgical resection of one or both ureters.*	ureterectomia
ureteritis *Inflammation of the ureter.*	ureterite
ureterocele *Protrusion of the distal portion of the ureter into the bladder.*	ureterocele
ureterolith *Presence of a stone in the ureter.*	ureterólito
ureterolithotomy *Removal of a ureteral stone.*	ureterolitotomia
ureterovaginal *Referring to the ureter and vagina.*	ureterovaginal
ureterovesical *Referring to the ureter and urinary bladder.*	ureterovesical
urethra *The canal connecting the urinary bladder with the outside of the body.*	uretra
urethral *Referring to the urethra.*	uretral
urethritis *Inflammation of the urethra.*	uretrite
urethrocele *A prolapse of the urethra through the meatus.*	uretrocele
urethrography *Imaging of the urethra after instillation of contrast media.*	uretrografia
urethroplasty *Surgical repair of the urethra.*	uretroplastia

English	Portuguese
urethroscope *A scope used to visualize the inside of the urethra.*	uretroscópio
urethrotomy *A surgical opening of the urethra.*	uretrotomia
urgency *Emergency or priority.*	urgência
uric acid *Uric acid is a purine-derived product of nitrogen metabolism that can increase the risk of gout and calculi.*	ácido úrico
urinal *Device used by men to void while in bed or sitting.*	urinol
urinalysis *Chemical and microscopic examination of the urine.*	urinálise
urinary *Referring to the urine.*	urinário
urinary bladder *The organ collecting urine from the ureters prior to discharge via the urethra.*	vesícula urinária
urinary casts *A protein precipitated from renal tubules and excreted in the urine.*	cilindro urinário
urinary incontinence *Involuntary micturition.*	incontenência urinária
urinary sediments *The debris that settles in a urine sample when left undisturbed.*	sedimento urinário
urinary tract *The organs and canals associated with urine secretion including the kidneys, ureters, bladder and urethra.*	trato urinário
urine *The fluid concentrated by the kidneys and expelled via the urethra.*	urina
urinometer *A device for measuring urine specific gravity.*	urinômetro
urobilin *A brownish pigment that is an oxidized form of urobilinogen.*	urobilina
urobilinogen *A colorless substance produced in the intestines when bilirubin is reduced.*	urobilinogênio
urochrome *A yellow pigment in the urine that gives urine its color.*	urocromo
urodynamics *A study done to determine whether a person has the contractile capacity in the bladder to void spontaneously.*	urodinâmica
urogenital *Referring to the urinary and genital systems.*	urogenital
urography *Roentgenography of the urinary tract after administration of contrast media.*	urografia
urolith *Urinary calculi.*	urólito
urology *Surgical specialty involving medical and surgical treatment of the urogenital system.*	urologia
urticaria *A diffuse pruritic macular rash, caused by an allergy.*	urticária
usual *Typical or normal.*	usual
uterine *Referring to the uterus.*	uterino
uterine bleeding *Bleeding that emanates from the uterus.*	sangramento uterino
uterine fibroids *Benign tumors made up of muscular and fibrous tissue in the uterus. This is an older term for what is now known as leiomyoma.*	fibróide uterino; leiomioma uterino
uterine prolapse *Protrusion of the uterus out the vagina.*	prolapso uterino
uterovesical *Referring to the uterus and urinary bladder.*	uterovesical; vesicouterino
uterus *The hollow organ in the female pelvis where a fertilized ovum embeds and grows.*	útero
utricle *A small sac. It can refer to a division of the membranous labyrinth.*	utrículo
uveitis *Inflammation of the uvea.*	uveíte
uvula *A fleshy pendent at the back of the soft palate.*	úvula
uvulectomy *Excision of the uvula.*	uvulectomia
uvulitis *Inflammation of the uvula.*	uvulite
vaccination *The act of receiving a vaccine.*	vacinação
vaccine *A solution of attenuated microorganisms given to prevent or treat a disease.*	vacina

English	Portuguese
vaccine certificate *A document that denotes what vaccines have been received by the holder.*	cartão das vacinas
vacuole *A cavity that develops in a cell.*	vacúolo
vagal *Referring to the vagus nerve.*	vagal
vagina *The canal in a female that extends from the vulva to the cervix.*	vagina
vaginal *Referring to the vagina.*	vaginal
vaginismus *Involuntary contraction of the vagina muscles that causes a painful spasm.*	vaginismo
vagitus *An infant cry that can be further defined as vagitus vaginalis in which the infant cries while its head is in the vaginal canal.*	vagido
vagotomy *Incision of the vagus nerve.*	vagotomia
vagus nerve *The tenth cranial nerve that supplies the heart, lungs visceral organs; its function is tested by assessment of elevation of the uvula.*	nervo vago
valgus *Refers to a joint being abnormally angulated away from the midline of the body.*	valgo
valine *An essential amino acid that assists with nitrogen equilibrium.*	valina
Valsalva's maneuver *A technique in which one attempts to exhale with the mouth and nose closed; this equalizes pressure in the ears.*	manobra de Valsalva
valvulotomy *Surgical incision of a valve.*	valvotomia
varicella *A virus that causes chickenpox and shingles. Also called herpes zoster.*	varicela
varicocele *A cluster of varicose veins in the scrotum.*	varicocele
varicose *Referring to an abnormally distended, irregular vein.*	varicoso
varix *A twisted, distended vein, artery or lymph vessel.*	variz
varus position *Refers to a joint being abnormally angulated toward the midline of the body.*	posição varo
vascular *Referring to a blood vessel.*	vascular
vasculitis *Inflammation of a blood vessel.*	vasculite
vasectomy *The surgical separation of each vas deferens with the intent of producing a sterile person.*	vasectomia
vasoconstriction *The process of making the blood vessels smaller which increases blood pressure.*	vasoconstrição
vasodilatation *The process of making the blood vessels larger which decreases blood pressure.*	vasodilitação
vasomotor *Referring to the constriction or dilation of vessels.*	vasomotor; angiocinético
vasopressin *A hormone secreted by the pituitary that facilitates the retention of sodium and water and also increases blood pressure.*	vasopressina
vasospasm *The abrupt constriction of a blood vessel.*	vasoespasmo
vasovagal *Referring to overstimulation of the vagus nerve, exhibited by hypotension, pallor, nausea and diaphoresis.*	vasovagal
vector *An organism that transmits disease.*	vetor
vegetation *Abnormal growth, such as cardiac valve vegetations as found in endocarditis.*	vegetação
vein *A vessel carrying blood back toward the heart.*	veia
velum *A veil-like part or covering of the palate; soft palate; Velum palatinum.*	véu
vena cava *The large vein that carries deoxygenated blood to the right atrium.*	veia cava

English	Portuguese
vena cava filter *A screen placed in the inferior vena cava to prevent blood clots from causing a pulmonary embolism.*	filtro em veia cava inferior
venereal disease *A condition transmitted via sexual intercourse.*	doença venérea
venereal wart *Common term for condyloma acuminatum.*	verruga venérea
venography *Roentgenography of a vein after administration of contrast media.*	venografia
venom *A term used to describe the toxin injected via a bite or sting.*	veneno
venous *Referring to the veins.*	venoso
ventilation *The movement of air into the lungs; generally meant to suggest by an artificial process.*	ventilação
ventral *Referring to the underside but in humans, a ventral hernia, for example, refers to an abdominal hernia.*	ventral
ventricle *1. One of two chambers of the heart. 2. The four interconnected cavities in the center of the brain.*	ventrículo
ventricular septal defect *An abnormal communication between the right and left ventricles via a hole in the septum.*	defeito septal ventricular
ventriculography *Roentgenography of the ventricles after administration of contrast media.*	ventriculografia
ventriculostomy *A tube placed into the third ventricle to relieve increased intracranial pressure.*	ventriculostomia do terceiro ventrículo
venula *The vessels that connect the capillary plexuses to veins.*	vênula
verminous *Referring to presence of worms.*	verminoso
verminous ileus *Obstruction due to masses of intestinal parasites.*	íleo por verme
verruca *A hyperplastic epidermal lesion, sometimes referred to as plantar wart.*	verruga
vertebra *A term for each bone surrounding the spine.*	vértebra
vertebral column *The cervical, thoracic and lumbar vertebrae.*	coluna vertebral
vertebrobasilar insufficiency *Diminished flow to the vertebral and basilar arteries causing posterior fossa symptoms.*	insuficiência vertebrobasilar
vertex *The crown of the head.*	vértice
vertigo *A sensation of imbalance with many possible causes.*	vertigem
vesical *Referring to the urinary bladder.*	vesical
vesicovaginal *Referring to the urinary bladder and vagina.*	vesicovaginal
vesiculitis *Inflammation of the urinary bladder.*	vesiculite
vestibular *Referring to a vestibule.*	vestibular
vestigial *Rudimentary.*	vestigial
viable *Referring to a fetus that can survive childbirth.*	viável
vial *A small cylindrical container typically used to hold liquid medicine.*	frasco
vibration *An instance of oscillation of parts.*	vibração
villous *Covered with many villi.*	viloso
villus *A small vascular prominence from a membrane surface.*	vilo; vilosidade
virilization *The result of androgen; a process of development of masculine characteristics.*	virilização
virology *The study of viruses.*	virologia
virulence *The potential severity of a disease or poison.*	virulência
visceral *Referring to the organs in the abdominal or thoracic cavity.*	visceral
viscometer *A device used to measure viscosity.*	viscosímetro
viscous *Having a thick, sticky consistency.*	viscoso
vision *State of being able to see.*	visão

English	Portuguese
vision, blurred *Haziness of the visual field.*	visão embaçado
visual field *The complete area a person can see with their eyes in a fixed position.*	campo visual
vital capacity (VC) *The maximal amount of air exhaled after a maximal inhalation.*	capacidade vital
vital signs *The designation for blood pressure, pulse, respirations and temperature.*	sinais vitais
vitamin B12 neuropathy *Abnormal sensation related to a chronic deficiency of cyanocobalamin; also called subacute combined degeneration of the spinal cord or Putnam-Dana syndrome.*	neuropatia por vitamina B12; degeneração subaguda combinada da medula espinhal
vitelline *Referring to the yolk of an egg or ovum.*	vitelino
vitiligo *The appearance of non-pigmented white patches on otherwise normal skin; hair is usually white in the affected areas.*	vitiligo; leucodermia
vitreous *Glass appearance; used to describe the vitreous body of the eye.*	vítreo
vivisection *Animal surgery done for purposes of research.*	vivissecção
vocal *Referring to that which emanates from the vocal cords.*	vocal
vocal cords *Paired folds of mucous membranes stretched across the larynx.*	cordas vocais; pregas vocais
voice *The sound produced through the larynx and out the mouth.*	voz
voiding *The act of urinating.*	micação
voiding cystography *Roentgenography of the bladder and urethra after administration of contrast media.*	cistograma miccional
volunteer *A person who performs work without expecting compensation.*	voluntário
volvulus *Twisting of the bowel leading to obstruction and sometimes perforation.*	vóvulo
vomit *The gastric contents that are expelled through the mouth.*	vômito
vomit, to *To expel gastric contents out the mouth.*	vomitar
vulval cleft *The area between the labia majora where the vagina and urethra rest.*	rima pudenda; fenda urogenital
vulvectomy *Surgical resection of the vulva.*	vulvectomia
vulvitis *Inflammation of the vulva.*	vulvite
vulvovaginitis *Inflammation of the vulva and vagina.*	vulvovaginite
waddling gait *Walking in short steps in a swaying fashion.*	marcha gingada
walker *A metal frame used to facilitate walking.*	estrutura para pacientes que precisam de mais sustentação na marcha
walking cast *A cast used for simple fractures of the lower leg.*	molde gessado por ambulação
ward *A section of a hospital where patients reside.*	enfermaria
wart *A flesh colored growth that is also called verruca.*	verruga
wasp *Any one of a winged hymenopterous insects.*	vespa
water *A colorless, odorless liquid.*	água
wax *Cerumen.*	cerúmen; cera do ouvido; cerume
weak *Feeble or deconditioned.*	débil
weakness *Feebleness.*	debilidade
weekly *That which occurs every seven days.*	semanalemente
weep, to *To ooze fluid, such as from a wound.*	exudar
weep, to *To shed tears.*	chorar
wet *Covered in moisture.*	umidade
wheal *A circumscribed urticarial lesion.*	pápula; placa de urticária

English	Portuguese
wheelchair *A wheeled device used for propulsion.*	cadeira de rodas
wheezing *A whistling or musical sound made by air passing through a narrowed airway.*	sibilos devido a respiração ofegante (P), respirar com dificuldade (B)
whiplash *Common term for cervical strain following a sudden deceleration.*	pescotapa; semelhente à chicotada
whipworm *A parasitic, intestinal nematode worm of the genus Trichuris.*	trichuris trichiura; tricuro
whisper *Speech in a volume that is barely discernible.*	sussurro
whispered pectoriloquy *The sound heard through the stethoscope when listening to a person's lungs. The sound resonates as it would when listening over a bronchus if there is an area of consolidation.*	pectorilóquia sussurrada
whisper test *The examiner whispers into one ear while blocking the other ear to see if the patient can hear in the ear whispered into.*	testo de sussurro
whisper, to *To speak in a volume that is barely discernible.*	sussurrar
whistle, to *To make a high pitch noise by forcing air through the lips.*	assobiar
white *Of the color of snow.*	branco
white matter *The brain tissue consisting of myelin sheaths and nerve fibers.*	substância branca
whitlow *An abscess occurring on the palmar surface of the fingertips.*	paroníquia
whooping cough *Pertussis*	coqueluche
wick *A drain using a thin piece of cloth or tubing.*	pavio; fio
widespread *Encompassing or spanning.*	difundido
width *Side to side measurement.*	largura
wisdom tooth *Third molar.*	dente do siso
wise *Possessing much knowledge.*	prudente
withdrawal *The action of being without drugs or alcohol.*	supressão
withhold, to *To refuse to give something.*	negar
World Health Organization (WHO)	Organização Mundial de Saúde (da ONU em Geneva)
worm *Any of long, slender, legless, soft-bodied invertebrates.*	verme
worry, to *To fret or have unease.*	preocupar
worsen, to *To deteriorate.*	piorar
wound *A tissue injury of varying severity.*	ferida; ferimento
wound care *The treatment applied to a tissue injury.*	tratamento por ferida
wrist *The articulation of the hand and radius/ulna.*	punho; pulso
wrist drop *The inability to hyperextend the wrist due to radial nerve injury.*	punho caído
x-ray	raio-X (P)
xanthine *A purine derivative that is found in the blood and urine after the metabolism of nucleic acids to uric acid.*	xantina
xanthochromia *A yellow tone to the skin or spinal fluid.*	xantocromia
xanthoma *A lipid deposition on the skin exhibited by an irregular yellow patch.*	xantoma
xerodermia *A mild form of ichthyosis.*	xerodermia
xerophthalmia *A manifestation of Vitamin A deficiency exhibited by dryness of the cornea and conjunctiva.*	xeroftalmia
xeroradiography *A form of radiography using photoelectric cells.*	xerorradiografia
xerosis *Pathological dryness of the skin or mucous membranes.*	xerose

English	Portuguese
xerostomia *A dry mouth from salivary gland hypofunction.*	xerostomia
xiphoid process *The inferior segment of the sternum.*	processo xifóide
yawn *Opening one's mouth and inhaling deeply due to sleepiness/boredom*	bocejar
yaws *A tropical disease characterized by ulcers on the extremities, caused by Treponema pertenue.*	framboesia
year *A time period that covers 365 days.*	ano
yearly *Occurring once each year.*	anualmente
yeast *A unicellular fungus.*	levedura
yell, to *To speak in a loud tone.*	gritar
yellow *A color between green and orange in the spectrum*	amarelo
yellow fever *A viral, hemorrhagic fever transmitted by mosquitos.*	febre amarela
young *Having lived for a short period.*	jovem
youth *The time between childhood and being an adult.*	mocidade
zero *No quantity.*	zero
Ziehl-Neelsen carbolfuchsin stain *A stain used to detect acid-fast bacilli that appear red on the methylene blue background.*	método de Ziehl-Neelsen
zinc *A chemical with atomic number 30.*	zinco
zonula *A small zone or junction.*	zônula
zoology *The study of animals.*	zoologia
zoonosis *An animal-born disease that can be transmitted to humans, such as rabies.*	zoonose
zygomatic bone *The triangular cheek bone.*	osso zigomático
zygote *A fertilized ovum.*	zigoto
zymogen *An inactive compound that is metabolized to an active state.*	zimogênio

Portuguese	English
abaixa-lingua	**tongue depressor; tongue blade** *As the name implies, the stick pushes the tongue down so the posterior aspect of the mouth can be viewed more readily.*
abasia	**abasia** *Inability to walk due to impaired coordination.*
abcesso (P), abscesso (B)	**abscess** *A localized collection of pus.*
abdominocentese	**abdominocentesis** *Puncturing of the abdominal wall for drainage purposes.*
abdómen (P), abdômen (B)	**abdomen** *The portion of the body bordered by the diaphragm and the pelvis.*
abducente	**abducent** *Abducting or to separate.*
aberrante	**aberrant** *Different than normal.*
aberto	**gaping** *Wide open.*
abertura	**aperture** *An opening or hole, as in the hole the light passes through in a camera.*
abertura inferior da pelve	**inferior pelvis strait** *The pelvic outlet.*
ablação	**ablation** *Surgical removal or amputation.*
abortamento	**miscarriage** *Spontaneous abortion.*
abortio induzido	**induced abortion** *Surgical or medical evacuation of the fetus.*
aborto	**abortion** *Premature expulsion of the fetus from the uterus.*
abraço	**clasp** *Holding onto something with one's hand.*
abrupto	**abrupt** *Suddenly or hastily.*
abscesso amebiano de fígado	**amebic liver abscess** *A pus filled fluid collection within the liver caused by amoebe.*
abscesso anorético	**anorrectal abscess** *A localized collection of pus in the anorrectal region.*
abscesso de cordão espinhal	**spinal cord abscess** *A localized collection of purulent material in or adjacent to the spinal cord.*
abscesso de fígado	**liver abscess** *A localized collection of pus in the liver.*
abscesso intra-abdominal	**intraabdominal abscess** *A collection of pus in the abdomen.*
abscesso peritonsilar	**peritonsillar abscess**
abscesso piogênico de fígado	**pyogenic liver abscess** *A pus filled fluid collection in the liver.*
abscesso retrofaríngeo	**retropharyngeal abscess** *A collection of purulent material posterior to the pharynx.*
abscesso subareolar	**subareolar abscess** *A purulent fluid collection in the areolar gland.*
absoluto	**absolute**
absorção (absorção intestinal)	**absorption (intestinal absorption)**
abuso	**abuse (sexual abuse)**
abuso de substâncias	**drug dependence** *Addiction to a substance.*
abuso de substâncias e diagnóstico psiquiátrico	**dual diagnosis** *Term used to describe the presence of alcohol/ drug addiction associated with a psychiatric diagnosis such as depression.*
acalasia	**achalasia** *Inability to relax the smooth muscle fibers of the gastrointestinal tract. In the case of esophageal achalasia one has dilatation and hypertrophy of the esophagus.*
acalculia	**acalculia** *The inability to perform mathematical calculations.*
acamado	**bedridden** *Term used to indicate one is so ill they cannot get out of bed.*
acantoma	**acanthoma** *An adult cornifying squamous carcinoma.*
acantose	**acanthosis** *Hypertrophy of the prickle cell layer of the skin.*
acantose nigricans	**acanthosis nigricans** *A skin disorder characterized by dark, thick, velvety skin in the body folds and creases.*

Portuguese	English
acapnia	**acapnia** *A condition of lower than normal carbon dioxide level in the blood.*
acariciar	**pamper, to** *Indulge with comfort and kindness.*
acaricida	**acaricide** *A treatment for mite infestation.*
acatalasia	**acatalasia** *A condition characterized by the congenital absence of the enzyme catalase.*
acatisia	**akathisia** *A condition exhibited by motor restlessness and inability to sit quietly.*
acavalgamento	**overriding suture** *The overlapping of cranial sutures noted on vaginal exam when the head is descended.*
aceder	**comply, to** *Adhere to.*
acelerar	**accelerate** *(To accelerate the healing process).*
acesso	**access** *Means of entry.*
acessório	**accessory** *Complimentary or concomitant.*
acetaminofen	**acetaminophen** *Mild analgesic drug used for pain relief.*
acetábulo	**acetabulum** *The cup-shaped cavity with which the head of the femur articulates.*
acetábulo, relativo ao	**acetabular** *Referring to the acetabulum.*
acetilcolina	**acetylcholine** *A reversible acetic acid ester of choline.*
acetonemia	**acetonemia** *The presence of acetone in the blood.*
acetonúria	**acetonuria** *The presence of acetone in the urine.*
acéfalo	**acephalous** *A absence of a head.*
achatamento de eminência nasal	**low nasal bridge** *A flattening of the top part of the nose.*
acidemia	**acidemia** *A lower than normal pH in the blood.*
acidente	**accident**
acidente	**casualty** *A person who is killed or seriously injured.*
acidente vascular cerebral	**stroke** *Common term for cerebrovascular accident.*
acidente vascular cerebral (AVC)	**cerebrovascular accident (stroke)** *A decrease in level of consciousness and paralysis caused by a cerebrovascular thrombosis, hemorrhage or vasospasm.*
acidente vascular cerebral amnésico	**amnesic stroke** *Cerebral infarct exhibited by loss of memory.*
acidez	**acidity** *Referring to an acid state.*
acima de	**above**
acinesia	**akinesia** *An absence of movement or sparsity of movement.*
acinestesia	**akinesthesia** *Lack of perception of movement.*
aclimatação	**acclimatization** *The process of becoming adapted to a new environment.*
acloridria	**achlorhydria** *The absence of hydrochloric acid in gastric secretions.*
acne	**acne** *Inflamed or infected sebaceous glands.*
acne vulgar	**acne vulgaris** *Chronic acne occurring on the face, chest and back of youth.*
acolia	**acholia** *The lack of bile.*
acomodção	**accommodation** *A term used to describe the ability of the eye to adjust to various distances.*
acondroplasia	**achondroplasia** *A congenital inadequacy of enchondral bone formation resulting in a type of dwarfism.*
aconselhar	**advise, to** *To give counsel.*
acontecimento	**on going** *Continuing,*
acordo	**agreement** *Accordance in opinion or feeling.*
acoria	**acorea** *The absence of the pupil of the eye.*

Portuguese	English
acreção	**accretion** *The expected growth of tissue from the intake of nutrients.*
acrocefalia	**acrocephaly** *A condition characterized by a pointed head.*
acrocianose	**acrocyanosis, Raynaud's disease** *A benign condition in which the feet and hands are cyanotic, cold and sweating.*
acrodermatite	**acrodermatitis** *Inflammation of the skin of the hands and/or feet.*
acrodinia	**acrodynia** *An infantile condition exhibited by swollen bluish-red extremities and later polyarthritis..*
acrofobia	**acrophobia** *The morbid fear of heights.*
acromatopsia	**achromatopsia** *Inability to differentiate yellow, blue, red or their intermediates.*
acromegalia	**acromegaly** *Hyperplasia of the nose, jaw, fingers and toes.*
acrótico	**acrotic** *Referring to great weakness or absence of a pulse.*
acrômio	**acromion** *The flattened process extending laterally from the spine of the scapula which forms the most prominent point of the shoulder.*
actina	**actin** *A protein in the muscle that, along with myosin, facilitates muscle contraction and relaxation.*
actinomicose	**actinomycosis** *A chronic bacterial infection that effects the face and neck and is caused by Actinomyces israelii. In rare cases it can cause a pulmonary infection.*
actomiosina	**actomyosin** *Myosin and actin complex present in muscles.*
acuidade	**acuity** *1. Relating to accuracy of hearing, as in hearing acuity. 2. Severity of illness as in, "What is the patient's acuity?"*
acupunctura	**acupuncture** *Traditionally an aspect of Chinese medicine involving insertion of needles into the skin.*
acústico	**acoustic** *Referring to the auditory system.*
açúcar	**sugar** *A sweet crystalline substance made from a plant such as sugar cane.*
adactilia	**adactylia** *A congenital condition exhibited by the absence of toes and fingers.*
adaptação à luz	**light adaptation** *The pupillary adjustment after going from a dark environment to one of bright light.*
adaptação á escuridão	**dark adaptation** *Adjustment to low light by reflex dilation of the pupil.*
adenectomia	**adenectomy** *The removal of a gland.*
adenite	**adenitis** *The inflammation of a gland.*
adeno-hipófise	**adenohypophysis** *The anterior portion of the pituitary gland.*
adenocantoma	**adenocanthoma** *Malignant tumor comprised of glandular tissue.*
adenocarcinoma	**adenocarcinoma** *Cancer from glandular tissue.*
adenofibroma	**adenofibroma** *Connective tissue with glands that form a tumor.*
adenoidectomia	**adenoidectomy** *Removal of the adenoids.*
adenoidite	**adenoiditis** *Inflammation of the adenoids.*
adenolinfoma	**adenolymphoma** *A salivary gland tumor, also called Warthin's tumor.*
adenomioma	**adenomyoma** *A tumor characterized by the overgrowth of endometrial and uterine muscle tissue.*
adenomiose	**adenomyosis** *A condition characterized by the overgrowth of endometrial and uterine muscle tissue.*
adenopatia	**adenopathy** *Generally referring to a condition of the lymphatic glands.*
adenovírus	**adenovirus** *A type of a virus that can cause upper respiratory tract infections.*

Portuguese	English
adenóide	**adenoid** *Referring to a gland.*
adenóides	**adenoids** *Pharyngeal tonsils.*
adequado	**adequate** *Sufficient.*
adequado	**apt** *Suitable in the circumstances.*
aderência	**adherence** *To stick to something figuratively or literally.*
adesão	**adhesion** *The abnormal adherence of tissue exposed to inflammation or after surgery.*
adiadococinesia	**adiadochokinesia** *The inability to perform rapid alternating movements.*
adiante	**forwards** *Towards the front.*
adicção	**addiction** *An abnormal dependency.*
adicionar	**add, to** *To count.*
adiposo	**adipose** *Referring to fat. (adipose tissue)*
adipsia	**adipsia** *Absence of thirst which can be caused by SIADH, hydrocephalus or injury/tumor to/of the hypothalamus.*
adjuvante	**adjuvant** *Term used to describe the medical treatment after initial therapy, as in adjuvant radiation therapy after initial chemotherapy.*
administração	**management** *The process of dealing with things or people.*
admissão	**admission (to hospital)**
ADN ácido desoxirribonucléico	**DNA Deoxyribonucleic acid.** *The hereditary material in humans and almost all other organisms.*
adolescência	**adolescence**
adormecido	**asleep** *To be in a dormant or inactive state.*
adrenal	**adrenal** *Referring to being near the kidney.*
adrenalectomia	**adrenalectomy** *Excision of the adrenal gland.*
adrenalina	**adrenaline (epinephrine)** *A hormone secreted by the adrenal glands and a synthetic medication used for treatment of allergic reactions and cardiac arrest.*
adrenérgico	**adrenergic** *That which is activated or transmitted by epinephrine.*
adstringente	**astringent** *An agent causing contraction of the skin.*
adução	**adduction** *To bring toward the midline.*
adutor	**adductor** *A muscle that brings a part to the midline.*
adventícia	**adventitia** *Outermost.*
aerodontalgia	**aerodontalgia** *The dental pain that occurs with low atmospheric pressure, like during airflight.*
aerofagia	**aerophagy or aerophagia** *A condition associated with hysteria in which one swallow repeatedly swallows air and then belches.*
aerossol	**spray** *Liquid blown through the air in the form of fine droplets.*
aeróbio	**aerobe** *An organism that grows in the presence of oxygen.*
afacia; afaquia	**aphakia** *The congenital absence of the lens of the eye.*
afagia	**aphagia** *The lack of eating.*
afasia	**aphasia** *Diminished ability to communicate via speech or writing.*
aferente	**afferent** *Moving toward the center.*
afetado	**affected**
afeto	**affect** *The expression of emotions or feelings.*
afídio	**aphid** *A minute insect that feeds on plants.*
aflatoxina	**aflatoxin** *A toxin produced by Aspergillus flavus.*
aflição	**grief** *Deep sorrow.*
afogamento	**drowning** *The process of dying from submerging in and inhaling water.*

Portuguese	English
afonia	**aphonia** *The loss of voice.*
afribinogenemia	**afibrinogenemia** *Marked deficiency of fibrinogen in the blood.*
afta	**canker sore** *An ulceration, usually of the mouth or lips.*
afta; sapinho	**thrush** *Candida albicans*
agenesia	**agenesis** *The absence of an organ. (cerebellar agenesis)*
agitação	**agitation** *A state of extreme emotional disturbance.*
agitação	**flutter** *Used to describe a cardiac rhythm disturbance, as in atrial flutter.*
agitação atrial	**atrial flutter** *Sawtooth waves on an electrocardiogram with atrial rate of 250-330 per minute.*
agluntinação	**agglutination** *The process of adherence of a mass.*
aglutição	**aglutition** *The inability to swallow.*
agnatia	**agnathia** *Congenital abnormality characterized by the absence of the mandible.*
agnosia	**agnosia** *A condition exhibited by the loss of sensory stimuli.*
agnosia digital	**finger agnosia** *The inability to distinguish which finger is being touched.*
agnosia do auditivo	**auditory agnosia** *Caused by a temporal lobe lesion, it is characterized by inability to recognize sounds as words.*
agnosia gustativo	**gustatory agnosia** *The loss of the sense of taste.*
agonia	**agony** *Anguish or torment.*
agonia	**anguish** *Significant mental or physical pain.*
agonista	**agonist** *A synthetic compound that activates cells normally activated by natural chemicals.*
agorafobia	**agoraphobia** *The fear of being in a large open space.*
agrafia	**agraphia** *The inability to express one's thoughts in writing.*
agranulocitose	**agranulocytosis** *A condition characterized by leukopenia and neutropenia.*
agressão	**aggression** *Violent or hostile behavior.*
aguçado	**sharp (pain)** *When describing pain, a piercing sensation.*
agudo	**acute** *Abrupt onset.*
agulha	**needle** *The slender cylindrical device attached to a syringe.*
agulha de acupuntura	**needle for lumbar puncture**
agulha de biopsia	**needle biopsy** *Use of a needle to aspirate body contents for microscopic or pathologic examination.*
ainda	**beyond** *On the farther side.*
ajustamento	**adjustment** *A modification of a plan.*
ajustar	**adjust, to** *To modify a plan.*
akathisia	**acathisia** *The inability to sit quietly or to have motor restlessness.*
alantóide	**allantois** *A posterior portion of the hind-gut of an embryo.*
albinismo	**albinism** *Congenital absence of pigment in the eyes, skin and hair.*
albino	**albino** *A person who lacks pigment in the eyes, skin and hair.*
albumina	**albumin** *A protein that is soluble in water and coagulates if heated.*
albuminúria	**albuminuria** *The presence of albumin in the urine.*
alcalino	**alkaline** *Referring to something with properties of an alkali.*
alcalose	**alkalosis** *A condition in which the pH is increased.*
alcalóide	**alkaloid** *Plant derived nitrogenous organic compound.*
alcalúria	**alkalinuria** *The urine in an alkaline state.*
alcançar	**accomplish, to** *Achieve.*

Portuguese	English
alcaptonúria	**alkaptonuria** *A condition exhibited by the urine turning dark upon standing because of the presence of alkapton bodies in it.*
alcoolémia	**blood alcohol level** *A quantitative measurement of the amount of alcohol in the blood.*
alcoolismo	**alcoholism** *An addiction to alcohol.*
alcoólico	**alcoholic** *A person with alcohol dependence.*
aldeído	**aldehyde** *A substance derived by oxidizing and containing a CHO group from alcohol.*
aldosterona	**aldosterone** *A steroid secreted by the adrenal cortex that regulates electrolytes.*
aldosteronismo	**aldosteronism** *A condition characterized by the excessive secretion of aldosterone.*
aleijado	**cripple** *A person with a physical disability; not used in polite society.*
alelo	**allele** *A type of a gene; in humans there are two alleles per chromosome pair.*
alergia	**allergy** *An immune response by the body to a compound it is hypersensitive to.*
alerta	**alert** *Being in a watchful, ready state.*
alexia	**alexia** *Inability to read due to a central brain lesion.*
alérgeno	**allergen** *Compound that causes an allergic reaction.*
alfa-fetoproteínas	**alpha-fetoprotein** *A glycoprotein that has a high serum level in hepatocellular and nonseminomatous germ cell tumors.*
alga	**algae** *Nonflowering plants containing chlorophyll but without stems, roots, or leaves.*
algodão	**cotton wool** *Raw cotton.*
algofilia	**algophilia** *Sexual perversion; getting pleasure in giving or receiving pain.*
algoritmo	**algorithm** *Any procedure designed to solve a problem in a step-by-step or mechanical fashion.*
alimentação mamária	**breast feeding** *The process of giving milk to a baby via the nipple.*
alimentar	**alimentary** *Referring to the gastrointestinal tract.*
alimento	**food** *Nutrition.*
alisar	**flatten, to** *To make even.*
aliviar	**alleviate, to**
aliviar	**relieve, to (pain)** *To make less severe.*
alívio	**relief** *Alleviation from pain or discomfort.*
almofada	**cushion** *A pillow or stuffed pad used to sit on.*
almofada	**pad** *A thick piece of soft clothing.*
aloenxerto	**allograft** *A tissue transplant of from someone of the same species but different genotype.*
alongamento	**lengthening** *Becoming longer.*
alopatia	**allopathy** *Treatment of disease with minute amounts of natural substances.*
alopecia	**alopecia** *The absence of hair in areas where it normally exists.*
alta da hospital	**hospital discharge** *To leave the hospital.*
alteração	**alteration** *The process of change or modification.*
altura	**height** *Distance between the bottom of the foot and top of the head.*
alucinação	**hallucination** *A perception that is not based on reality.*
alucinógeno	**hallucinogen** *A substance that elicits hallucinations.*
alveolar	**alveolar** *Referring to the alveolus.*

Portuguese	English
alvéolo	**alveolus** *A small sac like structure commonly used for the pulmonary alveolus.*
alvo	**target** *An objective towards which efforts are directed.*
amalgamar	**amalgamate,to** *To make an amalgam by dissolving a metal in mercury.*
amamentar	**suckle, to** *An infant taking to his mother's nipple.*
amarelo	**yellow** *A color between green and orange in the spectrum*
amargo	**bitter (taste)** *Having a harsh, unpleasant taste.*
amastia	**amastia** *A development condition exhibited by the absence of breasts.*
amaurose	**amaurosis** *Blindness that occurs without an ocular lesion but may include the optic nerve.*
amaurose fugaz	**amaurosis fugax** *This transient monocular blindness is considered a sign of an impending stroke.*
amálgama	**amalgam** *An alloy that includes mercury as one ingredient.*
ambidextro	**ambidextrous** *Ability to use both hands equal ability.*
ambissexual	**ambisexual** *Referring to both sexes.*
amblipoia	**amblyopia** *Decreased vision without an ocular lesion.*
ambulatório	**ambulation** *Relating to walking.*
ameaçador vida	**life-threatening** *Potentially fatal.*
amebas	**ameba** *A one-celled protozoan.*
amebicida	**amebicide** *A compound used to treat amebiasis.*
amebíase	**amebiasis** *A condition in which one is infected with amebae, mostly commonly Entamoeba histolytica.*
ameboma	**ameboma** *A mass caused by inflammation as seen in amebiasis.*
amelia	**amelia** *A congenital anomaly exhibited by the absence of limbs.*
amenorréia	**amenorrhea** *The absence of menses.*
amentia	**amentia** *The absence of mental ability.*
ametria	**ametria** *Obsolete term for congenital uterine agenesis.*
ametropia	**ametropia** *Abnormal refractive ability of the eyes resulting in hypermetropia, myopia or astigmatism.*
amilase	**amylase** *An enzyme involved in the hydrolysis of starch.*
amiloidose	**amyloidosis** *The accumulation of amyloid in body tissues.*
aminoácido	**amino acid** *A compound containing a carboxyl and an amino group.*
amiotrofia	**amyotrophy** *Atrophy of muscle tissue.*
amígdala	**amygdala** *Any almond shaped structure such as the tonsil*
amnésia	**amnesia** *The inability to remember past events.*
amnésia anterógrada	**amnesia, antegrade** *The inability to remember events which occurred after the insult that caused the condition.*
amniocentese	**amniocentesis** *Transabdominal aspiration of amniotic fluid.*
amniografia	**amniography** *X-ray of the gravid uterus after insertion of opaque dye.*
amorfo	**amorphus** *A fetus with no heart and no definitive shape.*
amostragem	**sampling** *The taking of samples.*
amônia	**ammonia** *A colorless alkaline gas.*
ampola	**ampulla** *The dilated end of a duct.*
amputação	**amputation** *Typically referring to the surgical removal of a limb.*
anabolismo	**anabolism** *The formation of molecules in organisms from simpler molecules.*
anacrótico	**anacrotic** *Referring to a prominent bulge on the ascending portion of a pulse recording.*

Portuguese	English
anaeróbio	**anaerobe** *An organism that lives in the absence of oxygen.*
anafilaxia	**anaphylaxis** *An exaggerated response to a foreign substance.*
anaforese	**anaphoresis** *Reduced activity of the sweat glands.*
anal	**anal** *Near or referring to the anus.*
analéptico	**analeptic** *A medication used as a stimulant to the central nervous system.*
analgesia	**analgesia** *The absence of pain.*
analgésico	**analgesic** *A medication used to remove pain.*
anaplasia	**anaplasia** *The loss of normal differentiation of tumor cells.*
anastomose	**anastomosis** *Surgical formation of a connection between two previously separate parts.*
anatomia	**anatomy** *The study of body structure.*
anatômico	**anatomical** *Referring to the anatomy.*
anáfase	**anaphase** *A stage in mitosis following metaphase.*
análise	**assay** *A procedure for measuring the activity of a biological sample.*
análise sêmen	**semen analysis** *Evaluation of semen used as part of a fertility workup.*
análogo	**analogous** *To resemble or be similar to.*
anão	**dwarf** *Abnormally small person.*
anciloglossia	**ankyloglossia** *Limitation of tongue motion because of a short frenulum.*
ancilose	**ankylosis** *Abnormal immobility of a joint.*
ancilostomíase	**ancylostomiasis** *A type of nematode parasite, also called hookworm.*
ancilóstomo duodenal	**hookworm** *A parasitic infection of the family Strongylidae that can cause anemia.*
androgênio	**androgen** *A compound that produces masculinizing characteristics.*
androsterona	**androsterone** *A hormone excreted in the urine of men and women.*
andrógino	**androgynous** *Referring to a female pseudohermaphroditism (a genetic female with masculine characteristics).*
anel	**ring** *A small circular band.*
anel de Kayser-Fleischer	**pericorneal ring** *Also known as Kayser-Fleischer rings exhibited by presence of brown or grey-green rings on the cornea. This is from the deposition of copper and seen in Wilson's disease.*
anel inguinal profundo	**inguinal ring (deep)** *Indirect inguinal hernias exit the abdominal cavity via the deep inguinal ring.*
anel inguinal superficial	**superficial inguinal ring** *The opening of the aponeurosis of the external oblique muscle for the round ligament or spermatic cord.*
anemia	**anemia** *Lower than normal red blood cell count.*
anemia aplásica	**aplastic anemia** *Bone marrow failure causing a decrease in all types of blood cells.*
anemia de células falciformes	**sickle-cell anemia** *A hereditary type of anemia characterized by crescent shaped red blood cells.*
anemia hemolítico	**hemolytic anemia** *Reduced number of erythrocytes due to shortened survival and inability of the bone marrow to compensate.*
anemia por deficiência de ferro	**iron-deficiency anemia** *A microcytic anemia.*
anencefalia	**anencephaly** *The congenital absence of the cranial vault and cerebral hemispheres.*
aneróide	**aneroid** *The absence of liquid.*

Portuguese	English
anestesia	**anesthesia** *Loss of sensation.*
anestesia de bloqueio nervoso	**nerve block anesthesia** *Locally administered anesthesia.*
anestesia em luva	**glove anesthesia** *Absence of sensation of the hand and wrist.*
anestesia epidural	**epidural anesthesia** *Medication into this space produces analgesia for surgical procedures.*
anestesista	**anesthetist** *A person who administers anesthesia.*
anestésico	**anesthetic** *A chemical that produces anesthesia.*
aneurisma	**aneurysm** *A condition exhibited by the dilatation of the walls of an artery or vein to form a blood-filled sac.*
aneurisma dissecante	**dissecting aneurysm** *A condition in which blood is present between the layers of an artery.*
anexo	**adnexa** *The appendages, for example, of the uterus are the ovaries, fallopian tubes and the ligaments of the uterus.*
angiectasia	**angiectasia** *Dilation of a blood or lymph vessel.*
angiite	**angitis or angiitis** *The inflammation of a lymph or blood vessel.*
angina do peito	**angina pectoris** *Exercise induced myocardial ischemia.*
angina por esforço	**exercised induce angina** *Chest pain noted during exertion related to coronary artery disease.*
angio-plastia	**angioplasty** *Surgical alteration of blood vessels.*
angiofibroma juvenil	**juvenile angiofibroma** *A noncancerous growth in the nose or pharyngeal region.*
angiografia	**angiography** *Roentgenographic imaging of blood vessels.*
angiografia coronário	**coronary angiography** *Roentgenographic visualization of the coronary vessels after injection of dye.*
angiograma	**angiogram** *Radiologic imaging of blood vessels.*
angioma	**angioma** *A tumor comprised of blood or lymph vessels.*
angioneurótico	**angioneurotic** *Caused by a neurosis affecting the blood vessels, like vasospasm.*
angiospasmo; vasoespasmo	**angiospasm** *A spasm of a blood vessel.*
angiossarcoma	**angiosarcoma** *A sarcoma comprised of blood vessels.*
angiotensina	**angiotensin** *A blood protein that increases aldosterone secretion.*
anidro	**anhydrous** *Lacking water.*
anidrose	**anhidrosis** *A condition exhibited by reduced quantity of sweat.*
anidrótico	**anhidrotic** *Something the reduces the quantity of sweat.*
animal de estimação	**pet** *An animal kept for companionship.*
aniseiconia	**aniseikonia** *A condition in which the ocular image of an object is viewed differently by each eye.*
anisocitose	**anisocytosis** *Variation in size of erythrocytes.*
anisocoria	**anisocoria** *Pupillary diameter inequality.*
anisomelia	**anisomelia** *Unequal size of arms or legs.*
anisometropia	**anisometropia** *Refractive power inequality between the two eyes.*
ano	**year** *A time period that covers 365 days.*
anomia	**anomia** *Inability to name or recognize familiar objects.*
anomolia congênito	**birth defect** *A congenital anomaly.*
anoniquia	**anonychia** *Congenital absence of fingernails or toenails.*
anoperíneo	**anoperineal** *Referring to the anus and perineum.*
anorexia	**anorexia** *The loss of appetite.*
anorexia nervosa	**anorexia nervosa** *A mental disorder characterized by the desire to avoid eating and to lose weight.*
anorético	**anorectal** *Referring to the anus and rectum.*
anorquia	**anorchous** *The absence of testicles.*

Portuguese	English
anosmia	**anosmia** *Lack of the sense of smell.*
anovulatório	**anovulatory** *Lack of ovulation.*
anoxemia	**anoxemia** *Reduction in blood oxygen concentration.*
anoxia	**anoxia** *Reduced oxygen levels in body tissues.*
anómalo (P) anormal (B)	**abnormal**
ansiedade	**anxiety** *Nervousness or unease.*
ansiedade neurose	**anxiety neurosis** *Abnormal presence of anxiety.*
ansioso	**anxious** *Experiencing nervousness or unease.*
antagonista	**antagonist** *A muscle or agent that acts in counteract to effects of another muscle or agent.*
antebraço	**forearm** *Segment of the arm from the elbow to wrist.*
antemão	**beforehand** *In advance or previously.*
antenatal	**antenatal** *Refers to events before birth.*
anterior	**anterior** *Toward the front.*
anterógrado	**anterograde** *Moving forward.*
antes da morte	**antemortem** *Refers to: before death.*
anteversão	**anteversion** *The forward leaning of an organ.*
anti-hemicrânia	**antimigraine** *Medication used to treat headaches.*
anti-histamina	**antihistamine** *Medication used to treat conditions exhibited by a histamine response*
anti-inflamatório	**anti-inflammatory agents** *Medications used to reduce inflammation.*
anti-linfocito	**antilymphocyte** *A serum globulin that has antibodies to lymphocytes.*
anti-séptico	**antiseptic** *A substance that inhibits microorganism growth.*
anti-soro	**antiserum** *A substance that contains antibodies to specific antigens.*
antiácido	**antacid** *A medication, usually with a calcium or magnesium base that binds with acid in the stomach.*
antibiótico	**antibiotic** *A medication that inhibits or kills microorganisms.*
anticoagulante	**anticoagulant** *Medication used to inhibit coagulation.*
anticolinesterase	**anticholinesterase** *Cholinesterase blocker.*
anticolinérgico	**anticholinergic** *Parasympathetic blocker.*
anticoncepcional oral	**oral contraceptive** *Tablet taken by mouth to prevent pregnancy.*
anticonvulsivante	**anticonvulsant** *Medication used to treat seizures.*
anticorpo	**antibody** *A protein that combines with and counteracts foreign substances.*
anticorpo antenuclear	**antinuclear factor** *Also called antinucleic antibody (ANA); it is found in conditions such as lupus and rheumatoid arthritis.*
anticódon	**anticodon** *A series of three nucleotides that form a unit of genetic code for transfer RNA.*
antidepressor; antidepressivo	**antidepressant** *Medication used to treat depression.*
antiemético	**antiemetic** *A medication used to control nausea.*
antiesposmódico	**antispasmodic** *Medication used to treat muscle spasm.*
antigénio (P), antígeno (B)	**antigen** *A foreign substance, like bacteria, that induces an immune response.*
antigo	**long-standing** *Having existed for a long time.*
antihelmíntico	**anthelmintic** *An agent used to destroy worms.*
antimalárico	**antimalarial** *Medication used to treat malaria.*
antimetabólito	**antimetabolite** *A substance that impedes metabolism.*
antimicótico	**antimycotic** *Inhibition of fungal growth.*
antimitótico	**antimitotic** *Impeding mitosis.*

Portuguese	English
antiperistáltico	**antiperistaltic** *An agent that impedes normal peristalsis.*
antipirético	**antipyretic** *Medication used to treat fever.*
antiprurítico	**antipruritic** *Medication used to treat pruritus.*
antiquado	**outdated** *Something that has passed the expiration date.*
antitireóde	**antithyroid** *A substance inhibiting the effect of the thyroid.*
antitoxina	**antitoxin** *A substance that inhibits the effect of a toxin.*
antitrombina	**antithrombin** *A substance that inhibits thrombin, thus decreasing the body's ability to coagulate.*
antitussivo	**antitussive** *Medication used to diminish a cough.*
antiveneno	**antivenin** *An antitoxin formulated for various types of snake bites.*
antídoto	**antidote** *A medication that neutralizes a toxin.*
antracose	**anthracosis** *Pneumoconiosis caused by coal dust.*
antraz	**anthrax** *An infectious disease caused by Bacillus anthracis; there are cutaneous, inhalation and gastrointestinal syndromes.*
antro	**antrum** *Referring to a cavity or chamber.*
antrotomia	**antrotomy** *To cut open the antrum.*
anualmente	**yearly** *Occurring once each year.*
anular, anelar	**annular** *Referring to a ring.*
anúria	**anuria** *The lack of urine excretion.*
aorta	**aorta** *The large artery originating at the left ventricle and going to the pelvis where it bifurcates.*
aórtica	**aortic** *Referring to the aorta.*
aparecimento global	**general appearance** *The overall look of a patient.*
aparelho	**splint** *A rigid support used to immobilize and extremity.*
aparelho justaglomerular	**juxtaglomerular apparatus** *Cells located in the tunica media of the afferent glomerular arterioles.*
aparência	**appearance** *The way someone looks or presents.*
apatia	**apathy** *Lack of interest in one's environment or indifference.*
apendectomia	**appendectomy** *Surgical excision of the appendix.*
apendicite	**appendicitis** *Inflammation of the appendix.*
apercepção	**apperception** *The ability to interpret sensory impressions.*
aperistaltismo	**aperistalsis** *Lack of intestinal peristalsis.*
aperto de mão	**grip strength** *Quantitative measurement of the force of a hand grip.*
apesar de	**regardless of** *Without consideration of.*
apêndice	**appendix** *An appendage of the cecum.*
apicectomia	**apicectomy** *Removal of the apex of the petrous portion of the temporal bone.*
aplicador	**applicator** *A device used to apply a topical medication.*
apnéia	**apnea** *Absence of respiration.*
apnéia do sono	**sleep apnea** *Episodic apnea during sleep that is exhibited by daytime symptoms of fatigue, difficulty concentrating and sleepiness.*
aponeurose	**aponeurosis** *A tendinous expansion that connects with muscle to move a part.*
aponta-caminho	**milestone** *An event indicative of a certain stage of development.*
apoplexia	**apoplexy** *Extravasation of blood within an organ.*
apófise	**apophysis** *Generally a bony outgrowth that forms a process or tubercle.*
apraxia	**apraxia** *The inability to carry out intentional movements when paralysis is not present.*
apreensivo	**apprehensive** *A fear that something unpleasant will happen.*

Portuguese	English
apresentação de fronte	**brow presentation** *The term used to describe which part of the body (forehead) is being delivered first in childbirth.*
apresentação de nádegas	**breech presentation** *Position of the feet or buttocks near the cervix.*
apresentação facial	**face presentation** *Referring to the part of the body coming out of the cervix first during childbirth.*
aprovação	**approval** *Accepting something as satisfactory.*
aproximadamente	**approximately** *Nearly but not completely.*
aproximado	**approximate** *Nearly but not totally accurate.*
aproximar	**approximate, to** *To bring together, as in wound margins.*
aptialia	**aptyalism** *Diminished or absence of saliva.*
aptidão	**aptitude** *A natural talent for something.*
apyretic; apirético	**afebrile** *Absence of fever.*
aquilia	**achylia** *The absence of chyle.*
aquiliodinia	**achilliodynia** *Pain around the calcaneal tendon.*
aquilobursite	**achillobursitis** *Inflammation around the calcaneal tendon.*
aquoso	**aqueous** *Use of water as a solvent or medium.*
ar	**air**
aracnodactilia	**arachnodactyly** *A condition exhibited by abnormally long and slender fingers.*
aracnóide	**arachnoid** *Refers to that which resembles a spider web.*
arbovírus	**arbovirus** *Virus that is transmitted by arthropods; responsible for diseases such as Yellow fever and dengue fever.*
arco	**arcus** *Narrow opaque band.*
arco superciliar	**superciliary arch** *The area superior to the upper border of each orbit.*
aréola	**areola** *The pigmented skin surrounding a nipple.*
argininssuccinicacidúria	**argininosuccinicaciduria** *Presence of arginosuccinic acid in the urine; associated with mental retardation.*
argiria	**argyria** *The greyish discoloration of the skin and conjunctiva.*
arguir	**argue, to** *To debate or reason. (quarrel)*
aritenóide	**arytenoid** *Referring to the cartilage in the posterior larynx.*
ARN ribossômico	**ribosomal RNA** *Four chains designated by their appropriate coefficients.*
arranhadura	**scratch** *A long, narrow superficial wound.*
arrebentar	**burst, to** *To rupture.*
arrenoblastoma	**arrhenoblastoma** *An ovarian tumor that results in masculine secondary sex characteristics.*
arritmia	**arrhythmia** *An abnormal heart rhythm.*
artefato	**artifact** *An aberration from the normal.*
artelho em martelo	**hammer toe** *A condition characterized by extension of the proximal phalanx and flexion of the second and distal phalanges.*
arterial	**arterial** *Referring to an artery.*
arteriectomia	**arteriectomy** *Surgical excision of an artery.*
arteriografia	**arteriography** *Roentgenography of an artery after infusion of contrast media.*
arterioplastia	**arterioplasty** *Surgical repair of an artery.*
arteriosclerose	**arteriosclerosis** *Hardening and thickening of arterial walls.*
arteriotonia	**arteriotomy** *Creation of an opening in an artery.*
arterite	**arteritis** *Inflammation of an artery.*
artéria	**artery** *Vessel that carries oxygenated blood from the heart to the periphery.*

Portuguese	English
artéria braquial	**brachial artery** *A continuation of the axillary artery and branches into the radial and ulnar among others.*
artéria femoral	**femoral artery** *Continuation of the external iliac to the popliteal artery.*
artéria inominada	**innominate artery** *The first branch off the aortic arch that branches into the right common carotid and right subclavian arteries.*
articulação	**joint** *Articulation of two adjacent bones.*
articulação acromioclavicular	**acromioclavicular joint** *Referring to the junction of the acromion and clavicle.*
articulação coxofemoral	**hip joint** *The lateral eminence of the pelvis from the waist to the thigh; it is formed by the iliac crest and greater trochanter.*
articulação em sela	**saddle joint** *A joint that exhibits two saddle type surfaces at a 90 degree angle to each other, such as the carpometacarpal joint.*
articulação talocrural	**ankle joint** *The articulation of the tibia/fibula and talus.*
articulação temporomandibular	**temporomandibular joint** *The hinged joint of the temporal bone and mandible.*
articular	**articular** *Referring to a joint.*
artificial	**artificial** *Not natural produced.*
artralgia	**arthralgia** *Joint pain.*
artrite	**arthritis** *Joint inflammation.*
artrite gonorréica	**gonorrheal arthritis** *A type of arthritis caused by the gram negative diplococcus Neisseria gonorrhoeae.*
artrite reumatóide	**rheumatoid arthritis** *A symmetric peripheral polyarthritis.*
artrodese	**arthrodesis** *Surgical fusion of a joint.*
artrodinia	**arthrodynia** *Joint pain.*
artrografia	**arthrography** *Joint roentgenography.*
artropatia hemofílico	**hemophilic arthropathy** *The permanent joint disease caused by recurrent bleeding into the joint.*
artroplastia	**arthroplasty** *Plastic surgery involving a joint.*
artroplastia do quadril	**hip replacement** *Both joint surfaces are replaced by high density material such as plastic or metal.*
artroscopia	**arthroscopy** *Viewing of the inside of a joint with a specially designed scope.*
artrotomia	**arthrotomy** *Surgical opening of a joint.*
asbesto	**asbestos** *A heat resistant silicate material.*
asbestose	**asbestosis** *Lung disease caused by the inhalation of asbestos.*
ascaricida	**ascaricide** *Agent that destroys ascaris.*
ascite	**ascites** *Serous fluid in the abdominal cavity.*
asfixia	**asphyxia** *A condition exhibited by a lack of oxygen and subsequent loss of consciousness or death.*
aspermia	**aspermia** *Absence of sperm.*
aspiração mecônio	**meconium aspiration** *Presence of meconium on the newborn indicating there was fetal distress in-utero.*
aspirador	**aspirator** *A device used to remove fluid from a cavity.*
aspirina; ácido acetilsalicílico	**aspirin** *Common name for acetylsalicylic acid.*
assegurar	**ensure, to** *To make certain of.*
assepsia	**asepsis** *Lack of infection.*
assexual	**asexual** *Without sex or sex organs.*
asséptico	**aseptic** *Being free of septic matter.*
assimetria	**asymmetry** *Lack of symmetry.*
assinclitismo	**asynclitism** *Oblique presentation of the head during delivery.*

Portuguese	English
assintomático	**asymptomatic** *The absence of symptoms.*
assistência	**assistance** *The act of helping.*
assistência ventilação	**assisted ventilation** *The act of helping one breathe through artificial means.*
assobiar	**whistle, to** *To make a high pitch noise by forcing air through the lips.*
asteatose	**asteatosis** *A condition exhibited by diminished sebaceous secretion.*
astenia	**asthenia** *Diminished strength and energy.*
astenopia	**asthenopia** *Visual fatigue accompanied by ocular pain.*
asterixe	**asterixis** *Commonly known as a flapping tremor, it is characterized by involuntary jerking movements of the hands and is seen commonly in hepatic encephalopathy.*
astrágalo	**astragalus** *Synonym of talus.*
astrocitoma	**astrocytoma** *A tumor comprised of astrocytes.*
astróglia	**astroglia** *The neurologic tissue which is composed of astrocytes.*
ataque	**attack** *A fit or paroxysm.*
ataque de pânico	**panic attack** *Sudden, profound anxiety.*
ataque isquêmico transitório	**transient ischemic attack** *Cerebral ischemic changes resulting from transitory hypoperfusion.*
ataque; convulsão	**seizure** *An episode of tonic/clonic movement noted in epilepsy.*
atar	**brace, to** *Application of a splint.*
atavismo	**atavism** *The inheritance of characteristics from remote rather than immediate ancestors.*
ataxia	**ataxia** *Lack of muscular coordination.*
atelectasia	**atelectasis** *Incomplete expansion or collapse of a lung.*
aterogênico	**atherogenic** *Something that causes atheromatous lesions in arterial walls.*
ateroma	**atheroma** *Degenerative arteriosclerosis.*
atetose	**athetosis** *An involuntary symptom exhibited by continuous slow, writhing movements, mostly in the hands.*
atividade	**activity**
atípico	**atypical** *Not usual.*
atlas	**atlas** *The first cervical vertebra.*
atomizador	**atomizer** *A device for propelling a fine mist.*
atonia	**atony** *Absence of normal muscle tone.*
ator natriurético atrial	**atrial natriuretic factor** *A chemical secreted by the right atrium that promotes sodium excretion in the urine.*
atresia	**atresia** *Closure of a body orifice as in atresia ani in which there is a congenital imperforate anus.*
atresia das coanas	**choanal atresia** *A congenital condition characterized by blockage of the nasal passages by tissue.*
atrial	**atrial** *Referring to the atrium.*
atrioventricular	**atrioventricular** *Referring to the atrium and ventricle.*
atrito	**rub** *A sound heard at times with pericarditis called more specifically a pericardial friction sound.*
atrito de fricção	**friction rub** *A noise heard during cardiac auscultation in patients with pericarditis, for example.*
atrofia	**atrophy** *A diminution in the size of a part.*
atrofia peroneiro	**peroneal atrophy** *Progressive muscle atrophy in the peroneal region.*
atropina	**atropine** *A parasympathetic agent derived from Atropa belladonna.*

Portuguese	English
atrófico	**atrophic** *Referring to atrophy.*
audição	**hearing** *Auditory perception.*
audiograma	**audiogram** *The recording of a one's hearing in decibels.*
audiologista	**audiologist** *A specialist in the field of hearing.*
audiômetro	**audiometer** *A device used to measure hearing.*
auditivo	**auditory** *Referring to hearing.*
aumento	**enlargement** *Becoming bigger.*
aural	**aural** *Referring to the ear.*
auricular	**auricular** *Referring to the auricle.*
auriculotemporal	**auriculotemporal** *The area of the ear and temple.*
aurícula	**auricle** *The external portion of the ear.*
ausculta; auscultação	**auscultation** *The act of listening to sounds emanating from the body.*
ausência de	**absence of**
autismo	**autism** *A mental condition exhibited by difficulty in forming relationships, communicating and uses abstract thought.*
autista	**autistic** *Referring to autism.*
auto-anticorpo	**autoantibody** *An antibody that acts against the organism's own tissue.*
auto-antígeno	**autoantigen** *A normal tissue constituent that prompts a cell-mediated response.*
auto-enxerto	**autograft** *Grafting tissue from one part of person to another part of the same person.*
auto-hipnose	**autohypnosis** *Self-hypnosis.*
auto-imunização	**autoimmunization** *The body's ability to promote an immune response without external resources.*
autoclave	**autoclave** *A device used for sterilization with the use of steam under pressure.*
autogênese	**autogenous** *Self-generated.*
autolíse	**autolysis** *A state of self destruction of cells within a body.*
autossômico	**autosomal** *Referring to an autosome.*
autotransfusão	**autotransfusion** *The reinfusion of one's own blood.*
autôpsia	**autopsy** *Examination of a body post-mortem in an attempt to determine cause of death.*
auxílio auditivo	**hearing aid** *A device that fits in the ear used to amplify sound.*
avaliação	**assessment** *An medical evaluation.*
avaliação	**evaluation** *Assessment or evaluation.*
avascular	**avascular** *An area with no blood supply.*
averiguar	**ascertain, to** *Synonym of "to determine".*
aviária	**avian** *Referring to birds.*
avitaminose	**avitaminosis** *A state of vitamin deficiency.*
avulsão escalpo	**scalp avulsion** *An injury causing the skin along with some subcutaneous tissue to be pulled from the skull.*
axila	**axilla** *The hollow beneath the arm.*
axilar	**axillary** *Referring to the axilla.*
axônio	**axon** *The structure along which nerve impulses are transmitted from the cell body to other cells.*
azia	**heartburn** *Synonym of pyrosis.*
azoospermia	**azoospermia** *The absence of spermatozoa in the semen.*
azotemia	**azotemia** *Prerenal disease.*
azotúria	**azoturia** *An excess of urea in the urine.*
azul	**blue** *A color between green and violet.*

Portuguese	English
ácarus	**acarus** *A mite.*
ácido	**acid** *Substance with a pH less than 7.*
ácido acetilsalicílico	**acetylsalicylic acid** *The chemical name for common aspirin.*
ácido ascórbico	**ascorbic acid** *Commonly known as vitamin C; a deficiency of this vitamin causes scurvy.*
ácido clorídrico	**hydrochloric acid** *A solution with a low pH formed by dissolving hydrogen chloride in water.*
ácido desoxirribonucléico	**deoxyribonucleic acid (DNA)** *The carrier of genetic information.*
ácido fólico	**folic acid** *Also called pteroylglutamic acid; a deficiency can cause megaloblastic anemia.*
ácido graxo	**fatty acid** *A carboxylic acid occurring as a an ester in fats and oils.*
ácido nicotínico	**nicotinic acid** *A deficiency of this substance results in pellagra.*
ácido nuclear	**nucleic acid** *An organic compound found in living cells; its molecules contain nucleotides linked in long chains.*
ácido para-aminobenzóico	**para-aminobenzoic acid** *A natural product (not FDA approved) reportedly beneficial for Peyronie's disease and scleroderma. It is a component of folic acid.*
ácido para-aminohipúrico	**para-aminohippuric acid (PAH)** *A chemical used for calculation of renal plasma flow.*
ácido ribonucléico	**ribonucleic acid** *An acid present in all living cells, it is a messenger for DNA.*
ácido taurocólico	**taurocholic acid** *A bile acid composed of cholic acid and taurine.*
ácido úrico	**uric acid** *Uric acid is a purine-derived product of nitrogen metabolism that can increase the risk of gout and calculi.*
ácino	**acinus** *A very small grape shaped portion of an acinous gland.*
ádito	**aditus** *The entrance to an organ or part.*
ágar	**agar** *Media used for bacterial cultures.*
água	**water** *A colorless, odorless liquid.*
água potável	**drinking water** *Water clean enough to ingest orally.*
água sanitária	**bleach** *A solution that includes sodium hypochlorite.*
ágüe	**ague** *A term used to describe recurrent fever and shivering typically associated with malaria.*
álcali	**alkali** *A class of compounds that form soluble carbonates.*
álcool	**alcohol** *Ethanol or ethyl alcohol.*
ápex cardíaca	**apex of heart** *Normally found 8cm to the left of the midsternal line in the 5th intercostal space.*
ápice; ápex	**apex** *The highest point of something.*
áscaris; lombriga	**ascaris** *A nematode from genus intestinal lumbricoid parasite, also called round worm.*
átrio	**atrium** *Referring to a chamber used as an entrance, as in the entrance to the heart.*
âmnio	**amnion** *The membrane lining the placenta which produces the amniotic fluid.*
ântero-inferior	**anteroinferior** *Toward the front and lower part.*
ântero-lateral	**anterolateral** *Toward the front and away from the midline.*
ântero-mediano	**anteromedian** *Toward the front and toward the midline.*
ântero-posterior	**anteroposterior** *From front to the back. (An AP x-ray has the beam directed from the front to the back.)*
ântero-superior	**anterosuperior** *Toward the front and the upper part.*
ânus	**anus** *The body opening distal to the rectum.*
bacalhau	**cod** *A large marine fish, also called codfish.*

Portuguese	English
bacia rasa de desenho curvo	**emesis basin** *A small bowl used to catch vomitus.*
bacilar	**bacillary** *Referring to bacilli.*
bacilo	**bacillus** *A rod-shaped bacterium.*
bacteriano	**bacterial** *Referring to bacteria.*
bactericida	**bactericidal** *An agent that destroys bacteria.*
bacteriemia	**bacteremia** *The presence of bacteria in the blood.*
bacteriostático	**bacteriostatic** *An agent that impedes bacterial growth.*
bacteriúria	**bacteriuria** *The presence of bacteria in the urine.*
bactérias	**bacteria** *Plural for any organism of the order Eubacteriales.*
baço	**spleen** *The visceral organ that is involved with production and removal of blood cells.*
bafômetro	**breath test (for alcohol)** *A check of alcohol level by testing exhaled air.*
bagaçose	**bagassosis** *A pulmonary disorder contracted from inhalation of the waste of sugar cane (bagasse dust).*
bainha	**sheath** *A covering.*
balança por bebé	**baby-scale** *A device used to weigh an infant.*
balanço ácido-básico	**acid-base balance** *The equilibrium of the electrolytes in the body.*
balanite	**balanitis** *Inflammation of the glans of the penis.*
balbucio	**lisping** *A speech problem in which "s" and "z" are pronounced "th".*
baloteamento	**ballottement** *Presence of movement of a floating object by palpation.*
banco de sangue	**blood bank** *An area where blood products are stored for later use.*
bandagem elástico	**elastic bandage** *A stretch gauze used for compression of an extremity.*
bandagem; atadura	**bandage** *A strip of gauze used to immobilize or support.*
baqueteamento	**clubbing** *Increase in the mass of the soft tissue of the terminal phalanges.*
barata	**cockroach** *A beetle-like insect with long legs and antennae.*
barreira hematocerebral	**blood brain barrier** *A matrix of capillaries that move blood between the blood and brain, as well as, limiting some substances from passing.*
barriga	**abdomen, lower**
basal	**basal** *Referring to the base.*
basia	**basin** *A small bowl used for washing.*
basilar	**basilar** *Referring to the base or lower segment.*
basófilo	**basophil** *A polymorphonuclear granulocyte.*
batimento	**beat** *As in heart beat.*
batimento cardíaco	**heart beat** *A single contraction of the heart.*
bálsamo	**balm** *A topical medical preparation.*
beber	**drink, to** *To imbibe.*
bebericar	**sip, to** *To slowly take small drinks of a fluid.*
bebé (P); bebê (B)	**baby** *A newborn.*
benigno	**benign** *Not harmful.*
berço	**cradle** *A bed for an infant.*
beriliose	**berylliosis** *A lung exhibited by granulomas and caused by inhalation of beryllium.*
bexiga distensão	**distended bladder** *Urinary bladder filled beyond the normal capacity.*

Portuguese	English
bezoar	**bezoar** *A concretion composed of either hair, vegetable/fruit fibers or hair and vegetable/fruit fibers that is found in the stomach.*
biblioteca	**library**
bicho	**bug** *Insect.*
bicho-do-pé	**chigger** *A parasitic mite of the genus Trombicula.*
bicúspide	**bicuspid** *Having two points as in bicuspid valve or a premolar tooth.*
bifurcado	**bifurcate** *When one branch divides into two branches.*
bigorna	**incus** *The middle ear bone between the stapes and malleus.*
bilateral	**bilateral** *Referring to both sides.*
bile	**bile** *An alkaline fluid secreted by the liver to aid digestion.*
Bilhárzia	**Bilharzia** *Historical name of a genus of flukes or nematodes now known as Schistosoma.*
biliar	**biliary** *Referring to bile, bile ducts or gallbladder.*
bilioso	**bilious** *Something that contains bile.*
bilirrubina	**bilirubin** *A pigment found in bile that is responsible for the yellow color seen in patients with elevated serum levels of bilirubin.*
biliverdina	**biliverdin** *A green pigment formed by oxidation of bilirubin.*
bilúria	**biliuria** *The presence of bile in the urine.*
bimanual	**bimanual** *Use of two hands, as in bimanual pelvic examination in which the right hand touches the cervix uteri and the left hand presses above the mons pubis.*
binauricular	**binaural** *Referring to both ears.*
binocular	**binocular** *Referring to both eyes.*
binovular	**binovular** *Derived from two different ova.*
biodisponibilidade	**bioavailability** *The portion of a drug that is able to be utilized by the body after it is introduced to the body.*
bioensaio	**bioassay** *A laboratory test determination as compared to normal.*
biologia	**biology** *The study of living organisms.*
biopsia	**biopsy** *The removal and examination of bodily tissues or fluids.*
biopsia por escova	**brush biopsy** *The process of tissue sampling using a brush.*
bioquímica	**biochemistry** *The study of chemistry and physiochemical processes in living organisms.*
biotina	**biotin** *A vitamin involved in the synthesis of fatty acids and glucose.*
bissinose	**byssinosis** *A disease caused by inhalation of cotton dust; a type of pneumoconiosis.*
bisturi	**bistoury; scalpel** *A surgical knife.*
bíceps	**biceps** *A muscle with two heads usually referring to the biceps brachii which is used for forearm flexion.*
bífido	**bifid** *Presence of two branches.*
biópsia excisional	**excisional biopsy** *Surgical removal of tissue for pathologic examination.*
biópsia por aspiração	**aspiration biopsy** *Removal of fluid from a cavity for pathologic analysis.*
blastomicose	**blastomycosis** *Infection caused by organisms of genus Blastomyces.*
blefarite	**blepharitis** *Inflammation of the eyelids.*
blefaroespasmo	**blepharospasm** *A spasm of the orbicularis oculi muscle that causes closure of the eyelid.*

Portuguese	English
blenorragia	**blennorrhea** *Discharge from the mucous membranes, usually referring to gonorrhea.*
bloqueador ß	**betablocker** *A substance that inhibits adrenergic stimulation. It is used to reduce pulse, blood pressure and to treat angina.*
bloqueadores do canal de cálcio	**calcium channel blocker** *A medication used to treat angina, supraventricular arrhythmias and hypertension; it works by blocking calcium influx into myocytes and vascular smooth muscle cells.*
bloqueio atrioventricular	**atrio-ventricular block** *An interruption of the electrical conduction at the atrio-ventricular node.*
bloqueio cardíaco	**heart block** *An alteration in the cardiac electrical conduction system.*
bloqueio de ramo	**bundle branch block** *A cardiac dysrhythmia produced by a blockage of a branch of the bundle of His.*
boca	**mouth** *The orifice on the lower part of the face.*
boca de trincheira	**trench mouth** *Inflammation and ulceration of the gingivae.*
bocado	**mouthful** *A large quantity of something in one's mouth.*
bocejar	**yawn** *Opening one's mouth and inhaling deeply due to sleepiness/boredom*
bocejo	**chemosis** *Swelling of conjunctival tissue adjacent to the cornea.*
bochecha	**cheek** *Lateral facial tissue.*
bojo	**bulge** *A protuberance on a flat surface.*
bolha	**bulla** *A large cutaneous serous filled vesicle.*
bolo	**bolus** *A fluid bolus is a phrase used for rapid infusion of fluid.*
bolsa de colostomia	**colostomy bag** *A pouch attached to the skin with a mild adhesive that collects stool emitted from a colostomy.*
bolsa de Douglas	**Douglas' pouch** *A recess in the peritoneum between the rectum and the uterus. Also called the rectouterine pouch.*
bolsas faríngeas	**pharyngeal pouch** *A lateral diverticulum of the pharynx.*
bócio	**goiter** *Swelling of the thyroid gland.*
braço	**arm** *One of two upper extremities.*
braço fraturado	**broken (arm)** *Fracture of the arm.*
bradicardia	**bradycardia** *Lower than normal cardiac rate measured in beats per minute.*
bradicinina	**bradykinin** *A peptide that causes contraction of smooth muscle and dilation of blood vessels.*
branco	**white** *Of the color of snow.*
branquial	**branchial** *Referring to or resembling the gills of a fish.*
braquial	**brachial** *Referring to the arm.*
braquicefalia	**brachycephaly** *The presence of a short broad skull.*
bregma	**bregma** *Located at the convergence of the coronal and sagittal sutures.*
brilhante	**bright** *Giving out a lot of light.*
broca	**drill** *Cylindrical metal tool uses for creating a hole in bone in surgery.*
bromidrose	**bromidrosis** *Foul smelling perspiration.*
bromismo	**bromism** *Poisoning caused by excessive intake of bromine.*
broncogênico	**bronchogenic** *Referring to the bronchi.*
broncografia	**bronchography** *Roentgenography of the bronchi after administration of contrast media.*
broncopneumonia	**bronchopneumonia** *Pneumonia that starts in the distal bronchioles.*
broncoscopia	**bronchoscopy** *Use of a scope to visualize the bronchi.*
broncospasmo	**bronchospasm** *Bronchial smooth muscle spasm.*

Portuguese	English
bronquiectasia	**bronchiectasis** *The presence of abnormally wide bronchi or branches.*
bronquiolar	**bronchial** *Referring to the bronchus.*
bronquiolite	**bronchiolitis** *Inflammation of the pulmonary bronchioles.*
bronquite	**bronchitis** *Inflammation of the mucous membranes of the bronchioles that causes bronchospasm and cough.*
bronquílo	**bronchiole** *A small branch that a bronchus divides into.*
brônquio	**bronchus** *The major air channels that bifurcate from the distal trachea.*
brucelose	**brucellosis** *A gram-negative bacteria in cattle that causes persistent fever in humans.*
bubão	**bubo** *An inflamed, swollen lymph node in the axilla or inguinal region.*
bucal	**buccal** *Referring to the cheek.*
bucinador	**buccinator** *A thin, flat muscle in the cheek wall.*
bulimia	**bulimia** *Pathologic increase in hunger.*
buraco trépano	**burr hole** *A treatment of subdural hematoma that involves drilling a hole into the cranium to release the hematoma.*
bursite	**bursitis** *Inflammation of the bursa.*
cabeça	**caput** *The head.*
cabeça	**head**
cabeça sucedânea	**caput succedaneum** *Edema that occurs in the scalp of an infant during child-birth.*
cabelo da cabeça	**hair (of head)**
cabelo de corpo	**hair (of body)**
cabelo pubiano	**pubic hair** *Hair present in the perineal area.*
cada	**every** *Each or all possible.*
cada dio	**every day** *Each day.*
cadáver	**cadaver** *A dead body.*
cadeira de rodas	**wheelchair** *A wheeled device used for propulsion.*
caduceu	**caduceus** *An ancient herald's wand with two serpents twined around that is a symbol of the medical arts.*
cagegoria	**grade** *A level of rank or quality.*
calafrio	**chill** *Sensation of coldness.*
calazar	**kala-azar** *A disease caused by Leishmania donovani that is exhibited by weight loss, fever, anemia and hepatosplenomegaly.*
calcanhar	**heel** *Proximal portion of the plantar aspect of the foot.*
calcário	**calcareous** *Referring to something containing lime or calcium.*
calcâneo	**calcaneus** *Commonly called the heel bone.*
calciferol	**calciferol** *It is formed when egesterol is exposed to ultraviolet light; a D vitamin.*
calcificação	**calcification** *Deposition of calcium salts causing hardening of an organic tissue.*
calcitonino	**calcitonin** *A thyroid hormone that lowers serum calcium levels.*
calibração	**calibration** *The process of calibrating an instrument.*
calibrador	**gauge** *The size or thickness of something. An 18gauge needle.*
calibrar	**calibrate, to** *To adjust an instrument using a standard.*
calo	**callus** *Thickened hardened skin.*
calor	**heat** *The quality of being hot.*
calor pruriginoso	**prickly heat** *A rash with small vesicles that is pruritic and associated with a warm moist environment.*
caloria	**calorie** *A unit of heat.*

Portuguese	English
calosidade	**callosity** *Callus; thickened hardened skin.*
calosidade	**clavus** *A corn or horny protrusion.*
calvária	**calvaria** *The portion of the skull that is composed of the superior aspects of the occipital, parietal and frontal bones.*
camada	**layer** *A stratum or thickness.*
camada granular	**granular layer** *A deep layer of the cerebellum.*
cambalear	**stagger, to** *To walk in an unsteady fashion.*
came	**flesh** *The tissue between the skin and bones.*
camisa-de-força	**strait-jacket** *A device used to temporarily restrain the arms of patients who are psychotic and violent.*
campo	**drape** *The fabric used as a sterile covering in the OR.*
campo visual	**visual field** *The complete area a person can see with their eyes in a fixed position.*
canabis	**cannabis** *A plant from the Cannibidaceae family that is known for its psychotropic effects.*
canal iônico	**ion channel** *A selectively permeable cell membrane to certain ions.*
canal sacro	**sacral canal** *The portion of the vertebral canal that progresses into the sacrum.*
canal semicircular	**semicircular canal** *The anterior, posterior and lateral canals in the inner ear that assist in balance control.*
canalículo	**canaliculus** *A term for various small channels.*
cancelar	**cancel, to** *To stop or revoke.*
cancro	**chancre** *The initial ulcer that is the source of entry for a pathogen.*
cancro (P) câncer (B)	**cancer; carcinoma** *A disease of uncontrolled abnormal cell growth.*
cancróide	**cancroid** *A tumor occurring in the stomach, small or large bowel.*
cancróide	**chancroid** *A sexually transmitted disease caused by Haemophilus ducreyi that is exhibited by ulcers without indurated margins.*
candidatura	**application** *The forms one fills out to obtain a grant.*
canela	**shin** *Refers to the anterior tibial region.*
canhoto	**left-handed** *The preference of using the left hand for common tasks.*
cano sangüínea	**blood tubing** *(used for infusion of blood)*
cansado	**tired** *Fatigued.*
capacidade pulmonar total	**lung capacity, total** *The amount of air in the lungs after a maximal inhalation.*
capacidade vital	**vital capacity (VC)** *The maximal amount of air exhaled after a maximal inhalation.*
capacidade vital forçada (CVF)	**forced vital capacity** *Vital capacity measured as the patient is exhaling as rapidly as possible.*
capilar	**capillary** *A vessel that connects arterioles to venules.*
capsulite	**capsulitis** *Inflammation of a capsule.*
capsulite adesiva	**adhesive capsulitis** *Also known as frozen shoulder.*
capsulotomia	**capsulotomy** *Incision of a capsule as in with eye surgery.*
caquexia	**cachexia** *Generalized weakness and severe wasting.*
carboxiemoglobina	**carboxyhemoglobin** *A compound formed from hemoglobin when it is exposed to carbon monoxide.*
carbroidratos	**carbohydrate** *A group of organic compounds including sugar and starch.*
carcingênico	**carcinogenic** *That which causes cancer.*

Portuguese	English
carcinmatose	**carcinomatosis** *Dissemination of cancer throughout the body.*
carcinoma	**carcinoma** *A malignant growth.*
carcinoma bronquiolar	**bronchial carcinoma** *A general term for a malignancy of the bronchi.*
carcinóide	**carcinoid** *A tumor occurring in the stomach, intestine and colon.*
cardiologia	**cardiology** *A specialty of medical practice involve treatment and prevention of heart disease.*
cardiomiopatia	**cardiomyopathy** *Chronic cardiac muscle disease.*
cardiovascular	**cardiovascular** *Referring to the heart or circulatory system.*
cardite	**carditis** *Inflammation of the heart.*
cardíaco	**cardiac** *Referring to the heart.*
carético	**cathartic** *To be cleansed or evacuated, referring to thought or the cleansing of the bowels.*
carência	**need** *A want or obligation.*
carina	**carina** *The protrusion of the lowest tracheal cartilage.*
cariocinese	**karyokinesis** *A part of mitosis involving the cell nucleus division.*
cariótipo	**karyotype** *The arrangement of chromosomes in a single cell.*
carnoso	**carneous** *Synonym of fleshy.*
caroteno	**carotene** *A hydrocarbon that can be converted to vitamin A.*
carotídeo	**carotid** *Referring to the large artery on each side of the neck.*
carpo	**carpus** *The joint between the hand and wrist.*
carpometacárpico	**carpometacarpal** *Referring to the carpus and metacarpus.*
carrapato das patas pretas	**deer tick** *Ixodes scapularis.*
carraspear	**clear one's throat, to** *To cough lightly in attempt to speak more clearly.*
cartão das vacinas	**vaccine certificate** *A document that denotes what vaccines have been received by the holder.*
cartilago cricóide	**cricoid cartilage** *The ring-shaped cartilage of the larynx.*
carúncula	**caruncle** *A small fleshy protuberance.*
caseína	**casein** *The principal protein in milk, a phospholipid.*
caspa	**dandruff** *Dead skin found in the hair.*
castanho	**brown** *Coffee-colored.*
castração	**castration** *Excision of the gonads.*
catabolismo	**catabolism** *The reduction of complex molecules to more simple ones in living organisms.*
cataforese	**cataphoresis** *The use of an electric field to move charged particles in fluid.*
catalepsia	**catalepsy** *A condition exhibited by rigidity and the person maintains the same position if he is moved by another.*
cataplexia	**cataplexy** *A condition exhibited by rigidity and immobility.*
catarata	**cataract** *An opacity of an eye lens or the capsule.*
catarro	**catarrh** *Inflammation of a mucous membrane.*
catarse	**catharsis** *The act of cleansing or purging, usually referring to thought.*
catatonia	**catatonia** *Seen in schizophrenia, it is a state of stupor or excitability and abnormal movements.*
cateter de demora	**indwelling catheter** *Continuous use tube usually referring to a tube in the urinary bladder.*
cateter; sonda	**catheter** *A flexible tube inserted into the body.*
caudal	**caudal** *Referring to a cauda.*
caudato	**caudate** *Referring to the caudate nucleus.*

Portuguese	English
causativo	**causative** *Something that induces an effect.*
cautério	**cautery** *Application of an electric current to cut something.*
cavidade	**cavity** *Pouch or chamber.*
cavidade	**hollow** *An indentation.*
cavidade timpânico	**tympanic cavity** *The air chamber medial to the tympanic membrane in the temporal bone, between the external acoustic meatus and the inner ear.*
caxumba	**mumps** *A contagious viral disease that is exhibited by parotid swelling and puts males at risk for sterility. Also called epidemic parotitis.*
cálcio	**calcium** *A chemical element that is an essential component in teeth and bone.*
cálculo	**calculus** *A stone of minerals that can lead to the blockage of the bile duct or ureters.*
cálculo dentário	**dental calculus** *Calcium phosphate and carbonate adhered to the teeth.*
cálice	**calyx** *A cup shaped organ or cavity.*
câmara hiperbárica	**hyperbaric chamber** *A device used to treat decompression illness.*
cânula	**cannula** *A tube inserted into the body.*
cápsula	**capsule** *A membranous sheath that covers an organ or structure.*
cárie	**caries** *Referring to decay or death of a tooth.*
cárie dentária	**dental caries** *Decay of teeth.*
cáustico	**caustic** *Abrasive or corrosive.*
câmara posterior do olho	**posterior chamber of the eye** *An aqueous filled space between the cornea and the lens.*
câibras por estômago	**stomach cramps** *Sensation of muscle contraction in the epigastric area.*
ceco	**cecum** *The portion of the bowel between the ileum and and the ascending colon.*
cefaléia em cacho	**cluster headache** *A unilateral, severe, recurrent headache.*
cefaléia; cefalalgia	**headache** *Cephalgia.*
cefálico	**cephalic** *Towards the head.*
cego	**blind** *Absence of sight.*
cego	**blunt** *Having a flat or rounded end.*
cegueira	**blindness** *Absence of visual perception.*
cegueira nocturna	**night blindness** *Common term for nyctalopia, it refers to low vision with reduced illumination, often seen with Vitamin A deficiency.*
cegueira para cores; daltônico	**color blindness** *The inability to distinguish colors.*
celíaco	**celiac** *Referring to the abdominal cavity.*
celulite	**cellulitis** *Infection characterized by diffuse, subcutaneous inflammation.*
celulose	**cellulose** *A polysaccharide that occurs naturally in fibrous products.*
centígrado	**centigrade** *A scale with 100 gradations, usually referring to a temperature scale.*
centímetro	**centimeter** *One hundredth of a meter.*
centrífuga	**centrifuge** *Machine used to separate substances of different weights.*
centrípeto	**centripetal** *The movement toward the center.*
centro	**center** *A point equidistant from all sides.*
cepa	**strain** *As in a muscle strain.*

Portuguese	English
ceratectomia	**keratectomy** *Excision of a portion of the cornea.*
ceratina	**keratin** *A protein found in the skin, hair, nails and enamel of the teeth.*
ceratoectasia	**keratectasia** *Obtrusion of the cornea.*
ceratoma	**keratoma** *A protuberance of horny tissue.*
ceratomalacia	**keratomalacia** *Softening of the cornea.*
ceratose	**keratosis** *A growth of keratin such as a wart or callosity.*
cerático	**keratic** *Referring to the cornea.*
cerca	**around** *On every side of.*
cercária	**cercaria** *Larval trematode worm that live in a molluscan.*
cerebelo	**cerebellum** *The part of the brain in the posterior portion of the skull that controls muscle coordination and movement.*
cerebração	**cerebration** *Operating activity of the cerebrum.*
cerebral	**cerebral** *Referring to the cerebrum.*
cerume; cerúmen	**cerumen** *Waxy substance found normally in the external ear canals.*
cerúmen; cera do ouvido; cerume	**wax** *Cerumen.*
cervical	**cervical** *Referring to the neck or the cervix.*
cervicectomia	**cervicectomy** *Excision of the cervix uteri.*
cervicite	**cervicitis** *Inflammation of the cervix.*
cesariana	**cesarean section** *Incision of the abdominal and uterine walls in order to deliver a fetus when natural delivery is not possible.*
cestóide	**cestode** *A class of parasitic flatworms.*
cetoacidose	**ketoacidosis** *Usually referring to diabetic ketoacidosis in which ketones are broken down, causing a decrease in blood pH.*
cetonemia	**ketonemia** *Presence of ketone in the blood.*
cetonúria	**ketonuria** *Presence of ketone in the urine.*
cetose	**ketosis** *The presence of an abnormally high level of ketones in the blood and body tissues.*
célula	**cell** *The smallest functional unit of an organism.*
célula parietal	**parietal cell** *Acid secreting cells of the stomach.*
célula alvo	**target cell** *An abnormal cell that is present in liver disease and certain hemoglobinopathies.*
célula calciforme	**goblet cell** *Aids in the secretion of respiratory and intestinal mucous.*
célula mastócito	**mast cell** *A cell containing basophilic granules that releases histamine and other substances during allergic reactions.*
célula pilosas	**hair cell** *Epithelial cells with hairlike projections.*
célula plasma	**plasma cell** *A cell that produces only one type of antibody.*
célula sangüínea	**blood cells** *A common term that does not differentiate between erythrocyte or leukocyte.*
célula sangüínea branca diferential	**differential leukocyte count** *The percentage of different types of leukocytes.*
cérebro	**brain** *A common term for cerebrum.*
cérebro anterior	**forebrain** *The part of the brain that includes the thalamus, hypothalamus and cerebral hemispheres.*
cérebro médio	**midbrain** *The portion of the brainstem superior to the pons.*
cérvix incompotente	**Cervical insufficiency (formerly incompetent cervix)** *Painless changes in the cervix that result in recurrent second semester pregnancy loss.*
chato	**flat** *Level or even; without bulges.*
chifre	**horn** *A keratinized outgrowth.*

Portuguese	English
cholagogo	**cholagogue** *A compound used to stimulate flow of bile from the liver.*
choque	**shock** *A condition characterized by systemic hypoperfusion.*
choque medular	**spinal shock** *Hypotension related to injury or intervention of the spine.*
chorar	**weep, to** *To shed tears.*
chumaço	**pledget** *A small plug of cotton or other synthetic material inserted into a wound.*
chumaço de algodão	**swab** *An absorbent material used for cleaning wounds or applying ointment.*
chumbo	**lead** *An element with an atomic number of 82.*
chuvoso	**moist** *Damp or humid.*
cianocobalmino	**cyanocobalamin** *Also called B12; used to treat pernicious and other macrocytic anemias.*
cianose	**cyanosis** *Bluish discoloration of the skin and mucous membranes.*
ciática	**sciatica** *Pain radiating from the buttock down the back of the leg; it is caused by a compressed spinal nerve root.*
cicatricial	**cicatricial** *Referring to cicatrix.*
cicatriz	**cicatrix (scar)** *New tissue in a healed wound.*
ciclite	**cyclitis** *Inflammation of the ciliary body.*
ciclo anovulatório	**anovulatory cycle** *A menstrual cycle in which no ovum is released.*
ciclo de Krebs	**Krebs cycle** *The process of aerobic respiration by which living cells generate energy.*
ciclo pilonidal	**pilonidal cyst** *A small cone-shaped cluster of tissue situated posterior to the third ventricle of the brain.*
ciclodiálise	**cyclodialysis** *The surgical creation of a communication between the anterior chamber of the eye and the suprachorodial space for the purpose of treating glaucoma.*
cicloplegia	**cycloplegia** *Paralysis of the ciliary muscle.*
ciclotimia	**cyclothymia** *Manic-depressive tendencies.*
ciclotomia	**cyclotomy** *Surgically creating an opening in the ciliary body.*
cifoescoliose	**kyphoscoliosis** *An abnormal outward and lateral curvature of the spine.*
cifose	**kyphosis** *Abnormal outward curvature of the spine.*
cilindro epitelial	**epithelial cast** *Debris found in the urine composed of columnar renal epithelium.*
cilindro urinário	**urinary casts** *A protein precipitated from renal tubules and excreted in the urine.*
cinase	**kinase** *An enzyme that facilitates movement of phosphate from ATP to another molecule.*
cinchonismo	**cinchonism** *The toxic effects induced by ingestion of cinchona bark; it is exhibited by tinnitus, deafness and cognitive changes.*
cineplastia	**kineplasty** *An amputation done in a fashion to facilitate ambulation.*
cinese	**kinesis** *Movement of a part in response to a stimulus.*
cinto	**belt** *A strap used to hold clothing up.*
circadiano	**circadian** *Referring to a 24 hour period.*
circulante	**currently** *Presently.*
circuncisão	**circumcision** *Surgical excision of the foreskin.*
circunferência	**circumference** *The distance around an object or part.*
circunscrito	**circumscribed** *To have well defined borders.*
cirro	**scirrhus** *A cancer that is hard to palpation.*

Portuguese	English
cirrose	**cirrhosis** *A liver disease characterized by destruction of liver cells and increased connective tissue.*
cirsóide	**cirsoid** *Similar to a tortuous vein, artery or lymph vessel.*
cirurgia	**surgery** *The incision of a body part using sterile technique in order to treat disease or injury.*
cirurgião (P)	**surgeon** *A physician who performs surgery.*
cirúrgico	**surgical** *Referring to surgery.*
cistadenoma	**cystadenoma** *Adenoma associated with cysts of neoplastic origin.*
cistectomia	**cystectomy** *Surgical removal of a cyst or the bladder.*
cisterna do quilo	**ampulla chyli** *Also called cisterna chyli; it is a dilated area of the thoracic duct that collects lymph from several areas.*
cisticerose	**cysticercosis** *The state of being infected with a type of tapeworm.*
cistinose	**cystinosis** *A congenital disorder of increased cystine that leads to renal insufficiency, rickets and dwarfism.*
cistinúria	**cystinuria** *The presence of cystine in the urine.*
cistite	**cystitis** *Inflammation of the urinary bladder.*
cisto de Baker	**Baker cyst** *A synovial fluid collection in the popliteal fossa.*
cisto de Bartholin	**Bartholin's cyst or abscess** *This is a purulent fluid collection in the Bartholin cysts which are located in the perivaginal area.*
cisto de Meibômio	**meibomian cyst** *An enclosed fluid collection along a sebaceous gland of the eyelid.*
cisto de tireoglosso	**thyroglossal cyst** *A common congenital growth in the thyroglossal duct.*
cisto dermóide	**dermoid cyst** *An abnormal growth containing hair follicles, skin and sebaceous glands.*
cisto hidático	**hydatid cyst** *A cyst produced by and containing tapeworm larvae.*
cisto ovariano	**ovarian cysts** *Generally used to describe benign tumors.*
cistocele	**cystocele** *Protrusion of the urinary bladder through the vaginal wall.*
cistografia	**cystography** *Roentgenographic visualization of the urinary bladder after insertion of contrast media.*
cistograma miccional	**voiding cystography** *Roentgenography of the bladder and urethra after administration of contrast media.*
cistolitíase	**cystolithiasis** *Presence of a calculus in the urinary bladder.*
cistoscopia	**cystoscopy** *Direct visualization of the urinary bladder with a cystoscope.*
cistoscopio	**cystoscope** *A device used to visualized the urinary bladder.*
citologia	**cytology** *The study of cells, their function and structure.*
citoplasma	**cytoplasm** *The protoplasm of the cell except for the nucleus.*
citotoxina	**cytotoxin** *That which is harmful to cells.*
citotóxico	**cytotoxic** *Referring to being harmful to cells.*
cíbalo	**scybalum** *A hard, dry formation of stool in the bowel.*
cílio; pestana	**eyelash** *Each of the short hairs on the eyelid.*
cístico	**cystic** *Referring to a cyst.*
clamidiose	**chlamydiosis** *A disease caused by the species Chlamydia.*
claro	**clear** *Transparent.*
claudicação	**claudication** *Intermittent claudication is a phrase used to describe pain experienced in the leg from arterial insufficiency.*
claustrofobia	**claustrophobia** *An unreasonable fear of being in an enclosed environment.*
clavícula	**clavicle** *A bone that articulates with the sternum and scapula.*

Portuguese	English
clavícula	**collarbone** *Common term for the clavicle.*
cleidotomia	**cleidotomy** *A procedure used in difficult deliveries in which the clavicle is broken to facilitate childbirth.*
clitóris	**clitoris** *A small erectile body in the anterosuperior aspect of the vulva.*
clivagem	**cleavage** *A sharp division or demarcation.*
clínica	**clinic** *A building where patients are evaluated.*
clínica	**health center** *A physical location where patients are treated.*
cloasma	**chloasma** *Brown or black macula that occur on the face during pregnancy or when there is ovarian dysfunction.*
clono calcâneo	**ankle clonus** *An abnormal response exhibited by alternating plantar- and dorsiflexion noted after the examiner rapidly dorsiflexes the foot.*
cloreto de sódio	**sodium chloride** *A colorless, crystalline compound; also table salt.*
cloridrato	**hydrochloride**
clorofórmio	**chloroform** *A colorless, sweet smelling liquid formerly used as a general anesthetic.*
cloroma	**chloroma** *A malignant tumor associated with myelogenous leukemia.*
clônico	**clonic** *Referring to a spasm that alternates in rigidity and relaxation.*
cnemial	**cnemial** *Referring to the shin.*
coagulação	**coagulation** *The formation of a clot.*
coana	**choanae** *The two openings between the nasal cavity and the nasopharynx.*
coarctação aórtica	**coarctation of the aorta** *A stricture, as in narrowing of the aorta.*
coágulo	**clot** *A thrombus or embolus.*
coágulo sangüíneo	**blood clot** *A mass of coagulated blood.*
cobalto	**cobalt** *A metal that with causes polycythemia with increased ingestion.*
cobre	**copper** *A chemical element with atomic number of 29.*
cocáina	**cocaine** *A highly addictive opiate derivative.*
coccidinia	**coccydynia** *Coccygeal pain.*
coco	**coccus** *A spherical shaped bacterium.*
codéina	**codeine** *A morphine derived analgesic.*
cogelação	**freezing (as in ambient temperature)** *Below 0 Celsius.*
cognição	**cognition** *The process of acquiring thought or understanding.*
coisa	**sour** *An acid or bitter taste.*
coito	**coitus** *Sexual intercourse between members of the opposite sex.*
cola	**glue** *Plastic cements*
colangiograma	**cholangiogram** *Radiologic imaging of the gallbladder and bile ducts.*
colangite	**cholangitis** *Inflammation of the bile ducts.*
colágeno	**collagen** *The principal supportive protein bone, skin, tendon and cartilage.*
colchão	**mattress** *A fabric case filled with material, used for sleeping.*
colecistectomia	**cholecystectomy** *Surgical excision of the gallbladder.*
colecistenterotomia	**cholecystenterostomy** *Creation of a surgical anastomosis between the intestine and the gallbladder.*
colecistite	**cholecystitis** *Inflammation of the gallbladder.*
colecistolitíase	**cholecystolithiasis** *The presence of gallstones in the gallbladder.*

Portuguese	English
colectomia	**colectomy** *Surgical removal of part of the colon.*
coledocolitotomia	**choledocholithotomy** *Creation of an incision in the bile duct for the purpose of removing a stone.*
colelitíase	**cholelithiasis** *Presence or creation of gallstones.*
colemia	**cholemia** *Bile or bile products in the blood.*
colesteatoma	**cholesteatoma** *A cystic mass that has a lining made of keratinizing material and cholesterol.*
colesterol	**cholesterol** *A compound or its derivatives are found in cell membranes and precursors to hormones but high levels can cause atherosclerosis.*
colélito	**gallstone** *Calculus produced in the bile duct or gallbladder.*
colher de chá	**teaspoon** *A measure instrument that holds 5 milliliters of fluid.*
colher de sopa	**tablespoon** *An eating utensil that holds 15milliliters of fluid.*
colherada	**spoonful** *A measurement that does not specify teaspoon or tablespoon.*
colinesterase	**cholinesterase** *An esterase used to cleave acetylcholine into choline and acetic acid.*
colinérgico	**cholinergic** *Referring to the stimulation, activation or transmission of acetylcholine.*
colite	**colitis** *Inflammation of the colon.*
colite ulcerativa	**ulcerative colitis** *Recurrent episode of inflammation of the membranous layer of the colon.*
colo do fêmur	**neck of the femur** *The portion of the femur between the shaft and head.*
colo rígido	**stiff-neck** *Cervical sprain with reduced range of motion.*
colo uterino	**cervix uteri** *The narrow end of the uterus.*
coloboma	**coloboma** *A congenital defect that involves a fissure of the eye.*
colonoscopia	**colonoscopy** *Inspection the color, ideally to the cecum, with a lighted scope.*
colostomia	**colostomy** *Surgically creating an opening in the colon that is extended to outside the abdominal wall.*
colostro	**colostrum** *The fluid secreted by the mammary glands a few days around parturition.*
colódio	**collodion** *A product of the breakdown of colloid.*
colóide	**colloid** *A solution used for infusion, such as albumin or hetastarch, that are more likely to remain in the intravascular space than crystalloids.*
colpite	**colpitis**; vaginitis *Inflammation of the vagina.*
colpocele	**colpocele** *A hernia into the vagina.*
colporrafia	**colporrhaphy** *A surgical procedure that involves suturing the vagina.*
colporrexe	**perineal laceration** *Tearing of the tissue adjacent to the vaginal that can occur during childbirth.*
colposcopia	**colposcopy** *Use of a scope to visualize the vagina and cervix.*
colposcópio	**colposcope** *A scope used to visualize the vagina.*
coluna posterior	**posterior columns** *The dorsal portion of the gray matter of the spinal cord.*
coluna vertebral	**vertebral column** *The cervical, thoracic and lumbar vertebrae.*
coluria	**choluria** *Term indicating the presence of bile in the urine.*
coma	**coma** *A state of unconsciousness.*
comadre; arrasterdeira	**bedpan** *A metal or plastic vestibule one sits on while in bed to defecate.*
comatose	**comatose** *Referring to a coma.*
começo	**onset** *The beginning of an event.*

Portuguese	English
começo do trabalho de parto	**labor onset** *The time when a pregnant woman begins uterine contractions in the process of childbirth.*
comedão	**comedone** *The medical term (singular) for blackheads.*
comensal	**commensal** *Living in or on another organism without being a detriment.*
comentário	**comment** *A remark providing an opinion.*
comer	**eat, to** *To consume food.*
comparação	**matching** *Corresponding in pattern or style.*
compatível	**compatible** *To coexist without problems.*
compêndio	**compendium** *A concise summary about a subject.*
complacência	**compliance** *The act of going along with a plan.*
comportamento alimentação	**feeding behavior** *How a child is tolerating breast or cup feeding.*
composto	**compound** *A substance formed by covalent union of two or more atoms.*
compreensão	**comprehension** *Understanding.*
compressão	**compression** *Squeezing together.*
compressão de cordão espinhal	**cord compression** *Pressure being applied to the spinal cord.*
comprimento	**length** *The end to end measurement.*
comprimido com revestimento entérico	**coated tablet** *A pill covered with a substance to slow absorption or reduce gastric irritation.*
comprimido de ação prolongada	**sustained release tablet** *Describes a medicine that is slowly dispersed so it has a lasting effect.*
comprimido; tablete	**tablet** *A small disk of a compressed solid substance.*
comprimir	**squeeze, to** *To apply pressure.*
comum	**common** *That which is usual.*
comum	**general** *Common or expected.*
comum	**trivial** *Of little importance or value.*
concavidade	**concavity** *The state of being concave.*
concavidade	**socket** *An anatomical hollow that is part of an articulation. (eyeball socket)*
concentração	**concentration** *The quantity of a substance per unit volume.*
concepção	**conception** *The act of an egg being fertilized by sperm.*
concêntrico	**concentric** *Referring to circles or arcs that share the same center.*
concha	**concha** *A part of the body that is spiral shaped. Nasal concha are the small bones in the sides of the nasal cavity.*
concreção	**concretion** *A hard solid mass.*
concussão	**concussion** *Head trauma resulting in temporary loss of consciousness.*
condiloma	**condyloma** *A warty papule near the anus or vulva.*
condralgia	**chondralgia** *Cartilaginous pain.*
condrite	**chondritis** *Cartilaginous inflammation.*
condroma	**chondroma** *Cartilaginous hyperplastic growth.*
condromalacia	**chondromalacia** *Excessive softening of the cartilages.*
condrossarcoma	**chondrosarcoma** *Cartilaginous tumor which exhibits rapid growth.*
cone	**cone** *A light sensitive cell in the retina.*
confabulação	**confabulation** *The fabrication of experiences to compensate for memory loss.*
confiança, de	**reliable** *Trustworthy.*
confiánca	**confidence** *Self-assurance.*
confinatmento	**confinement** *As in confined to bed.*

Portuguese	English
conflito	**conflict** *Dispute or disagreement.*
conforme	**according to**
confusão	**confusion** *Disorientation.*
congestivo	**congestive**
congênito	**congenital** *A disease or anomaly present from birth.*
conhecer	**acquaint, to** *To make someone familiar with something.*
conjuntiva	**conjunctiva** *The membrane that lines the eyelid.*
conjuntivite	**conjunctivitis** *Inflammation of the conjunctiva.*
conjuntivite	**pink eye** *Common term for acute contagious conjunctivitis.*
consangüinidade	**consanguinity** *The relationship by blood.*
consciência	**conscious** *Being award and being able to respond to one's surroundings.*
consciência, perdir	**loss of consciousness** *Unresponsive to verbal and tactile stimuli.*
conselheiro marital	**marital counseling** *Therapy aimed at marriage reconciliation.*
conservador	**conservative** *Control rather than elimination of a disease.*
consistente	**consistent** *Compatible with something or congruous with.*
consolidação	**consolidation** *An area of fixed secretions in the lung.*
constipação (B); prisão de ventre (P); obstipação	**constipation** *A condition exhibited by difficulty in having a bowel movement due to hard stools.*
constrição	**constriction** *Circumferential tightening*
consulta genético	**genetic counseling** *A discussion of the concerns related to genetic testing.*
consumo	**intake** *An amount of food taken into the body.*
consumo de alimento	**food intake** *Quantitative record of nutritional intake.*
consumo de fluido	**fluid intake** *The amount of oral consumption plus the amount of intravenous fluids administered.*
consumo oxigênio	**oxygen consumption** *The body's utilization of oxygen per unit of time.*
conta-gotas	**dropper** *A device used to administer medicines one drop at a time.*
contagem sangüínea completa	**complete blood count** *An assay that includes white blood cell, red blood cell, platelet count, hemoglobin, hematocrit and white blood cell differential.*
contagioso	**contagious** *Description of a disease that can be spread by direct or indirect contact.*
contaminar	**contaminate, to** *To make impure by exposing to an polluted agent.*
contar	**count, to** *To determine a number.*
contato; contacto	**contact** *The touching of two bodies or a person who has been exposed to a contagious disease.*
contracepção	**birth control** *Any method of limiting contraception.*
contraceptivo	**contraceptive** *A device or medication used to prevent pregnancy.*
contradição	**contraindication** *A situation in which two elements are inconsistent.*
contraditório	**contradictory** *Two elements that are inconsistent.*
contrair espasmodicamente	**twitch** *A sudden jerking movement.*
contratura de Dupuytren	**Dupuytren's contracture** *A disease of the palmar fascia causing a flexion contracture of the fourth and fifth fingers.*
contratura isquêmica	**ischemic contracture** *A muscle's resistance to passive stretch that is related to a decrease in arterial flow from any reason.*
controlar por	**check for, to**
controle de natalidade	**family planning** *Birth control.*

Portuguese	English
contusão	**bruise** *Common term for ecchymosis.*
contusão	**contusion** *An area of broken capillaries in the skin causing discoloration; commonly called a bruise.*
conveniente	**convenient** *Opportune or well-timed.*
convexo	**convex** *Having an exterior curved the outside of a sphere.*
convulsão	**convulsion** *An involuntary series of tonic and clonic movements.*
convulsão	**epileptic seizure** *A convulsion related to abnormal brain activity (as opposed to being precipitated by hypoglycemia.)*
coqueluche	**pertussis** *Synonym for whooping cough.*
coqueluche	**whooping cough** *Pertussis*
coracóide	**coracoid** *A prominence on the scapula to which the biceps is attached.*
coração	**heart** *Muscular organ that pumps blood thru the circulatory system.*
coração pulmonar	**cor pulmonale** *Heart disease that is secondary to lung disease.*
corcunda	**hunchback** *Synonym of kyphosis.*
corda	**chorda** *A cord or sinew.*
corda venérea	**chordee** *Downward bending of the penis.*
cordas vocais; pregas vocais	**vocal cords** *Paired folds of mucous membranes stretched across the larynx.*
cordão espermático	**spermatic cord** *The structure containing the ductus deferens, testicular artery, and nerves that goes from the inguinal ring to the testis.*
cordão espinhal	**spinal cord** *The bundle of nerves that with the brain comprise the central nervous system.*
cordão umbilical	**umbilical cord** *The stalk between the placenta and the unborn infant.*
cordite	**chorditis** *Inflammation of a vocal or spermatic cord.*
cores de conjunctiva	**color of conjunctiva** *A point of assessment to check for pallor.*
coréia	**chorea** *Involuntary, continuous rapid, jerking movements.*
coréia de Sydenham; coréia menor	**Saint Vitus' dance** *Historic name for chorea minor characterized by hypotonia and emotional lability months after a streptococcal infection.*
coréia de Sydenham; coréia menor	**Sydenham chorea** *Historically known as Saint Vitus' dance, it is a childhood chorea associated with rheumatic fever.*
coriza	**coryza** *An acute condition exhibited by copious nasal discharge.*
coriza (B); constipação (P)	**cold** *Viral upper respiratory tract infection.*
corneano	**corneal** *Referring to the cornea.*
coroidite	**choroiditis** *Inflammation of the choroid.*
coroidociclite	**choroidocyclitis** *Inflammation of the ciliary processes and choroid.*
coronóide	**coronoid** *Crown-shaped.*
coróide	**choroid** *Similar to the chorion (fertilized ovum or zygote)*
corpo caloso	**corpus callosum** *A point of connection between the two cerebral hemispheres.*
corpo carotídeo	**carotid body** *Carotid artery receptors that are sensitive to blood chemistry changes.*
corpo celular	**cell body** *The portion of the cell containing the nucleus.*
corpo cetônico	**ketone body** *One ketone with a decarboxylation product of acetone.*
corpo ciliar	**ciliary body** *The connection between the iris and the choroid.*

Portuguese	English
corpo estranho	**foreign body** *Term used to describe an object found in a body orifice that is not part of the body.*
corpo geniculado	**geniculate body** *Protrusions on the thalamus that relay visual and auditory signals to the brain.*
corpo inclusão	**inclusion body** *Variably shaped bodies in the nuclei of cells found in infections such as rabies and herpes.*
corpo lúteo	**corpus luteum** *A structure that is discharged from an ovary; it degenerates if it is not impregnated.*
corpo superfícies área; fórmula de Dubois	**body surface area** *Dubois formula is: (weight in kilograms)to the 0.425th power x (height in centimeters) to the 0.725th power x 0.007184.*
corpos quadrigêmeos	**quadrigeminal bodies** *The cranial and caudal colliculi.*
corpulência	**corpulence** *Fatness.*
corpúsculo	**corpuscle** *A red or white blood cell.*
corrente	**current** *Flow or stream.*
corrente	**stream** *The flow of a liquid.*
corrente sangüínea	**blood stream** *Common term or the arterial or venous systems.*
corte transversal	**cross-section** *A transverse section through a specimen or structure.*
cortical	**cortical** *Referring to the cortex.*
corticoropina	**corticotropin** *A hormone of the adrenal cortex.*
corticosteróide	**corticosteroid** *A hormone developed in the adrenal cortex.*
cortisol	**cortisol** *An adrenal cortical hormone, also called hydrocortisone.*
cortisona	**cortisone** *An adrenal cortical hormone responsible for carbohydrate regulation.*
costela	**rib** *A series of curved paired boney articulations protecting the thorax.*
costocondrite	**costochondritis** *Inflammation of the rib and or its cartilage.*
coto	**stump** *Term used to designate what remains of an amputated extremity.*
cotovelo (cotovelo direito, cotovelo esquerdo)	**elbow** *The joint between the humerus and radius/ulna.(right elbow, left elbow)*
cotovelo do tenista; epicondilite umeral lateral	**tennis elbow** *Inflammation at the lateral aspect of the epicondyle where the muscle and tendon join; lateral epicondylitis.*
coxa	**thigh** *The body region between the inguinal crease and knee.*
coxodinia	**coxalgia** *Pain in the hip.*
cóccix	**coccyx** *The small bone formed by the natural fusion of rudimentary vertebrae.*
cóclea	**cochlea** *The essential organ of hearing which is in a spiral form.*
códon	**codon** *A series of three nucleotides that form a unit of genetic code.*
cólera	**cholera** *An infectious disease exhibited by vomiting and diarrhea and caused by Vibrio cholerae.*
cólico	**colic** *Acute abdominal pain.*
cólico renal	**renal colic** *Pain caused by passage of a calculus through the ureter.*
cólon	**colon** *The portion of the large intestine that goes from the cecum to the rectum.*
cólon ascendente	**ascending colon** *The portion of the colon between the cecum and the right colic flexure.*
cópula	**copulation** *Sexual relations.*

Portuguese	English
córnea	**cornea** *The transparent segment located at the anterior part of the eye.*
córtex	**cortex** *An external layer.*
córtex adrenal	**adrenal cortex** *The outer layer of the adrenal gland.*
côndilo	**condyle** *A rounded protrusion of a bone.*
cranial; craniano	**cranial** *Referring to the skull.*
cranioclasto	**cranioclast** *An instrument used to crush a fetal skull.*
craniofaringioma	**craniopharyngioma** *A tumor that originates in the hypophyseal stalk.*
craniossinostose	**craniosynostosis** *Closure of the sutures of the skull that occurs prematurely.*
craniotabe	**craniotabes** *Softening of the skull bones causing widened sutures; this occurs in rickets.*
craniotomia	**craniotomy** *Surgical creation of a hole in the skull.*
craurose vulvar	**kraurosis vulvae** *Dryness and shrinkage of the vulva.*
cravo; pino	**pin** *Hardware used in surgery.*
crânio	**cranium** *The skeleton of the head.*
creatina	**creatine** *A compound involved with muscle contraction.*
creatinina	**creatinine** *A compound excreted in the urine that is produced by the metabolism of creatine.*
crenoterapia	**crenotherapy** *A form of treatment from mineral springs.*
crepitação	**crepitus** *A noise heard when one auscultates the lungs that is similar to the sound of rubbing hair between one's fingers. It is also considered the sound of two broken bones rubbing together.*
crescimento	**growth** *The increase in physical size.*
cretinismo	**cretinism** *A chronic condition caused by diminished thyroid hormone secretion.*
criança; menino	**child** *A person aged 1 to 8 years old.*
cribriforme	**cribriform** *Like a sieve; the olfactory nerves pass through the cribriform plate of the ethmoid bone.*
criestesia	**cryesthesia** *Abnormal sensitivity to cold.*
criocirurgia	**cryosurgery** *The application of extreme cold to destroy tissue.*
crioterapia	**cryotherapy** *The use of cold for therapeutic purposes.*
criptorquismo	**cryptorchism** *A condition characterized by the failure of the testes to descend into the scrotum.*
criptosporidiose	**cryptosporidiosis** *A parasitic related diarrhea seen in AIDS.*
crise	**crisis** *A turning point in the treatment of a disease.*
crista acústica	**acoustic crest** *A prominence on ampulla of the semicircular ducts.*
crista ilíaca	**iliac crest** *The upper border of the ilium.*
cristalóide	**crystalloid** *A substance that can pass through a semipermeable membrane; not a colloid.*
cristalúria	**crystalluria** *The presence of crystals in the urine.*
cromossoma	**chromosome** *A structure in the nucleus of living cells that carries genetic information.*
cromtina	**chromatin** *A desocyribose nucleic acid that carries the genes of inheritance.*
crosta	**crust** *Dried serous exudate covering a wound.*
crônico	**chronic** *When referring to an illness, it means recurring or persistent.*
cruciforme	**cruciform** *Shaped like a cross.*
crupe	**croup** *An acute laryngeal condition that is accompanied by a hoarse, barking cough.*

Portuguese	English
crural	**crural; femoral** *Referring to the femur or leg.*
cuidado de sanatório	**long-term care** *Generally referring to nursing home care.*
cuidados enfermagem	**nursing care** *The assessment and treatment provided by nurses.*
cuidados intensiva	**intensive care** *Vigorous treatment of the acutely ill.*
cuidados pré-natal	**prenatal care** *Medical care received while one is pregnant.*
culdoscopia	**culdoscopy** *Examination of the female pelvic viscera with a scope inserted through the posterior vaginal fornix.*
cultura	**culture** *The growth of bacteria in artificial medium.*
cuneiforme	**cuneiform** *The three bones between the navicular bone and the metatarsals.*
cura	**cure** *A remedy for a medical illness.*
curador	**healing** *The process of becoming healthy again.*
curare	**curare** *A toxic botanical substance used at one time in poison darts in South America. Curare derivatives have been used in general anesthesia.*
curativo	**curative** *A remedy capable of healing completely.*
curativo	**dressing** *The gauze applied to a wound.*
curativo compressivo	**pressure dressing** *A dressing used for compression to reduce bleeding.*
curativo oclusivo	**occlusive dressing** *A synthetic covering for a wound that has a semipermeable membrane.*
cureta	**curette** *The instrument used during a curettage.*
curetagem	**curettage** *Removal of tissues from a cavity.*
cutâneo	**cutaneous** *Referring to the skin.*
cutícula	**cuticle** *The dead skin at the base of the toenail or fingernail, also called the eponychium.*
cúspide	**leaflet** *Cusp.*
dacrioadenite	**dacryoadenitis** *Inflammation of the lacrimal gland.*
dacriocistite	**dacryocystitis** *Inflammation of a lacrimal sac.*
dacriocistorrinostomia	**dacryocystorhinostomy** *Surgical reaction of a communication between the lacrimal sac and nasal cavity.*
dacriólito	**dacryolith** *A stone in the lacrimal sac or duct.*
dador de cuidado	**caregiver** *A person who provides care to another.*
daqui	**hence** *Thus.*
data de admissão	**date of admission** *Beginning date of hospitalization.*
data de alta	**discharge date** *The day a patient is released from the hospital.*
data de expiracão	**expiration date** *The date when a medication should no longer be used.*
data de nascimento	**date of birth**
de fato	**indeed** *As a matter of fact.*
de fora	**free from** *Without or clear of.*
debaixo	**under; infra** *Sometimes used when indicating a patient is "under treatment" for a condition (active treatment).*
debilidade	**debility** *Physical weakness.*
debilidade	**weakness** *Feebleness.*
debilidade muscular	**muscle weakness** *Decreased muscular function.*
debridamento	**debridement** *Trimming the dead tissue adjacent to a wound.*
decapitação	**decapitate, to** *The physical separation of the head from the body.*
decibel	**decibel** *A unit used in the measurement of sound.*
decídua	**decidua** *The mucous membrane lining the uterus during pregnancy.*
declaração	**statement** *A written or oral commentary.*

Portuguese	English
declínio	**decline** *As in a decrease in status or health.*
decréscimo	**decrease** *Becoming smaller or fewer.*
decussação	**decussation** *An area of intersection.*
dedo	**finger** *Any of the five digits on the hand.*
dedo (do pé)	**toe** *Any of the digits of of the feet.*
dedo em gatilho	**trigger finger** *A condition in which one's finger gets stuck in the flexed position and when extended it snaps like a trigger. Also called stenosing tenosynovitis.*
dedo em martelo; dedo de beisebol	**mallet finger** *Flexion contracture of the distal phalanx.*
defecação	**defecation** *The discharge of feces from the rectum.*
defeito	**defect** *A shortcoming or imperfection.*
defeito septal atrial	**atrial septal defect** *An abnormal communication between the atria of the heart.*
defeito septal ventricular	**ventricular septal defect** *An abnormal communication between the right and left ventricles via a hole in the septum.*
defeito; mancha	**blemish** *A small mark on one's skin.*
defesa	**guarding** *A symptom used to describe a patient resisting an examination because of severe pain; often seen in patients with peritonitis.*
deficiência	**deficiency** *Insufficiency or deficit.*
deformidade	**deformity** *A malformation or imperfection.*
deglutição	**deglutition** *The process of swallowing.*
deglutir	**swallow, to** *To cause something to pass down the esophagus.*
delirante	**delusional** *Referring to a delusion.*
delírio	**delirium** *An acute mental state exhibited by altered thought processes and restlessness.*
delírio por supressão álcool	**delirium tremens** *A condition seen when alcohol is withdrawn which is exhibited by restlessness, hallucinations and tremors.*
delírio; ilusão	**delusion** *A belief that is contradictory to rational thought.*
deltóide	**deltoid** *A term referring to "three". The deltoid muscle has its origin at three areas: clavicle, acromion, and spine of the scapula.*
demarcação	**demarcation** *Having a fixed boundary.*
demência	**dementia** *A chronic brain disorder exhibited by memory loss, personality changes and faulty reasoning.*
demografia	**demography** *The study of the structure of human populations.*
demulcente	**demulcent** *Something that relieves irritation or inflammation.*
dendrito	**dendrite** *Impulses are transmitted along a dendrite to a nerve cell body.*
dengue	**dengue** *A mosquito-borne viral disease exhibited by fever and joint pain.*
densidade	**density** *The denseness of an object.*
dentado	**dentatum** *Also referred to as dentate nucleus of cerebellum.*
dentadura	**denture** *A frame that holds artificial teeth.*
dental	**dental** *Referring to teeth.*
dente	**tooth** *One of a set of hard, bony enamel coated structure in the jaw.*
dente do siso	**wisdom tooth** *Third molar.*
dente molar	**molar tooth** *Any of the most posterior teeth bilaterally which includes 8 deciduous and usually 12 permanent teeth.*
dentes canino	**canine teeth** *Located between the incisors and premolars.*
dentes decíduo	**deciduous teeth** *The first teeth.*

Portuguese	English
dentes permanente	**permanent teeth** *Dentition that comes in after the primary teeth.*
dentes pré-molar	**premolar** *The teeth anterior to the molars.*
dentição	**dentition** *The natural teeth.*
dentista	**dentist** *A professional capable of treating diseases of the teeth and gums.*
dependência cocáina	**cocaine addiction** *Physical habituation to cocaine.*
dependência do inalação de cola	**glue sniffing addiction** *Habituation of plastic cement fumes inhalation which includes toluene, xylene and benzene.*
depilatório	**depilatory** *An agent used to remove hair.*
depliação	**epilation** *Removal of hair and the roots.*
depressão	**depression** *A medical condition exhibited by profound despondency.*
deprimido	**depressed** *Melancholy.*
depuração	**clearance** *The process of removing something.*
derivação	**shunt** *An alternate path for blood or fluid.*
derivção padronizada; derivção indireta	**chest leads** *Leads going from the skin to an electrocardiographic device.*
dermatite	**dermatitis** *Non-specific inflammation of the skin.*
dermatografia	**dermatography** *A description of the skin.*
dermatologia	**dermatology** *The medical profession involving the treatment of skin conditions.*
dermatologiststa	**dermatologist** *A physician specializing in dermatology.*
dermatomicose	**dermatomycosis** *An infection of the skin by Trichophyton, Microsporum or Epidermophyton fungi.*
dermatomiosite	**dermatomyositis** *Inflammation of the skin, subcutaneous tissue and adjacent muscle.*
dermatose	**dermatosis** *Any skin disease.*
dermatose actinico	**actinic dermatosis** *A skin disease caused by exposure to radiation from the sun, ultraviolet waves or gamma radiation.*
dermatófito	**dermatophyte** *A fungal parasite living on the skin.*
dermátomo	**dermatome** *The area of sensation of the skin supplied by a single posterior spinal root.*
dermografia	**dermographia** *A raised, pale line with hyperemic borders is elicited upon scratching the skin with a dull instrument, in this condition.*
desabamento	**collapse** *A physical or mental breakdown.*
desabrigado	**homeless** *Having nowhere to live.*
desanimado	**down** *In a lower position.*
desaparecimento	**disappearance** *An instance of something/someone gone missing.*
desarticulação	**disarticulation** *The separation or amputation of a joint.*
descamação	**desquamation** *The shedding of skin in flakes or sheets.*
descamação	**exfoliation** *The shedding of scales.*
descarga ótico	**discharge, ear** *Otic secretions.*
descarga rinal	**discharge, nasal** *Nasal secretions.*
descarga vaginal; corrimento vaginal	**discharge, vaginal** *Vaginal secretions.*
descendente	**descending** *Moving toward the inferior portion.*
descendência	**offspring** *One's children.*
descerebrar	**decerebrate** *The removal of the brain.*
descolamento prematuro da placenta	**abruptio placentae** *The premature detachment of a normally implanted placenta resulting in maternal decompensation.*

Portuguese	English
descompensação	**decompensation** *The inability of an organ to respond to functional overload.*
descompressão	**decompression** *The surgical procedure relieving pressure on a part.*
desconforto	**discomfort** *A feeling of physical or mental unease.*
desconforto fetal	**fetal distress** *Term used to describe an abnormal heart rate or rhythm in a fetus indicating the need for urgent childbirth.*
desconhecido	**unknown** *Uncertain or undisclosed.*
desejo	**craving** *An unusually strong urge for something.*
desequilíbrio	**disequilibrium** *The absence of stability.*
desfibrilação	**defibrillator** *A device used to convert an abnormal cardiac rhythm (ventricular fibrillation) into a normal rhythm with use of electrical stimulation.*
desidratação	**dehydration** *The status of having a decrease in total body water.*
desinfetante	**disinfectant** *A substance that kills bacteria.*
deslocação	**dislocation** *The displacement of a bone when referring to an articulation.*
deslocamento	**displacement** *Movement from normal position.*
desmaio; síncope	**faint** *Weak and dizzy.*
desmóide	**desmoid** *A tumor typically found in the abdomen which contains. muscle and connective tissue.*
desnervação	**denervation** *The removal of nerve supply.*
desnutrição	**malnutrition** *Lack of appropriate nutrition.*
desorientação	**disorientation** *Mental confusion.*
despeito	**despite** *Notwithstanding.*
despersão	**scatter** *The degree to which repeated measurements differ.*
despertar	**awakening** *The state of being conscious.*
despojar	**disrobe, to** *To remove clothing.*
desprezo	**slight** *Minor or small.*
dessecação	**desiccation** *The act of drying up.*
dessensibilizar	**desensitize, to** *To gradually expose a person to an offending agent to prevent an abnormal response upon a secondary exposure.*
destro	**dexter**; *right; straight; erect*
destro	**right-handed** *Having a preference to use the right hand.*
desvendar um segredo	**blurt out, to** *To speak without considering the repercussions.*
desvio	**bypass** *An alternate route, typically referring to an arterial bypass.*
desvio	**deviation** *Away from the norm.*
deterioração	**deterioration** *Worsening in one's medical condition.*
detoxicação	**detoxification** *The process of removing toxins from the body.*
detrito	**detritus** *Particulate matter produced by the decomposition of an organic substance.*
detrusor da urina	**detrusor urinae** *Smooth muscle fibers that extend from the urinary bladder to the pubis.*
deuteranomalia	**deuteranomaly** *Abnormal color vision sometimes called "green weakness".*
devido à	**owing to** *On account of.*
dextrana	**dextran** *A high glucose polymer used as a plasma substitute.*
dextrocardia	**dextrocardia** *Location of the heart in the right hemithorax.*
débil	**weak** *Feeble or deconditioned.*

Portuguese	English
débito cardíaco	**cardiac output** *Amount of blood pumped by the heart in liters per minute.*
década	**decade** *Ten years.*
diabete insípido	**diabetes insipidus** *Caused by a deficiency in vasopressin, it is exhibited by great thirst and large volume urine output (and normal blood sugar).*
diabete melito	**diabetes mellitus** *A disease exhibited by a deficiency of the pancreatic hormone insulin.*
diabético	**diabetic** *A person who has diabetes mellitus.*
diaforético	**diaphoretic** *Exhibited by profuse perspiration.*
diafragma	**diaphragm** *The muscular separation between the thoracic and abdominal cavities.*
diagnóstico	**diagnostic** *A specific symptom or characteristic.*
diagnóstico diferencial	**differential diagnosis** *A list of possible alternative diagnoses for a patient who is ill.*
diametro conjugado	**conjugate diameter** *A pelvic inlet measurement used to determine whether a woman is capable of delivering a fetus vaginally.*
diapasão	**tuning fork** *A device used to distinguish between perceptive and conductive hearing loss.*
diapedese	**diapedesis** *The outward passage of blood elements through an intact vessel wall.*
diarréia	**diarrhea** *Increase in frequency and a loose consistency of the stools.*
diartrose	**diarthrosis** *An articulation allowing free movement.*
diastase	**diastase** *Amylase.*
diatermia	**diathermy** *The use of heat produced from high-frequency electric currents to medically or surgically treat someone.*
diáfise	**diaphysis** *The central part of a long bone.*
diástole	**diastole** *The period of dilatation of the heart; between the first and second heart sounds.*
diátese	**diathesis** *A medical tendency to develop a specific condition.*
dieta	**diet** *The kinds of food a person eats.*
diferencial	**differential** *A term used to refer to the various options for diagnoses.*
difosfato de adenosina	**adenosine diphosphate** *A product of hydrolysis of ATP.*
difteria	**diphtheria** *A contagious bacterial disease characterized by a grey membrane on the pharynx along with respiratory or cutaneous symptoms; caused by Corynebacterium diphtheriae.*
difundido	**widespread** *Encompassing or spanning.*
digestão	**digestion** *The process of enzymatic breakdown of food in the alimentary canal.*
digital	**digitalis** *Cardiac medication derived from the leaf of Digitalis purpurea.*
dilatação	**dilatation** *The process of becoming wider or larger.*
dilatador	**dilator** *An instrument that dilates.*
diluição	**dilution** *The process of making a weaker solution.*
dimercaprol	**dimercaprol** *A medication used as a binding agent for heavy metal poisoning.*
dioptria	**dioptre** *Referring to refraction or transmitted and refracted light.*
dióxido	**dioxide** *A compound containing two oxygen atoms.*
dióxido de carbono	**carbon dioxide gas** *A gas expelled during exhalation.*
diplegia	**diplegia** *The paralysis of both arms or both legs.*

Portuguese	English
diplococos	**diplococcus** *A bacterium that occurs in pairs including pneumococcus and Neisseria gonorrhoeae and Neisseria meningitidis.*
diplopia	**diplopia** *Double vision.*
diplopia monocular	**monodiplopia** *Double vision in only one eye.*
diplóide	**diploid** *A nucleus containing two complete sets of chromosomes.*
dipocondrodistrofia	**lipochondrodystrophy** *A congenital condition exhibited by short stature, kyphosis, mental deficiency and short fingers.*
dipsomania	**dipsomania** *Twins that are joined at some part of their bodies.*
direito	**right** *Opposite of left.*
disafia	**dysaphia** *Altered sense of touch.*
disartria	**dysarthria** *Difficulty in articulation of speech.*
disbarismo	**dysbarism** *Condition caused by a change in pressure, noted most commonly among scuba divers.*
discinesia	**dyskinesia** *Abnormal movement.*
disco óptico	**optic disk** *The area of the retina where the optic nerve enters.*
disco herniado	**herniated disc** *Prolapse of the nucleus pulposus into the spinal cord.*
discondroplasia	**dyschondroplasia** *The formation of cartilaginous and bony tumors near the epiphyses.*
discoria	**dyscoria** *A discordance in pupillary reaction.*
discrasia	**dyscrasia** *An abnormal condition, mostly referring to the blood.*
discreto	**discrete** *Separate and distinct.*
disdiadococinesia	**dysdiadocokinesia** *The inability to arrest one motor response and substitute its opposite.*
disenteria	**dysentery** *A severe form of diarrhea with blood and mucous in the stool.*
disestesia	**dysesthesia** *1. Impairment of the sense of touch. 2. The presence of persistent pain upon receiving a light touch.*
disfagia	**dysphagia** *Difficulty in swallowing.*
disfasia	**dysphasia** *Difficulty in speaking caused by cerebral dysfunction.*
disfunção	**dysfunction** *Abnormal function in a gland or body organ.*
disgenesia gonadal	**gonadal dysgenesis** *The lack of complete development of the gonads.*
dislalia	**dyslalia** *The absence of comprehensible speech articulation.*
dislexia	**dyslexia** *Difficulty in learning or reading written language with no effect on intelligence.*
dismenorréia	**dysmenorrhea** *Pain during menstruation.*
disodrose	**dyshidrosis** *Disregulation of sweating*
disostose cleidocraniana	**cleidocranial dysostosis** *A congenital condition exhibited by abnormal ossification of the cranial bones and absence of clavicles.*
dispareunia	**dyspareunia** *Pain during sexual intercourse.*
dispepsia	**dyspepsia** *Indigestion.*
displasia	**dysplasia** *The increase in organ size due to an increase in the number of abnormal cell types.*
dispnéia	**dyspnea** *Difficult breathing.*
dispnéia por esforço	**exercise-induced dyspnea**
disponibilidade	**availability** *A person or thing that is available.*
disponível	**available** *Attainable, obtainable.*
dispositivo contraceptivo intra-uterino (DIU)	**intrauterine contraceptive device (IUD)** *A device used to physically prevent the implantation of a fertilized ovum.*

Portuguese	English
dispositivo lanceta	**fingerstick device** *A device used to project a lancet into the skin so a drop of blood can be obtained for analysis.*
disquezia	**dyschezia** *Pain experienced during defecation.*
disritmia atrial	**sinus arrhythmia** *Cardiac dysrhythmias related to sinoatrial nodal dysfunction.*
dissacarídeo	**disaccharide** *A type of sugar that yields two monosaccharides upon hydrolysis.*
dissecção	**cut** *An incision.*
dissecção	**dissection** *Autopsy or postmortem exam.*
disseminação	**dissemination** *To be spread or dispersed widely.*
dissolução	**dissolution** *Disintegration.*
distal	**distal** *Situated away from the center of the body.*
distância, à	**apart** *Separated by a distance.*
distensão	**distension** *Swollen.*
distiquíase	**distichiasis** *Presence of two rows of eyelashes on one eyelid which are turned inward toward the globe.*
distocia	**dystocia** *Difficult birth caused by fetal position, narrow pelvis or lack of opening of the cervix.*
distribuição	**distribution** *The manner in which something is shared or spread out.*
distrofia muscular	**muscular dystrophy** *A hereditary condition exhibited by progressive muscular weakness and muscle atrophy.*
distúrbio	**disorder** *Impairment.*
distúrbio alimentar	**eating disorder** *General term for pathologic eating habits.*
distúrbio de cognição	**cognitive disorders** *Any disease process that involves altered cognition.*
distúrbio de comportamento	**behavior disorder** *An abnormal mental state.*
distúrbio maníco-depressivo	**manic-depressive psychosis** *A mental disorder exhibited by alternating periods of depression and mania.*
distúrbios afetivos	**affective disorders** *Manic-depressive psychosis.*
disúria	**dysuria** *Difficulty or pain upon urination.*
diurese	**diuresis** *Increased excretion of urine.*
diurético	**diuretic** *Medication which causes an increased excretion of urine.*
diurno	**diurnal** *Occurring during the day.*
diverticulite	**diverticulitis** *Inflammation of the diverticulum.*
diverticulose	**diverticulosis** *Presence of diverticulum.*
divertículo	**diverticulum** *A sac or pouch created by herniation of a mucous membrane in the alimentary canal.*
dígito	**digit** *Finger.*
doador	**donor** *Referring to a person who donates tissue or an organ.*
doar	**endow, to** *To supply or provide for.*
dobra do pele	**skin fold** *An overlapping of skin formed by subcutaneous tissue.*
dobra glútea	**gluteal fold** *The horizontal crease between the buttock and upper thigh.*
doença	**disease** *Malady or disorder.*
doença	**sickness** *Illness or a state of disease.*
doença antecedentes	**past history** *Prior medical problems experienced by a patient.*
doença da arranhadura do gato	**cat scratch fever** *An infectious disease characterized by local inflammation a the site of the scratch, local lymph adenopathy and fever.*

Portuguese	English
doença da Floresta de Kyasnur	**Kyasanur Forest disease** *A viral fever noted in Mysore, India transmitted by Haemaphysalis spinigera. It is characterized by fever, headache, generalized pains, diarrhea, and intestinal bleeding.*
doença da urina em xarope de bordo; leucinose	**leucinosis; maple syrup urine disease** *A condition characterized by an enzyme defect causing an increase in leucine in the urine.*
doença da urina em xarope de bordo; leucinose	**maple syrup urine disease** *A condition characterized by an enzyme defect causing an increase in leucine in the urine.*
doença de Addison	**Addison's disease** *A disease of the adrenal gland exhibited by anemia, hypotension and a bronze tone to the skin.*
doença de Alzheimer	**Alzheimer's disease** *A dementia of unknown cause or pathogenesis.*
doença de Crohn	**Crohn's disease** *An inflammatory bowel disease.*
doença de Graves; doença de Basedow ou Parry	**Graves' disease** *A form of hyperthyroidism exhibited by a goiter and exophthalmos.*
doença de Hansen	**Hansen's disease** *Leprosy*
doença de Hodgkin	**Hodgkin's disease** *Also called Hodgkin's lymphoma, it is a cancer that begins in the lymphocytes.*
doença de Huntington	**Huntington's chorea** *A neurodegenerative disease characterized initially by behavioral changes and later by a movement disorder. Called Huntington's disease now.*
doença de Itai-Itai	**ouch-ouch disease** *Common term for Itai-Itai disease that is derived from "it hurts, it hurts" said by patients suffering from cadmium poisoning.*
doença de Köhler	**Köhler's disease** *A genetic disease characterized by osteonecrosis and subsequent collapse of the tarsal navicular bone.*
doença de Lobo; lobomycosis	**Lobo's disease** *A condition exhibited by small, red, hard papules in the sacral region caused by Lacazia loboi.*
doença de Milroy; doença de Nonne-Milroy	**Milroy's disease** *Hereditary disease exhibited by leg edema.*
doença de Parkinson	**Parkinson's disease** *A progressive neuromuscular disease exhibited by masklike facial expression, resting tremor, cogwheel rigidity and abnormal gait.*
doença de Peyronie; doença de van Buren; fibromatose peniana	**Peyronie's disease** *Curvature of the penis during an erection to to plaque.*
doença de Pott; espondilite tuberculosa	**Pott's disease** *Also referred to as tuberculous spondylitis it is caused by a spinal deformity caused by a tuberculosis infection of the spine.*
doença de Steinert; distrofia miotônica	**myotonia dystrophica; Steinert's disease** *A condition exhibited initially by hypertonic muscles followed by atrophy of the facial and neck muscles.*
doença de Strümpell; espondilite deformante	**Strümpell's disease** *Also known as spondylitis deformans, it is characterized by arthritis and osteitis deformans of the spinal cord with a rounded kyphosis and rigidity.*
doença de tsutsugamushi	**tsutsugamushi disease** *An acute febrile infectious disease caused by Rickettsia tsutsugamushi. It is characterized by fever, pain lymphadenopathy, small black lesions on the genitals, neck or axilla.*
doença desmielinizante	**demyelinating disease** *A condition characterized by the loss of myelin.*
doença do caixão	**caisson disease** *Decompression sickness.*
doença do movimento	**motion sickness** *Nausea associated with travel.*
doença do pé e boca; fata contagiosa	**foot and mouth disease** *A contagious viral disease exhibited by oral and digital vesicles.*

Portuguese	English
doença do sono; tripanossomíase gambiense	**sleeping sickness** *Also called Trypanosomiasis, this disease is caused by a parasitic protozoa and transmitted by the tsetse fly.*
doença dos Açores	**Azorean disease** *A form of hereditary ataxia found in peoples of Azorean descent. Also called Machado-Joseph disease or Portuguese-Azorean disease.*
doença dos legionários; legionelose	**legionnaires' disease** *The name was derived after an outbreak at a convention of the American Legion; it is manifested by fever, chills, dyspnea, and cough.*
doença fetalis cardíaca	**congenital heart disease** *A cardiac disorder present prior to birth.*
doença inflamatória pélvica	**pelvic inflammatory disease** *Generally a bacterial infection affecting a woman with potential involvement of the uterus, fallopian tubes, ovaries and cervix.*
doença isquémico cardíaco	**ischemic heart disease** *Inadequate blood supply to the heart.*
doença matinal	**morning sickness** *Nausea associated with pregnancy.*
doença periodontal	**periodontal disease** *Present around to a tooth.*
doença reumática do coração	**rheumatic heart disease** *A manifestation of rheumatic fever, frequently causing valvular dysfunction.*
doença transmitida sexualmente	**sexually transmitted disease (STD)** *A condition one obtains from another during sexual relations.*
doença venérea	**venereal disease** *A condition transmitted via sexual intercourse.*
doloroso	**painful** *Affected with pain.*
dopamina	**dopamine** *An intermediate product in the creation of norepinephrine.*
dor	**pain** *Physical suffering or discomfort.*
dor do afiado	**stabbing pain** *A sharp piercing quality to pain.*
dor do membro-fantasma	**phantom limb pain** *Pain sensed in an area where one has had an amputation as though the limb is still present.*
dor em região lombar	**low back pain** *Pain in the lumbar region.*
dor em região lombar	**lumbago** *Pain in the region of the lumbar spine.*
dor nas costas	**back pain** *Discomfort on the dorsal surface of the torso.*
dor referida	**referred pain** *Pain felt in an area distinct from the original source.*
dores do parto	**labor pains** *The intermittent pain associated with uterine contractions.*
dores pós-parto; dores puerperais	**after-pains** *The pain experienced after childbirth caused by uterine contractions.*
dorsal	**dorsal** *Referring to the back or back surface.*
dorsiflexão	**dorsiflexion** *Backward bending of the foot or hand.*
dorso	**dorsum** *The back part.*
dosa de manutenção	**dose, maintenance** *The chronic dose given after the initial bolus.*
dosagem	**dosage** *The amount and frequency a medication is given.*
dose	**dose** *The quantity of a medication.*
dose excessiva	**overdose** *An above normal dose of a medication.*
dose freqüência	**dosing interval** *The number of times per unit a medication is given.*
dose letal	**lethal dose** *The amount of a drug required to cause death.*
drástico	**drastic** *Having significant effect.*
droga	**drug** *A medication, sometimes with negative connotation.*
duas vezes	**two times** *One action being done on two occasions.*
ducha	**douche** *Cleansing of a canal; unless otherwise specified it refers to cleansing of the vaginal canal.*

Portuguese	English
ducto	**duct** *Hollow tubular tissue used to carry fluid from a secretory organ.*
ducto arterioso permeável	**patent ductus arteriosus** *A condition exhibited by failure of the ductus arteriosus (communication between the aorta the the pulmonary artery normally noted in a fetus) to close.*
ducto biliar	**bile ducts** *The structures that are conduits for passage of bile from the liver and gallbladder to the duodenum.*
ducto cístico	**cystic duct** *The duct connecting the gallbladder to the common bile duct.*
ducto de Botallo	**ductus arteriosus** *A fetal artery that communicates between the pulmonary artery and the descending aorta.*
ducto hepático	**hepatic duct** *The right and left hepatic ducts join the cystic duct to form the common bile duct.*
ducto lactífero	**lactiferous duct** *A canal that carries milk.*
duelo	**bereavement** *The sorrow one feels with the loss of a loved one.*
duodenal	**duodenal** *Referring to the duodenum.*
duodenectomia	**duodenectomy** *Excision of the duodenum.*
duodenite	**duodenitis** *Inflammation of the duodenum.*
duodeno	**duodenum** *The portion of the small bowel between the stomach and jejunum.*
duplicação	**duplication** *The process of duplicating something.*
duplo	**double** *Twice the size, quantity or strength.*
dura-máter	**dura mater** *The outermost covering of the brain and spinal cord.*
duro	**hard** *Rigid or very firm.*
eclâmpsia	**eclampsia** *A maternal condition characterized by convulsions and hypertension that can lead to maternal and fetal death.*
ecmnésia	**ecmnesia** *Memory loss for recent events but retained memory of remote events.*
ecocardiografia	**echocardiography** *The use of ultrasound waves to visualize the heart and its structures.*
ecolalia	**echolalia** *The meaningless repetition of the words spoken by another person.*
econdroma	**ecchondroma** *Hyperplastic growth of cartilage on the surface of other cartilage.*
ectasia	**ectasia** *Expansion or distension.*
ectoderma	**ectoderm** *The outermost layer of the three layers of the embryo.*
ectópico	**ectopic** *Abnormal position.*
ectrodactilia	**ectrodactylia** *A congenital anomaly exhibited by absence of one digit or part of a digit.*
ectrópio	**ectropion** *Eversion of the eyelid, usually the lower lid.*
eczema	**eczema** *A medical condition exhibited by pruritic, red, scaly patches on the scalp, cheeks and extensor surfaces.*
eczema disodrotica	**dyshidrotic eczema** *A dermatitis characterized by vescicobullous lesions.*
edema	**edema** *Extravascular fluid accumulation.*
edema angioneurótico	**angioedema** *Also called angioneurotic edema, it is caused by a histamine reaction. It can produce welts in mild cases but in severe cases can cause swelling of the lips and tongue.*
edema angioneurótico	**angioneurotic edema** *A condition exhibited by sudden edema of skin and mucous membranes.*
edema de declive	**ankle edema or dependent edema** *Extracellular fluid volume noted by swelling or pitting.*
edema de declive	**lower extremity edema** *Interstitial edema of the legs.*

Portuguese	English
edema depressível	**pitting edema** *Edema of the lower extremities characterized by an indentation being left when the examiner applies pressure with their thumb.*
edema pulmonar	**pulmonary edema** *Characterized by abnormal fluid buildup in the lungs.*
edema sólido	**nonpitting edema** *Subcutaneous swelling that cannot be indented with compression.*
edematoso	**edematous** *Referring to the presence of edema.*
educação	**education** *Instruction or guidance.*
efedrina	**ephedrine** *A chemical used to treat asthma because it expands bronchial passages and used to control spinal anesthesia associated shock because it constricts blood vessels.*
efeito adverso	**adverse effect** *In reference to medication use, it is an undesirable consequence of the drug.*
efeito colateral	**side effect** *An expected but unwanted effect of a medication.*
efeito cumulativo	**cumulative effect** *A consequence of successive additions.*
efetor	**effector** *An organ that responds to a stimulus.*
eficaz	**efficacious** *Effective.*
efusão	**effusion** *The accumulation of fluid in a body cavity.*
efusão pleural; pleurisia com derrame	**pleural effusion** *An abnormal collection of fluid between the internal chest wall and the pleura.*
egocêntrico	**egocentric** *Thinking of self without considering the feelings or thoughts of others.*
eixo	**axis** *The second cervical vertebra.*
ejaculação	**ejaculation** *The emission of semen at the moment of sexual climax in a male.*
elastina	**elastin** *A connective tissue-based glycoprotein.*
electivo	**elective** *Non-urgent and not life-saving.*
elefantíase	**elephantiasis** *A condition caused by nematode parasites leading to lymphatic obstruction and limb or scrotal swelling.*
eletrocardograma	**electrocardiogram** *Display of a person's heart beat that can be used in the diagnosis of cardiac disorders.*
eletrodo	**electrode** *A device used to facilitate conduction of electricity to or from a body.*
eletroencefalograma	**electroencephalogram (EEG)** *A display of brain waves used in the diagnosis of brain disorders, especially epilepsy.*
eletroforese	**electrophoresis** *The movement of charged particles in a fluid that is under the influence of an electric field. This is used in testing for various maladies in the form of serum protein electrophoresis.*
eletromiografia	**electromyography** *The display of the electrical activity of muscle.*
eletrólito	**electrolyte** *The ionized constituents including potassium, sodium, chloride and others.*
elevado	**high** *Elevated.*
elevador	**levator** *A muscle that raises part of the body; the levator labii superioris raised the upper lip.*
elixir	**elixir** *A medical solution.*
em aleatório	**at random** *Occurring by chance alone.*
em bandas	**banding** *The process of encircling with a thin piece of material.*
em série	**serial** *In a series.*
emaciação	**emaciation** *Abnormally thin and weak.*
emaptia	**empathy** *To be concerned for and share the feelings of another.*
embaixo de	**below** *Under.*

Portuguese	English
embolectomia	**embolectomy** *The removal of an embolus.*
embolia gordurosa	**fat embolism** *A deposit of fat that obstructs a vessel.*
embolismo pulmonar	**pulmonary embolism** *A sudden blockage of a lung artery frequently emanating from a blood clot in one's leg.*
embrião	**embryo** *The term used to describe a fertilized ovum in the first 8 weeks of development.*
embriologia	**embryology** *The study of the embryo.*
emergência	**emergency** *An urgent, life-threatening situation.*
emersão	**emergence** *Coming into prominence.*
emetropia	**emmetropia** *The normal correlation between eye refraction and the axial length of the eyeball.*
emético	**emetic** *An agent that induces vomiting.*
eminência tenar	**thenar eminence** *Formed by the bellies of the abductor pollicis brevis, flexor pollicis brevis and opponens pollicis.*
emissão noturno	**nocturnal emission** *Involuntary emission of semen at night.*
emoção	**emotion** *An intense feeling.*
emoliente	**emollient** *Having softening or soothing qualities.*
empiema	**empyema** *A collection of purulent material in a body cavity, usually referring to a thoracic empyema.*
emplastro; gesso	**plaster** *Dehydrated gypsum that has water added to it in order to immobilize fractured extremities.*
emulsão	**emulsion** *The dispersion of one liquid into another, but it is not dissolved.*
enartrose	**enarthrosis** *The type of joint in which a spherical bone is set into the socket of another bone.*
encefalinas	**enkephalin** *Peptide found in the brain that has similar effects as the endorphins.*
encefalite	**encephalitis** *Inflammation of the brain.*
encefalocele	**encephalocele** *The protrusion of the brain through a defect in the skull.*
encefalografia	**encephalography** *Roentgenography of the brain.*
encefalomalacia	**encephalomacia** *Abnormal softness of the brain.*
encefalomielite	**encephalomyelitis** *Inflammation of the brain and spinal cord.*
encefalopatia	**encephalopathy** *Degeneration of cerebral function.*
encefalopatia espongiforme bovina	**mad cow disease** *Bovine spongiform encephalopathy, a disease that cause cerebral degeneration exhibited by ataxia.*
encefálico	**encephalic** *Referring to the brain.*
encondroma	**enchondroma** *An abnormal increase in cartilage growth on the inside of bone or of other cartilage.*
encontro marcado	**appointment** *A previously scheduled time to see a person.*
encoprese	**encopresis** *Involuntary defecation.*
encravamento	**nailing** *Referring to placement of an intramedullary rod in a long bone in order to treat a fracture.*
encurtamento	**shortening** *Notable for having a shorter length.*
endarterite	**endarteritis** *Tunica intima inflammation.*
endcrinologia	**endocrinology** *The study of endocrine glands and hormones.*
endêmico	**endemic** *When a disease is commonly found in a location or in a people group.*
endireita	**bonesetter** *A person who sets bones without being a physician.*
endocardite	**endocarditis** *Inflammation of the endocardium.*
endocervicite	**endocervicitis** *Inflammation of the mucosal lining of the cervix.*
endoderma	**endoderm** *The innermost layer of the embryonic germ cell layers.*

Portuguese	English
endogênico	**endogenous** *Originating from within.*
endolinfa	**endolymph** *The fluid collection the labyrinth of the ear.*
endometrioma	**endometrioma** *An isolated benign mass containing endometrial tissue.*
endometriose	**endometriosis** *Presence of uterine mucosal tissue in the pelvis in abnormal locations.*
endometritie	**endometritis** *Inflammation of the endometrium.*
endométrio	**endometrium** *The mucous membrane lining of the uterus.*
endoneuro	**endoneurium** *The tissue in a peripheral nerve that separates the individual nerve fibers.*
endorfina	**endorphin** *Hormone secreted that activates the body's opiate receptors and acts as an analgesic.*
endoscópio	**endoscope** *A device used to view the interior of a hollow organ (sigmoidoscope, gastroscope)*
endotelioma	**endothelioma** *A mass that propagates from the endothelium of blood vessels, lymphatics or serous cavities.*
endotraqueal	**endotracheal** *Within the trachea.*
endócrino	**endocrine** *Referring to glands that secrete hormones and other chemicals into the blood.*
endurecimento	**induration** *An area that is abnormally hard.*
enema	**enema** *A procedure involving insertion of fluid into the rectum.*
enema de bário	**barium enema** *Administration of barium into the rectum followed by roentgenography to check for rectal or colon abnormalities.*
enfermaria	**ward** *A section of a hospital where patients reside.*
enfermaria isolamento	**isolation ward** *A ward where patients with infectious disease are housed.*
enfermeira	**nurse** *A person trained to care for the sick.*
enfermeira especializada	**nurse practitioner** *A person with advanced training capable of acting as a patient's primary care provider.*
enfermidade terminal	**terminal illness** *A disease with no viable treatment with death being inevitable.*
enfisema	**emphysema** *Abnormal enlargement of the airspaces distal to the terminal bronchioles.*
enfraquecimento	**impairment** *A specific disability.*
enoftalmia	**enophthalmos** *Posterior displacement of the eyeball in the orbit.*
enorme	**enormous** *Very large.*
enostose	**enostosis** *The abnormal bony growth inside a bone or on the cortex.*
entalhe	**nick** *A small groove or notch.*
enterectomia	**enterectomy** *Surgical resection of part of the intestine.*
enterite	**enteritis** *Inflammation of the intestines.*
enterobíase	**enterobiasis** *An infection caused by worms from the genus Enterobius.*
enterococo	**enterococcus** *A gram positive cocci that occurs naturally in the intestine but is pathogenic elsewhere in the body.*
enteroptose	**enteroptosis** *Inferior displacement of the intestines in the abdomen.*
enterotomia	**enterotomy** *A surgical opening of the intestines.*
enterólito	**enterolith** *A calculus of the intestine.*
entérico	**enteric** *Referring to the intestines.*
entorpecimento	**numbness** *Decreased sensation to tactile stimuli.*
entorse	**sprain** *A joint injury without fracture.*

Portuguese	English
enucleação	**enucleation** *Surgical removal of a globe.*
enurese	**enuresis** *Involuntary urination.*
envolvido	**involved** *Difficult to comprehend.*
enxerto	**graft** *A piece of tissue surgically transplanted.*
enxerto ósseo	**bone graft** *The transfer of bone to aid in the healing of a complex fracture.*
enxofre	**sulfur** *A chemical element with atomic number of 16.*
enzima	**enzyme** *A compound that acts as a catalyst for reactions within cells as assists with digestion outside of cells.*
eosinofilia	**eosinophilia** *An increased number of eosinophils in the blood.*
eosinófilo	**eosinophil** *A cell with eosin stain used to designate a type of leukocyte that is elevated during allergic reactions.*
ependimoma	**ependymoma** *A tumor composed of cells that line the ventricles of the brain.*
epêndima	**ependyma** *The glial lined covering of the cerebral ventricles and the central portion of the spinal cord.*
epibléfaro	**epiblepharon** *A condition exhibited by the eyelashes pressing against the eyeball.*
epicárdio	**epicardium** *The serous membranous, innermost lining of the pericardium.*
epicondilite	**epicondylitis** *Inflammation of the epicondyle.*
epicôndilo	**epicondyle** *A protrusion at the distal end of the humerus.*
epicrânio	**epicranium** *The skin, fibrous layer (aponeurosis), and muscles lining the scalp.*
epidemia	**epidemic** *Ubiquitous development of an infectious disease.*
epidemiologia	**epidemiology** *The study of the incidence, development and control of disease.*
epiderme	**epidermis** *The skin cells overlying the dermis.*
epidermofitose	**epidermophytosis** *A fungal skin infection caused by an organism from the genus Epidermophyton.*
epididimite	**epididymitis** *Inflammation of the duct that moves sperm from the testis to the vas deferens.*
epididimorquite	**epididymo-orchitis** *Inflammation of the epididymis and the testis.*
epidural	**epidural** *The space around the dura of the spinal cord.*
epifisite	**epiphysitis** *Inflammation of the end of a long bone that is separated from the shaft by a cartilaginous disc.*
epigástrio	**epigastrium** *The section of the abdomen that overlies the stomach.*
epiglote	**epiglottis** *Tissue at the base of the tongue that covers the trachea when one swallows.*
epilepsia	**epilepsy** *A condition associated with abnormal brain activity and exhibited by sudden, recurrent convulsions, sensory disturbances and loss of consciousness.*
epileptiforme	**epileptiform** *Being similar to epilepsy.*
epileptogênico	**epileptogenic** *That which induces seizures.*
epinefrina	**epinephrine** *A hormone secreted by the adrenal gland.*
episclerite	**episcleritis** *Inflammation of the tissue lying above the sclera.*
episiotomia	**episiotomy** *A surgical incision of the vagina used to aid childbirth.*
epispadia	**epispadias** *A congenital condition characterized by the urethral meatus being at the superior aspect of the penis*
epistaxe	**epistaxis** *Bleeding emanating from the nose.*
epitelial	**epithelial** *Referring to the epithelium.*

Portuguese	English
epitelioma	**epithelioma** *A malignant tumor composed of epithelial cells.*
epitélio	**epithelium** *The tissue lining the skin and the gastrointestinal tract that is derived from the embryonic ectoderm and endoderm..*
epitroclear	**epitrochlea** *The medial condyle of the humerus.*
epífise cerebral;corpus da glândula; corpo pineal	**epiphysis cerebri** *A small structure situated on the mesencephalon between the two sections of the thalamus.*
equilíbrio	**equilibrium** *When opposing forces are in balance.*
equimose	**ecchymosis** *Skin discoloration caused by bleeding beneath the epidermis.*
equinococo	**Echinococcus** *A tapeworm of the family Taeniidae that can cause hydatid cysts.*
equipamento	**equipment** *Apparatus or instrument.*
ergonomia	**ergonomics** *The study of workplace design that focuses on reducing work-related injuries.*
ergosterol	**ergosterol** *A compound converted to vitamin D2 upon exposure to ultraviolet light.*
ergômetro	**ergometer** *A device that measures energy expenditure.*
erguer	**lift, to** *Raise to a higher level.*
eritatoblasto	**erythroblast** *A nucleus containing immature erythrocyte.*
eritema multiforme	**erythema mutliforme** *A skin condition exhibited by purpuric lesions and bullae usually on the distal parts of extremities but can affect the face and trunk.*
eritema nodoso	**erythema nodosum** *The presence of red or purple nodules on the pretibial area.*
eritroblastose fetal	**erythroblastosis fetalis** *A hemolytic disease of the newborn.*
eritrocianose	**erythrocyanosis** *A condition exhibited by purple patches with asymmetric swelling, pruritus and burning.*
eritrocitopenia	**erythrocytopenia** *Low level of erythrocytes in the blood stream.*
eritrocitose	**erythrocytosis** *A higher than normal level of erythrocytes in the blood stream.*
eritropoiese	**erythropoiesis** *The production of red blood cells.*
eritrócito	**erythrocyte** *Called a red blood cell, it transports oxygen and carbon dioxide to and from the tissues.*
erliquiose	**ehrlichiosis** *A tickborne infectious disease.*
erosão	**erosion** *The gradual destruction of surface tissue.*
erro	**error** *Mistake or inaccuracy.*
eructação	**eructation** *Belch or burp.*
erupção	**outbreak (of a disease)** *A sudden start of a disease in a population.*
erupção cutâneo das fraldas	**diaper rash** *Macular rash in the inguinal/perineal region related to exposure to urine.*
erupção devida à infestação com o ácaro	**poultryman's itch** *Pruritus associated with the mite Dermanyssus gallinae.*
erupção por drogas	**drug eruption** *A diffuse rash caused by a medication.*
escabiose	**scabies** *A skin condition exhibited by intense pruritus and a macular rash commonly in the perineal and interdigital spaces.*
escabiose norueguesa	**Norway itch** *A severe pruritus caused by scabies and is associated with immune disorders such as AIDS.*
escafocefalia	**scaphocephaly** *A condition exhibited by a long narrow skull because of early closure of the sagittal sutures.*
escala	**scale** *A device to check a person's weight.*

Portuguese	English
escala de Glasgow do coma	**Glasgow coma scale** *A scale used to grade one's level of consciousness with a score of 3 being totally unresponsive and a score of 15 being normal.*
escaldadura	**scald** *A burn injury from extremely hot water.*
escalpelo	**scalpel** *A knife used during surgery for incision of skin and tissue.*
escalpo	**scalp** *The skin covering the head except for the face.*
escama	**squama** *A scale or platelike body.*
escamoso	**squamous** *Scaly.*
escaneamento ósseo	**bone scan** *Bone imaging using technetium 99m (99mTc) diphosphate.*
escara	**eschar** *Dry, hard, dead tissue commonly seen with a chronic pressure ulcer or anthrax.*
escarificação	**scarification** *Multiple small scratches of the skin, as is sometimes used for vaccine administration.*
escasso	**sparing** *Economical.*
escápula	**scapula** *Medical term for the shoulder blade.*
esclera	**sclera** *The white outer covering of the eyeball.*
esclerite	**scleritis** *Inflammation of the eyeball.*
esclerodactilia	**sclerodactylia** *Scleroderma of the digits.*
esclerodermia	**scleroderma** *A systemic disease of the connective tissues.*
esclerose lateral amiotrófica	**amyotrophic lateral sclerosis** *A progressive neurodegenerative disorder.*
esclerose múltipa	**multiple sclerosis** *A chronic neurologic disease exhibited by numbness, vision and speech problems, and motor incoordination.*
esclerose tuberosa	**tuberous sclerosis** *An inherited neurocutaneous disorder exhibited by benign hamartomas of the brain, lung, kidney, skin and other organs.*
esclerotomia	**sclerotomy** *Surgical incision of the sclera.*
escoar lentamente	**ooze, to** *To slowly leak.*
escoliose	**scoliosis** *A lateral curvature of the spine.*
escopofilia	**scopophilia** *Sexual please attained by viewing sexual organs.*
escorbuto	**scurvy** *A disease of vitamin C deficiency exhibited by bleeding gums.*
escore de Apgar	**Apgar score** *A scoring system for newborns that utilizes heart rate, respiratory effort, muscle tone, responsiveness and skin color.*
escotoma	**scotoma** *A blind spot within an otherwise normal visual field.*
escova	**brush** *Implement used for cleaning or for taking a tissue sample.*
escólex	**scolex** *The front end of a tapeworm.*
escrotal	**scrotal** *Referring to the scrotum.*
escroto	**scrotum** *The sac which contains the testes.*
escrófula	**scrofula** *Cervical tuberculous lymphadenitis.*
escudo	**shield** *A protective device, as in face shield.*
escurecimento; blecaute	**blackout** *Common term for loss of consciousness.*
escútulo	**scutulum** *A crust of tinea capitis.*
eserina	**eserine** *Physostigmine.*
esferocitose	**spherocytosis** *The presence of spherocytes in the blood.*
esferocitose hereditária	**hereditary spherocytosis** *A familial hemolytic disease exhibited by abnormally thick erythrocytes.*
esferócito	**spherocyte** *An erythrocyte without the usual central pallor; it is noted in spherocytosis and some hemolytic anemias.*

Portuguese	English
esfigmomanômetro	**sphygmomanometer** *Device for measuring blood pressure.*
esfincterotomia	**sphincterotomy** *Surgical incision of the anal sphincter.*
esfíncter	**sphincter** *A muscle the surrounds an orifice or duct so it closes when the muscle contracts.*
esforço	**effort** *Attempt or endeavor.*
esforço expulsivo de uma partuiente	**bearing down** *As in during labor.*
esfregaço	**smear** *Used to refer to a specimen smeared on a slide.*
esguichar	**squirt, to** *To eject a liquid from a small opening.*
esmegma	**smegma** *A thick curdled secretion found around the clitoris and the prepuce.*
esofagectomia	**esophagectomy** *Surgical removal of the esophagus.*
esofagite	**esophagitis** *Inflammation of the esophagus.*
esofagoscopia	**esophagoscopy** *Visual inspection the esophagus utilizing a scope.*
esofágico	**esophageal** *Referring to the esophagus.*
esotropia	**esotropia** *Medial deviation of the eyes at primary gaze.*
esôfago de Barrett	**Barretts's esophagus** *A condition characterized by varying degrees of esophageal injury from gastric acid.*
esôfago(B), esófago (P)	**esophagus** *The muscular tube that connects the throat to the stomach.*
espacticidade em faca de mola	**clasp knife reflex** *An abnormal response seen in the setting of a pyramidal tract lesion in which there is a rapid decrease in resistance during passive movement of a joint.*
espaço morto	**dead space** *The area in the respiratory tract where air is not exchanged.*
espaço morto anatômico	**anatomical dead space** *The area between the mouth and pulmonary alveoli.*
espaço morto fisiológico	**physiologic dead space** *The combination of anatomic and alveolar dead space.*
espaço no interior de uma estrutura tubular	**lumen** *A hollow cavity.*
espasmo	**spasm** *An involuntary contraction of muscles.*
espasmo carpopedal	**carpopedal spasm** *A spasm of the carpus and the foot.*
espasmo de torção	**torsion spasm** *Also called dystonia musculorum deformans, a genetic condition exhibited by twisting contortions sideways and forward while walking.*
espasmolítico	**spasmolytic** *A substance that diminishes spasms.*
espasticidade	**spasticity** *Refers to continuous spastic movement.*
espático	**spastic** *Stiff, awkward movement of the muscles.*
específico	**specific** *Clearly defined.*
espectrometria	**spectrometry** *The use of a device to measure spectra.*
espectroscópio	**spectroscope** *A device for producing and recording spectra.*
espelho	**mirror** *A device used for reflecting an image.*
esperar	**expect, to** *To suppose or presume.*
esperma	**sperm** *Short term for spermatozoon.*
espermatocele	**spermatocele** *A cyst in the epididymis containing spermatozoa.*
espermatogênese	**spermatogenesis** *The production of spermatozoa.*
espermatozóide	**spermatozoon** *A mature male germ cell that is capable of fertilizing an ovum.*
espermicida	**spermicide** *A substance capable of killing sperm.*
espernear	**kick, to** *To strike an object with one's foot.*
espécime	**specimen** *A sample for medical testing.*

Portuguese	English
espécime urinárais meso-corrente	**clean catch urine specimen** *A urine specimen obtained by having a patient cleanse the perineal area prior to voiding in a collection device.*
espéculo	**speculum** *A device used to open a canal for inspection. (vaginal speculum)*
espiga	**spica** *A figure of eight bandage.*
espinha	**spine** *The spinal column or a thorny protrusion.*
espinhal	**spinal** *Referring to the spine.*
espirógrafo	**spirograph** *A device used to record respiratory movements.*
espirômetro	**spirometer** *A device used to measure pulmonary capacity.*
espirrar	**sneeze, to** *To suddenly expel air from the nose and mouth because of nasal irritation.*
espícula	**spicule** *A sharp, slender part.*
esplenectomia	**splenectomy** *Surgical excision of the spleen.*
esplenomegalia	**splenomegaly** *An abnormally enlarged spleen.*
esplênico	**splenic** *Referring to the spleen.*
espondilite	**spondylitis** *Inflammation of the vertebrae.*
espondilite ancilosante	**ankylosing spondylitis** *A type of arthritis found in the spine that is exhibited by bony fusion.*
espondilolistese	**spondylolisthesis** *The overlapping of one vertebra over another.*
espondilólise	**spondylolysis** *Dissolution of the vertebra.*
espongiose	**spongiosis** *Edema of the spongy layer of the skin.*
esponja	**sponge** *Sterile fabric used to soak up fluid during surgery.*
espontâneo	**spontaneous** *Occurring without provocation.*
esporão calcâneo	**calcaneal spur** *A bony protrusion on the calcaneus.*
esporotricose	**sporotrichosis** *A Sporotrichum schenckii infection manifested by formation of lymphatic and subcutaneous nodules.*
espuma	**foam** *A mass of small bubbles in a liquid.*
espuma	**froth** *Covered with a mass of small bubbles.*
espumar por boca	**froth at the mouth, to** *To have a mass of saliva with small bubbles in it coming out of the mouth.*
esputo	**sputum** *A mixture of respiratory tract secretions and saliva.*
esqueleto	**skeleton** *Internal bony framework.*
esquema	**scheme** *A program or plan.*
esquerdo	**left**
esquimência	**quinsy** *Peritonsillar inflammation or abscess.*
esquistossomíase	**schistosomiasis** *A condition, sometimes known as bilharzia, which involves infestation with flukes of the genus Schistosoma.*
esquistócito	**schistocyte** *Part of a red blood cell seen in hemolytic anemia.*
esquizofrenia	**schizophrenia** *A chronic mental condition exhibited by delusions, hallucinations, and faulty perception.*
essencial	**essential** *Crucial or necessary.*
estadiamento	**staging** *Refers to a stratification of cancer for example.*
estado	**state** *Status.*
estado	**status** *Position or condition*
estado de equilíbrio	**steady state** *In equilibrium.*
estado nutricional	**nutritional status** *The relative state of one's nutrition.*
estado prévio	**prior status** *Referring to a person's previous state of health.*
estafiloma	**staphyloma** *Protrusion of the cornea due to inflammation.*
estafilorrafia	**staphylorrhaphy** *Surgical repair of a defect between the soft palate and uvula.*
estagnado	**standing** *Position or status.*

Portuguese	English
estalido	**click** *A sound heard by the sudden closure of a heart valve.*
estalido	**crackles or rales** *A crackling noised noted while auscultating the lungs.*
estapedectomia	**stapedectomy** *Surgical excision of the stapes.*
estase	**stasis** *Lack of movement.*
estágio final	**end stage** *Terminal stage. End stage cancer means there is no cure possible and death is imminent.*
estágio terminal	**advanced stage** *A late period of a disease.*
estático	**static** *Not changing.*
esteatoma	**steatoma** *A sebaceous cyst or lipoma.*
esteatorréia	**steatorrhea** *Excrement with an abnormally high fat content.*
esteatose	**steatosis** *Fatty degeneration; when referring to the liver it involves invasion of fat into hepatocytes.*
estender	**extend, to** *To expand or stretch out.*
estenose	**stenosis** *Narrowing of an orifice.*
estenose pulmonar	**pulmonary stenosis** *A stricture between the pulmonary artery and the right ventricle.*
estenose aórtica	**aortic stenosis** *Narrowing of the aortic orifice.*
estenose mitral	**mitral stenosis** *Narrowing of the left atrioventricular orifice.*
estercobilina	**stercobilin** *A substance created by the reduction of bilirubin and gives excrement the brown hue.*
estereognose	**astereognosis** *Lack of ability to recognize objects by touching them.*
esterilização	**sterilization** *A procedure done to prevent production of offspring.*
esternal	**sternal** *Referring to the sternum.*
esterno	**sternum** *Commonly called the breast bone, it consists of the corpus, manubrium and xiphoid process.*
esternocleidomastóide	**sternocleidomastoid** *The pair of muscles that connect the sternum, clavicle and mastoid process.*
esterognose	**stereognosis** *The ability to identify an object by touch.*
esterol	**sterol** *Unsaturated steroid alcohols such as cholesterol.*
estertor	**rale** *An abnormal lung sound noted during auscultation.*
estetoscópio	**stethoscope** *Device used to auscultate the heart, lungs and over arteries to assess for abnormalities.*
estéril	**sterile** *1. Infertile 2. Refers to equipment that is free of contamination.*
estilete	**stylet** *A thin wire within a catheter that is removed after the catheter is in place.*
estimulação cardíaco	**cardiac pacing** *Electromechanical stimulation of the heart.*
estímulo liminar	**liminal stimulus** *Referring to a stimulus of threshold strength.*
estomatite aftosa	**aphthous stomatitis** *Grouped small lesions that occur on the tongue or in the mouth.*
estomatite gangrenosa	**cancrum oris** *Gangrenous stomatitis.*
estourar nó dos dedos	**crack one's knuckles** *Moving the fingers side to side or with flexion in such a manner to cause a popping or crackling sound.*
estômago	**stomach** *Organ of digestion between the esophagus and small bowel.*
estrabismo	**strabismus** *An anomaly of ocular movement.*
estranho	**strange** *Unusual in an unsettling way.*
estreitamento	**stricture** *A narrowing of a canal or duct.*
estria	**stria** *A narrow bandlike body.*
estribo	**stapes** *This auditory ossicle is the innermost of three ossicles and is shaped like a stirrup.*

Portuguese	English
estribo	**stirrup** *An attachment to an exam table where a woman puts her legs to assist examination of the genitalia.*
estridor	**stridor** *An abnormal, high-pitched, musical sound caused by an obstruction in the larynx or stenosis of the vocal cords.*
estrogênio	**estrogen** *A hormone involved with developing and maintaining female sexual characteristics.*
estroma	**stroma** *A term used to describe the framework of an organ.*
estrutura para pacientes que precisam de mais sustentação na marcha	**walker** *A metal frame used to facilitate walking.*
estudo de controle de placebo	**placebo controlled study** *When a study is placebo controlled it means part of the group received an inactive treatment while the other group received active therapy.*
estupor	**stupor** *A reduced level of consciousness.*
estupro	**rape** *Forced sexual relations.*
etanol	**ethanol** *Synonym for ethyl alcohol.*
etiologia	**etiology** *The underlying cause of a problem.*
eunuco	**eunuch** *A man who has been castrated.*
eutanásia	**euthanasia** *Killing someone painlessly who is thought to have a terminal condition.*
evacuação	**evacuation** *The emptying of an organ of fluids or gas.*
evelhecimento	**aging** *Becoming older.*
eventração	**eventration** *Protrusion of the intestines from the abdomen.*
eversão	**eversion** *To turn outward.*
evidente	**evident** *Obvious.*
evisceração	**evisceration** *The removal of bowels from the body.*
evitável	**avoidable** *That which can be stopped or inhibited.*
evulsão	**evulsion** *Forcible extraction.*
exacerbação	**exacerbation** *Worsening of an existing problem.*
exacerbação	**flare-up** *A sudden worsening one's condition.*
exame	**examination** *Assessment or evaluation.*
exame clínico	**clinical examination** *Physical assessment data.*
exame físico	**physical exam** *Examination of a client to assess their medical status.*
exame retal digital	**rectal digital examination** *Use of a gloved finger to assess the rectal vault.*
exantema	**exanthema** *A rash that accompanies a disease or fever.*
exantema	**skin rash** *Dermal exanthema.*
exantema; erupção cutânea	**rash** *Exanthema or urticaria.*
exaustão de calor	**heat exhaustion** *A condition that occurs secondary to prolonged exposure to high ambient temperature; it is exhibited by subnormal temperature, dizziness and nausea.*
excesso	**excess** *Surplus or overabundance.*
excesso de peso	**overweight** *Defined as BMI over 25kilograms per meters squared.*
excipiente	**excipient** *An inactive substance used to deliver an active substance.*
excluir	**rule out, to** *To perform a test or exam to exclude an illness or disease.*
excoriação	**excoriation** *Superficial loss of skin.*
excreções	**excreta** *Fecal material.*
excremento; fezes	**excrement** *Feces.*
exenteração	**exenteration** *Complete surgical removal of an organ.*

Portuguese	English
exhumar	**exhumation** *To remove a dead body from a grave.*
exigente	**demanding** *Requiring a lot of skill or requiring a lot of others.*
exoftalmia; exoftalmo	**exomphalos** *Umbilical hernia.*
exostose	**exostosis** *A bony prominence growing from the surface of a bone.*
exotoxina	**exotoxin** *A toxin released from a living cell.*
exotropia	**exotropia** *A type of strabismus that is characterized by the eyes turned outward.*
exógeno	**exogenous** *Referring to external factors.*
expansão	**expansion** *Enlargement or increase in size.*
expectativa vida	**life expectancy** *The length of time a person is anticipated to live.*
expectoração	**expectoration** *The presence of sputum that has been coughed out.*
expectorante	**expectorant** *A substance that promotes the secretion of sputum.*
expiratório	**expiratory** *Referring to exhalation of air from the lungs.*
expressão (facial)	**facies** *A facial expression that is typical for a particular disease.*
expulsão	**expulsion** *Evacuation or elimination.*
expulsão placentário	**expulsion of placenta** *Passage of the placenta out the cervix after childbirth.*
exsudato	**exudate** *The fluid, cells, and debris found in the tissues or a cavity (like pleural space) during inflammation.*
extensão	**extension** *Going from a bent to straight position.*
extensor	**extensor** *Referring to the extension of an extremity or part of an extremity.*
externo	**external** *Outside of the body.*
extirpar	**extirpate, to** *To totally destroy.*
extra-sístole	**extrasystole** *Either a premature atrial or ventricular contraction.*
extracapsular	**extracapsular** *Situated outside a capsule.*
extracelular	**extracellular** *Outside the cell.*
extrato	**extract** *A substance in a concentrated form.*
extravasamento	**extravasation** *Referring to a situation in which blood or fluid goes out of a vessel it is normally flowing into.*
extremidade	**extremity** *Refers to one arm or one leg.*
extrínseco	**extrinsic** *Coming from outside or external sources.*
extubação	**extubation** *The removal of a tube that was in a body orifice.*
exudar	**weep, to** *To ooze fluid, such as from a wound.*
êmbolo	**embolus** *A blood clot, air bubble or fatty deposit that cause obstruction of a vessel.*
êmbolo de ar	**air embolism** *The blockage of an artery or vein by an air bubble.*
êmese	**emesis** *Vomiting.*
face	**face** *Anterior aspect of the head from the forehead to the chin.*
faceta	**facet** *A small flat surface of a bone.*
fadiga	**fatigue** *Tiredness and exhaustion.*
fagocitose	**phagocytosis** *The action of a phagocyte.*
fagócito	**phagocyte** *A cell capable of surrounding and digesting microorganisms.*
fala	**speech** *Oral articulation.*
falange	**phalanx** *One of the long bones of the fingers or toes.*

Portuguese	English
falciforme	**falciform** *Referring to something that is curved. The falciform ligament attaches the liver to the diaphragm.*
familial	**familial** *Referring to the family*
família	**family**
faradismo	**faradism** *The gradual increasing and decreasing of the amplitude of electricity.*
faringe	**pharynx** *The membranous cavity from the mouth to esophagus.*
faringectomia	**pharyngectomy** *Surgical excision of part of the pharynx.*
faringite	**pharyngitis** *Inflammation of the pharynx.*
faringite	**sore throat** *Common term for pharyngitis.*
faringolaríngectomia	**pharyngolaryngectomy** *Surgical removal of part of the pharynx and larynx.*
farínfeo	**pharyngeal** *Referring to the pharynx.*
farmacêutico	**pharmacist** *A professional who prepares and sells medicine through various systems, including governmental organizations like the Veterans Administration.*
farmacocinética	**pharmacokinetics** *The study of the distribution, absorption and excretion of drugs within the body.*
farmacologia	**pharmacology** *The study of all aspects of medicines.*
farmácia	**pharmacy** *A business that sells prescription medication.*
fasciculação	**fasciculation** *Involuntary contraction of muscle fibers.*
fascículo	**fascicle** *A bundle of nerve or muscle fibers.*
fasciíte	**fasciitis** *Inflammation of a fascia.*
fasciotomia	**fasciotomy** *Incision into a fascia.*
fatal	**fatal** *Lethal.*
fatia	**slice** *A sliver or shaving.*
fator anti-hemofílico	**antihemophilic factor** *Also called factor VIII. A deficiency of the factor causes hemophilia.*
fator de liberação do hormônio do crescimento	**growth hormone-releasing factor** *Released by the hypothalamus, it induces the release of somatotropin.*
fatura	**bill** *A financial statement that indicates how much one owes.*
favo	**favus** *Tinea capitis caused by Trichopyton schoenleini.*
fazer cócegas	**tickle, to** *To lightly touch a person to cause one to laugh.*
fáscia	**fascia** *The fibrous sheath enclosing a muscle or organ.*
FCE fluido cerebroespinhal	**CSF** *Abbreviation for cerebrospinal fluid.*
febre	**fever** *A temperature above the normal range.*
febre amarela	**yellow fever** *A viral, hemorrhagic fever transmitted by mosquitos.*
febre da mordida de rato	**rat bite fever** *As the name implies, it is a condition exhibited by fever, nausea and skin erythema after one is bitten by a rat.*
febre de feno	**hay fever** *An allergy exhibited by pruritus of the eyes and nose, rhinorrhea and excessive lacrimal secretion.*
febre de query	**Q fever** *A disease caused by rickettsiae from the ingestion of unpasteurized milk.*
febre de tifo	**mite fever** *Synonym of typhus fever.*
febre do mosquito-palha	**sandfly fever** *A febrile illness transmitted by a sandfly, from the genus Phlebotomus, and found in the Mediterranean.*
febre do navio; tifo epidêmico	**typhus fever** *A rickettsiae infection exhibited by rash, fever, headache and myalgia.*
febre do Vale Rift	**Rift valley fever** *A human febrile illness that is an endemic disease in sheep, transmitted by mosquitos and direct contact and caused by a virus of the family Bunyaviridae.*
febre dos arrozais	**rice-field fever** *An infection cause by a species of Leptospira, affecting rice workers in Italy and Sumatra.*

Portuguese	English
febre efêmera	**ephemeral fever** *A fever lasting no more than 24-48 hours.*
febre escaraltina	**scarlet fever** *A condition caused by streptococci that is exhibited by fever and a bright red (scarlet) rash.*
febre hemoglobinúrica	**blackwater fever** *A term used to describe the fever associated with malaria when the urine is reddish-black.*
febre ondulante; febre de Malta	**undulant fever** *Wave-like variations in the fever, going from very high to normal and back again, as seen in Brucellosis.*
febre quintã; febre das treincheiras	**quintan fever** *Also known as trench fever as it was first noted during trench warfare in WW I. It is a rickettsial fever caused by Bartonella quintana and transmitted by a louse; signs and symptoms are myalgia, headache, malaise, fever and chills.*
febre recorrente; febre da foma	**relapsing fever** *A recurrent bacterial infection, with fever, caused by Spirochetes.*
febre reumática	**rheumatic fever** *A febrile streptococcal disease causing pain and joint swelling.*
febre terçã	**tertian fever** *A febrile syndrome caused by Plasmodium vivax which produces a fever spike every 48 hours.*
febre tifóide	**typhoid fever** *A condition caused by ingestion of food or water containing salmonella typhi that is exhibited by fever and abdominal signs and symptoms.*
febre transmitida por carrapato	**tick-borne fever** *A relapsing fever caused by a spirochete of the genus Borrelia.*
febril	**febrile** *Presence of an supraphysiologic temperature.*
fecal	**feces** *Excrement.*
fechado	**closed**
fecundidade	**fecundity** *The capability of producing offspring quickly and frequently.*
fedor	**fetor** *A foul odor.*
feira	**fair** *Equitable.*
feixe de His	**atrioventricular bundle** *Also called bundle of His.*
feixe de His	**bundle of His** *The atrial contraction rhythm is facilitated by this bundle to the ventricles.*
fenda	**crevice** *A narrow opening.*
fenda palatina	**cleft palate** *A congenital abnormal opening in the palate.*
fenestração	**fenestration** *Usually referring to a surgical window.*
fenilcetonúria	**phenylketonuria** *A hereditary condition in which a person cannot excrete phenylalanine; untreated it causes brain and spinal cord dysfunction.*
fenótipo	**phenotype** *The visual expression exhibited by a person from the association of the genotype with the environment.*
ferida de bala	**gunshot wound** *An penetrating injury sustained from a bullet.*
ferida puntiforme	**stab wound** *An injury occurring with a sharp object.*
ferida; ferimento	**wound** *A tissue injury of varying severity.*
ferir	**injure, to** *To hurt or to wound.*
ferro	**iron** *An element found in hemoglobin.*
fertilidade	**fertility** *The ability of a person to contribute to contraception.*
fertilização	**fertilization** *The melding of male and female gametes to form a zygote.*
fetal	**fetal** *Referring to the fetus.*
fetichismo	**fetichism** *The glorification of an inanimate object.*
feto	**fetus** *Medical term for the infant prior to birth.*
fêmea	**female** *Feminine.*
fêmur	**femur** *The long bone in the thigh.*

Portuguese	English
fibras musgosas	**mossy fiber** *Nerve fibers that surround the nerve cells of the cerebellar cortex.*
fibrilação	**fibrillation** *Uncoordinated, ineffective contraction as in atrial fibrillation.*
fibrina	**fibrin** *An insoluble protein formed when fibrinogen is acted upon by thrombin.*
fibroadenoma	**fibroadenoma** *A benign breast mass composed of fibrous and glandular tissue.*
fibroblasto	**fibroblast** *A collagen producing cell in connective tissue.*
fibrocodrite	**fibrochondritis** *The inflammation of a structure composed of cartilage and fibrous tissue.*
fibroelastose	**fibroelastosis** *The abnormal increase in growth of fibrous and elastic tissue.*
fibromatose plantar	**plantar fibromatosis** *Deep fascia nodules on the plantar aspect of the feet.*
fibromioma	**fibromyoma** *A mass containing fibrous and muscle tissue.*
fibrose	**fibrosis** *Connective tissue that is scarred and thickened after injury.*
fibrose cística	**cystic fibrosis** *A congenital disorder exhibited by abnormal thick mucous which leads to problems in the intestines, pancreas and lungs.*
fibrosite	**fibrositis** *Fibrous connective tissue that is inflamed.*
fibrossarcoma	**fibrosarcoma** *A sarcoma composed primarily of malignant fibroblasts.*
fibróide	**fibroid** *A benign mass, typically uterine, composed of fibrous and muscle tissue.*
fibróide uterino; leiomioma uterino	**uterine fibroids** *Benign tumors made up of muscular and fibrous tissue in the uterus. This is an older term for what is now known as leiomyoma.*
fichário	**clinical record** *The ongoing medical summary.*
filamento terminal	**filum terminale** *The thin structure at the end of the conus medullaris which connects the spinal cord with the coccyx.*
filária	**filaria** *A parasitic nematode worm that is transmitted by flies and mosquitos causing filariasis.*
filha	**daughter**
filiforme	**filiform** *Threadlike.*
filtro em veia cava inferior	**vena cava filter** *A screen placed in the inferior vena cava to prevent blood clots from causing a pulmonary embolism.*
fimose	**phimosis** *Stricture of the prepuce preventing it from being pulled back over the glans penis.*
final	**last** *Final.*
fino	**thin** *Lean or slender.*
firma	**firm** *Hard or unyielding.*
fisiologia	**physiology** *A subspecialty of biology that studies the normal functioning of the body.*
fisioterapia	**physiotherapy** *Physical therapy.*
fissura	**fissure** *A general term for a cleft or deep groove. An anal fissure, for example, is a small ulcer adjacent to the anus.*
fita adesiva	**adhesive tape** *Tape used to secure dressings or intravenous lines to the body.*
fita métrica	**tape measure** *A long length of tape, marked at intervals for measuring.*
fitar	**gaze** *Steady, intent look.*
fixação	**fixation** *1. An obsessive interest. 2. The securing of a body part.*
fíbula; perônia	**fibula** *The smaller of two bones in the lower leg.*

Portuguese	English
fígado	**liver** *A large glandular organ in the right upper quadrant that functions in digestive processes, as well as, neutralizing toxins.*
fímbria	**fimbria** *A slender projection at the end of the fallopian tube near the ovary.*
fístula	**fistula** *An abnormal communication between two organs or an organ and the skin, as in rectovaginal fistula.*
fístula anal	**anal fistula** *An opening in the skin that tracts to the anal canal thus causing some fecal material to leak from the opening in the skin.*
flagelação	**flagellation** *1. The protrusion found on flagella. 2. Massage administered by tapping a body part with fingers.*
flagelo	**flagellum** *A slender appendage that allows protozoa to swim.*
flape	**flap** *A term used to describe a piece of tissue partially excised and placed over an adjacent surface.*
flato	**flatus** *Term for air that is expelled from the anus.*
flatulência	**flatulence** *The gas expulsed from the anus.*
flácido	**flaccid** *Limp. A term applied to an extremity one cannot move actively.*
flebectomia	**phlebectomy** *Surgical excision of a vein.*
flebite	**phlebitis** *Inflammation of a vein.*
flebotrombose	**phlebothrombosis** *Presence of a clot in a vein, without associated inflammation.*
flegmasia	**phlegmasia** *Inflammation or fever.*
flexor	**flexor** *A muscle that bends an extremity or part of an extremity.*
flexura	**flexure** *The action of bending.*
flexura direita do cólon	**hepatic flexure of the colon** *The junction of the ascending and transverse portion of the colon.*
flexura esplênica	**splenic flexure of the colon** *The portion of the colon that turns from the transverse to the descending colon.*
flexura sigmóide	**sigmoid flexure** *The S shaped curve located between the descending colon and rectum.*
flictenular	**phlyctenular** *Related to the formation of small vesicles on the cornea or conjunctiva.*
fluência	**flow** *Movement in a continuous stream.*
fluido amniótico	**amniotic fluid** *The fluid surrounding the fetus.*
fluido cerebroespinhal	**cerebrospinal fluid (CSF)** *The fluid between the pia mater and arachnoid membrane.*
fluido intra-ocular	**intraocular fluid** *Fluid within the globe.*
fluido lacrimal	**lacrimal fluid** *Fluid secreted by the lacrimal gland.*
fluido sinovial	**synovial fluid** *The fluid that surrounds, for example, the knee within a capsule.*
fluoresceína	**fluoresceine** *A fluorane dye used to check for corneal ulcers.*
fluorescência tela	**fluorescent screen** *A screen used to view x-rays.*
fluoretação	**fluoridation** *The addition of fluorine to something.*
fluoroscopia	**fluoroscopy** *The continuous viewing of roentgenographic images with a fluorescent screen.*
flutuante	**floating** *Buoyant or suspended.*
fluxo de ar	**air flow** *The rate of air movement.*
fluxo máximo	**peak flow** *A measurement of lung function used in asthma.*
flúor	**fluorine** *A chemical that causes severe burns if exposed to the skin.*
fobia	**phobia** *An profound fear of something.*
foice do cérebro	**falx cerebri** *A fold in the dura that separates the two cerebral hemispheres.*

Portuguese	English
folicular	**follicular** *Referring to a small secretory gland.*
folículo piloso	**hair follicle** *Tubelike invagination of the epidermis that the hair shaft develops from.*
fome	**hunger** *A sense of discomfort caused by a lack of food.*
fome aérea	**air hunger** *The sensation of shortness of breath.*
fonação	**phonation** *The vocalization of sounds.*
foniatria	**phoniatrics** *The treatment of speech abnormalities.*
fontanela	**fontanelle or fontanel** *The space between the bones in the skull that are separate at birth.*
fora de	**away from** *Separated from.*
forame	**foramen** *An opening in a bone.*
forame magno	**foramen magnum** *The hole in the skull that the spinal cord passes through.*
forame nutriente	**nutrient foramen** *A conduit for passage of nutrient vessels in the marrow of bone.*
forame oval	**foramen ovale** *A hole in the atrial septal wall in a fetus.*
forame oval permeável	**patent foramen ovale** *A congenital anomaly in which there is a defect in the wall between the right and left atria; this can be a benign condition or result in cryptogenic strokes.*
força	**strength** *Force, might or vigor.*
forense	**forensic** *Referring to the scientific method of studying crime.*
formador	**former** *Prior.*
formigamento	**tingling** *Prickling or stinging sensation.*
formulário	**formulary** *A list of medicines that are permissible to prescribe.*
forte	**strong** *Having the power to move heavy objects.*
fosfatase ácida	**acid phosphatase** *A phosphate derived chemical that is optimally active in an acidic environment.*
fosfatúria	**phosphaturia** *Presence of phosphates in the urine.*
fosfolipídeo	**phospholipid** *A substance, such as lecithin, that when hydrolyzed produces fatty acids, glycerin, and a nitrogen compound.*
fosfonecrose	**phosphonecrosis** *The breakdown of the mandible caused by excessive exposure to phosphorus.*
fossa	**fossa** *A shallow depression.*
fossa cubital	**cubital fossa** *The bend at the elbow.*
fossa popliteo	**popliteal fossa** *The hollow in the posterior aspect of the knee joint.*
fotofobia	**photophobia** *Abnormal sensitivity to light.*
fotossensibilização	**photosensitization** *The process of reacting to sunlight by developing edema and dermatitis.*
fotômetro de chama	**flame photometer** *A device used to measure the intensity of light.*
fórceps; pinça	**forceps** *A surgical instrument, commonly called tweezers.*
fórnice	**fornix** *A vaulted structure.*
fóvea	**fovea** *The area on the retina where the visual acuity is optimal.*
fraco de espírito	**feeble-minded** *Antiquated term used to describe a person unable to make seemingly simple decisions because of a cognitive impairment.*
fragilidade ósseo	**fragilitas ossium** *A condition exhibited by excessively brittle bones. Also called osteogenesis imperfecta.*
fralda	**diaper** *Undergarment worn to absorb urine in incontinent persons.*
framboesia	**framboesia; yaws** *An endemic tropical disease caused by Treponema pertenue.*

Portuguese	English
framboesia	**yaws** *A tropical disease characterized by ulcers on the extremities, caused by Treponema pertenue.*
frasco	**flask** *A narrow-necked container.*
frasco	**vial** *A small cylindrical container typically used to hold liquid medicine.*
fratura	**break** *A common term for a fracture in a bone.*
fratura	**fracture** *A broken bone.*
fratura aberta	**compound fracture** *Open fracture.*
fratura aberta	**fracture, open** *A fracture in which there is a break in the skin and bone is exposed.*
fratura afundamento	**fracture, depressed** *The presence of concavity associated with a fracture as in a depressed skull fracture.*
fratura cominutiva	**fracture, comminuted** *A broken bone where one segment overrides the other.*
fratura do crânio com afundamento	**depressed skull fracture** *Concave fracture deformity of the skull.*
fratura em galho verde	**fracture, greenstick** *A spiral fracture.*
fratura fechada	**fracture, closed** *A broken bone where there is no break in the skin.*
fratura patológico	**fracture, pathologic** *A fracture due at least in part to another condition, such as a fracture at a location where there is bone cancer.*
fratura por avulsão	**fracture, avulsion** *A broken bone associated with a ligament or tendon pulling a piece of the bone away.*
fratura por estresse	**fracture, stress** *A fracture associated with overuse.*
fratura por tensão	**stress fracture** *A long bone fracture caused by repetitive mechanical stress.*
frenicectomia	**phrenicectomy** *Surgical excision of the phrenic nerve.*
frenoplegia	**phrenoplegia** *Paralysis of the diaphragm.*
freqüência	**frequency** *Rate of occurrence.*
freqüência cardíaca	**heart rate** *Number or cardiac contractions per minute.*
freqüência respiratória	**respiratory rate** *The number of breaths per minute.*
fresco; frio	**cool** *Chilly or cold.*
frêmito	**fremitus** *A vibration that is appreciated with palpation.*
frênico	**phrenic** *Referring to the diaphragm.*
frênulo	**frenulum** *The tissue that connects the inferior portion of the tongue to the base of the mouth.*
friável	**friable** *Easily reduced to powder.*
fricção	**friction** *Grating or rasping.*
frio	**algid** *cold*
frio (temperatura baixa)	**cold** *Having a sense of being cold.*
frontal	**frontal** *Referring to the anterior aspect, as in frontal lobe.*
fronte	**forehead** *Section of the face from the hairline to the eyebrows.*
frouxidão	**laxity** *A description of a joint that is loose.*
frouxidão	**looseness** *Possessing a quality of not being tight.*
frutosúria	**fructosuria** *Presence of fructose in the urine.*
fuga de idéias	**flight of ideas** *Streams of unrelated ideas noted in a manic phase.*
fulminante	**fulminant** *Sudden and severe.*
fumar	**smoke, to** *To inhale on a cigarette.*
funcionamento prolongado	**long-acting** *Referring to a drug with long lasting effects.*
função	**function** *An activity natural to a person or thing.*
função, perdir	**loss of function** *Inability to complete routine activities.*

Portuguese	English
funda	**truss** *A synthetic device for containing a hernia within the abdomen.*
fundo de olho	**fundus oculi** *Portion of the interior eyeball in the posterior aspect which can be viewed by an ophthalmoscope.*
fundo do olho	**eyeground** *The fundus that is visualized with an ophthalmoscope.*
fundo gástrico	**fundus of the stomach** *Referring to the part of the stomach above the cardiac notch.*
fungada	**sniffing** *Short, rapid nasal inhalation.*
fungicida	**fungicide** *An agent that destroys fungus.*
fungo	**fungus** *A spore-producing organism that feeds on organic matter.*
funiculite	**funiculitis** *Inflammation of the funiculi.*
funículo da medula espinhal	**funiculus of the spinal cord** *The white matter of the spinal cord that is further defined by location.*
funículo lateral	**funiculus, lateral** *The lateral white column of the spinal cord between the anterior and posterior nerve roots.*
furunculose	**furunculosis** *The presence of multiple furuncles.*
furúnculo	**furuncle** *A painful erythematous nodule with a central core.*
fusiforme	**fusiform** *Spindle-shaped.*
fuso acromático	**achromatic spindle** *The threads between the poles of the spindle in karyokinesis.*
fúrcula	**fourchette** *The fork shaped fold of skin where the labia minora meet superior to the perineum.*
gagueira	**stammering** *The impulse to repeat the first letter of words and involuntary pauses while speaking.*
galactocele	**galactocele** *A milk-filled cyst in the mammary gland.*
galactorréia	**galactorrhea** *Excessive production of milk.*
galactose	**galactose** *A sugar that is a constituent of lactose.*
galactosemia	**galactosemie** *1. Galactose in the blood. 2. A congenital condition exhibited by impaired carbohydrate metabolism.*
galope	**gallop** *An abnormal heart sound.*
galvanismo	**galvanism** *The use of electric currents for medical treatment.*
galvanômetro	**galvanometer** *A device used to measure small electric currents.*
gamaglobulina	**gamma globulin** *A blood serum protein with little electrophoretic mobility.*
gameta	**gamete** *A germ cell that is able to unite with another germ cell of the opposite gender to form a zygote.*
ganglionectomia	**ganglionectomy** *The removal of a benign swelling on a tendon sheath.*
gangrena	**gangrene** *Tissue death from either impaired blood flow or an infection.*
gangrena gasosa	**gas gangrene** *A life and limb threatening disorder caused associated with tissue death and caused by an anaerobic bacterium in the genus of Clostridium.*
gara de macaco	**monkey-paw** *An appearance due to median nerve palsy causing atrophy of the thenar eminence with adduction and elevation of the thumb, resembling that of a simian.*
gargalhar	**laugh, to**
garganta	**throat** *The anterior aspect of the neck.*
gargarejar	**gargle, to** *To rinse one's mouth out and exhale through the liquid.*
gargulismo	**gargoylism** *A congenital defect, also known as Hurler syndrome, it is characterized by skeletal anomalies, mental retardation and gargoyle-like facial features.*

Portuguese	English
garrafa	**bottle** *A container used for the storage of liquids.*
garrote	**tourniquet** *A device tied tightly around an extremity to diminish blood flow or blood loss.*
gasimetria arterial	**arterial blood gas** *Measurement of the arterial concentration of carbon dioxide and oxygen.*
gastrectomia	**gastrectomy** *Complete or partial surgical resection of the stomach.*
gastrina	**gastrin** *Hormones that stimulates gastric secretions.*
gastrite	**gastritis** *Inflammation of the stomach.*
gastrocele	**gastrocele** *Protrusion of part of the stomach in the form of a hernia.*
gastrocnêmio	**gastrocnemius** *A large muscle in the lower leg, responsible for ankle plantar flexion, that is attached to the distal femur and achilles tendon.*
gastroenterite	**gastroenteritis** *A bacterial or viral infection that leads to vomiting and diarrhea.*
gastroenterostomia	**gastroenterostomy** *A surgical opening in the stomach or intestine.*
gastroesofagopatia por refluxo (GEPR)	**GERD gastroesophageal reflux disease** *A condition characterized by gastric contents being regurgitated into the esophagus or mouth.*
gastrojejunostomia	**gastrojejunostomy** *A surgical procedure that directly connects the stomach to the jejunum.*
gastropexia	**gastropexy** *Securing the stomach to the abdominal wall.*
gastroscopia	**gastroscopy** *Use of an endoscope to directly visualize the stomach.*
gastrostomia	**gastrostomy** *A surgical creation of an opening in the stomach.*
gavagem	**gavage** *The instillation of food into the stomach with use of a tube.*
gaze	**gauze** *A fabric used for dressing changes.*
gástrico	**gastric** *Referring to the stomach.*
gânglio da base	**basal ganglia** *Structures adjacent to the thalamus that are involved with coordination of movement.*
gânglio espinhal	**spinal ganglion** *The ganglion located on the dorsal root of each spinal nerve.*
gânglio estrelado	**stellate ganglion** *Formed by the seventh cervical, eighth cervical and first thoracic ganglia.*
gânglio geniculado	**geniculate ganglion** *The sensory ganglion of the facial nerve.*
gel; gelatina	**gel** *A jellylike substance.*
gelado	**frozen** *Past participle of to freeze. Freeze: turn a liquid into a solid.*
geladura	**frostbite** *Local tissue destruction after exposure to cold.*
gemente	**grunting** *A low guttural sound used to describe a person with profound respiratory difficulty.*
gemido	**groan** *A deep inarticulate sound made due to pain or despair.*
gene	**gene** *A unit of heredity that is passed on from parent to child.*
genético	**genetic** *Referring to genes or heredity.*
gengiva	**gum** *Gingiva.*
gengival	**gingival** *Referring to the gums.*
gengivite	**gingivitis** *Inflammation of the gums.*
geniculado	**geniculate** *Bent at a sharp angle.*
genitália	**genitalia** *Genitals.*

Portuguese	English
genitália ambigua	**genital ambiguity** *A disorder of sexual development in which the genitalia are not sufficiently developed to tell clearly if the person is male or female.*
genitourinário	**genitourinary** *Referring to the urinary system through the organs or urine excretion.*
genoma	**genome** *A full set of genetic information for an organism.*
genu valgum; joelho valgo	**knock knees** *Common term for genu valgum.*
genuflexão	**kneeling** *Being on one's knees as in the prayer position.*
geriatria	**geriatrics** *The study of the health of old people.*
germe	**germ** *Microorganism.*
gerontologia	**gerontology** *The study of old persons.*
gestação; gravidez	**gestation** *The development of a fetus from conception until birth.*
gêmeos	**twins** *Two infants born at the same birthing.*
gêmeos dizigóticos	**dizygotic twins** *Twins from two separate zygotes (non-identical twins).*
gêmeos idênticos	**identical twins** *Twins from the same zygote.*
giardíase	**giardiasis** *A flagellate protozoa, Giardia lamblia, that causes diarrhea.*
gigante	**giant** *Huge or massive.*
ginecologia	**gynecology** *The branch of medicine associated with the reproductive system of women.*
ginecomastia	**gynecomastia** *Enlargement of the breasts.*
giro	**gyrus** *Convolutions of the brain where there is infolding.*
gínglimo	**ginglymus** *A joint that allows movement in one direction only.*
glabela	**glabella** *The area of the forehead above and between the eyebrows.*
glande mamária	**mammary gland** *The mass of tissue posterior to the nipples which has the essential task of milk production.*
glande peniana	**glans penis** *The distal aspect of the penis.*
glande pineal	**pineal gland** *A small body posterior to the third ventricle of the brain.*
glande pituitário	**pituitary gland** *A gland at the base of the hypothalamus.*
glande salivar	**salivary gland** *The parotid, submandibular and sublingual glands that secrete saliva.*
glande sebáceo	**sebaceous gland** *A gland in the skin that secretes sebum.*
glaucoma	**glaucoma** *A condition characterized by increased intraocular pressure.*
glândula acinosa	**acinous gland** *The exocrine part of the pancreas.*
glândula apôcrina	**apocrine gland** *A gland that releases some of its cytoplasm in secretions; an example is axillary sweat glands.*
glândula endócrino	**endocrine gland** *A gland that secrete hormones and other substances into the blood.*
glândula supra-renal	**adrenal gland** *A gland located on the superior aspect of both kidneys.*
glenóide	**glenoid** *Referring to the fossa that is a shallow depression, such as the hollow of the scapula where the humeral head sets.*
glicemia	**glycemia** *The amount of glucose in the blood.*
glicerina	**glycerin** *A byproduct in the manufacture of soap that is used as a laxative.*
glicogênio	**glycogen** *A compound that stores glucose and when it undergoes hydrolysis forms glucose.*
glicoproteína	**glycoprotein** *A protein that has a carbohydrate attached to its polypeptide chain.*

Portuguese	English
glicosúria	**glycosuria** *Presence of glucose in the urine.*
glicólise	**glycolysis** *The production of energy and pyruvic acid when glucose is broken down by enzymes.*
gliocogênese	**glycogenesis** *The production of glycogen from glucose.*
glioma	**glioma** *A neural malignant tumor of glial cells.*
gliomiome	**gliomyoma** *A mass with gliomatous and myomatous characteristics.*
globo pálido	**globus pallidus** *A portion of the lentiform nucleus in the brain.*
globulina anti-linfocito	**antilymphocyte globulin** *The gamma globulin portion of antilymphocyte serum.*
glomerulonefrite	**glomerulonephritis** *Inflammation of the renal glomeruli, usually from hemolytic streptococcus.*
glomérulo	**glomerulus** *A grouping of capillaries where waste is filtered from the blood.*
glossal	**glossal** *Referring to the tongue.*
glossectomia	**glossectomy** *Surgical resection of the whole or part of the tongue.*
glossina; moscas tsé-tsé	**tsetse fly** *An insect that transmits the protozoa trypanosoma and can cause sleeping sickness.*
glossite	**glossitis** *Inflammation of the tongue.*
glossodinia	**glossodynia** *Tongue pain.*
glossofaríngeo	**glossopharyngeal** *The name for cranial nerve IX that supplies the tongue and pharynx.*
glote	**glottis** *Essentially the vocal structure, including the true vocal cords and the opening between them.*
glóbulo líquido, um	**drop** *A single bit of fluid as in a drop seen while giving IV fluids.*
glucagon	**glucagon** *A pancreatic enzyme responsible for breakdown of glycogen to glucose.*
glúteo	**gluteal** *Referring to the gluteus.*
gnático	**gnathic** *Referring to the jaws.*
gnose	**gnosia** *Ability to recognize things and people.*
godura	**fat** *A greasy or oiling substance naturally occurring in the body.*
goiva	**gouge** *A chisel with a concave blade used in surgery.*
golpe de vista	**glance** *A brief look at something.*
goma de mascar	**gum (chewing gum)**
goma; sifiloma	**gumma** *A soft granulomatous tumor of the skin or cardiovascular system seen in tertiary syphilis.*
gonadotrofina	**gonadotrophin** *Pituitary hormone that promotes gonadal activity.*
gonococo	**gonococcus** *A diploccocal bacteria that is the causative agent in gonorrhea, formally Neisseria gonorrhoeae.*
gonorréia	**gonorrhea** *A sexually transmitted disease that is exhibited by purulent discharge from the vagina or penis.*
gorduroso	**fatty** *Greasy or oily.*
gota	**gout** *Monosodium urate crystal deposition disease.*
gota a gota	**drop by drop** *Expression meaning little by little.*
gotas oftalmológicas	**eye drops** *Liquid applied to eyes for various medical problems.*
gotas por minuto	**drops per minute** *Refers to iv fluid rate.*
gotejamento pós-nasal	**post-nasal drip** *The descent of sinus drainage.*
gotejar	**dribble, to** *To slowly, drip-by-drip, release urine for example.*
gônada	**gonad** *A testis or an ovary.*
gradeado	**cancellous** *A bony mesh-like structure with many pores.*

Portuguese	English
grama	**gram** *A unit of mass, 1/1000th of a kilogram.*
grampo	**cramp** *A painful contraction of muscles.*
grande lábio pudendo	**labium majus (plural= labia majora)** *The folds of skin forming the lateral borders of the pudendal cleft.*
granuloma	**granuloma** *A mass of granulation tissue.*
granulócito	**granulocyte** *A white blood cell with cytoplasmic secretory granules.*
gravidez	**pregnancy** *The period of being pregnant.*
gravidez e parto	**bear, to** *To give birth to a child.*
gravidez ectópica	**ectopic pregnancy** *A pregnancy that is not intrauterine.*
gráfico anatômico	**anatomical chart** *A pictorial diagram of part of the anatomy.*
gráficos coloridos de Ruess	**color chart** *A card used to check for color blindness.*
grávida	**gravida** *Pregnant.*
gritar	**yell, to** *To speak in a loud tone.*
grosa	**gross** *Distended; not well defined.*
grude	**paste** *A thick, soft moist substance usually with medicine mixed in.*
guáiaco	**guaiac** *A substance derived from guaiacum trees used to test for trace amounts of blood, in stool for instance.*
gustativo	**gustatory** *Referring to sense of taste.*
guteral	**guttural** *Having a harsh quality; coming from the back of the throat.*
halitose	**halitosis** *Foul odor emanating from the mouth.*
hamartoma	**hamartoma** *A nodule of superfluous tissue.*
hamato; uncinado	**hamate bone; uncinate bone** *The medial bone in the distal row of carpal bones adjacent to the fifth metacarpal.*
haplóide	**haploid** *Either a single set of chromosomes or a set of nonhomologous chromosomes.*
hapteno	**hapten** *The molecular component that determines immunologic specificity.*
hábito	**habit** *A custom or inclination.*
hálux valgo	**hallux valgus** *Also called bunion, it is the lateral deviation of the great toe.*
hálux varo	**hallux varus** *Medial deviation of the great toe.*
hebefrenia	**hebephrenia** *A type of schizophrenia exhibited by hallucinations and inappropriate laughter.*
hedonismo	**hedonism** *Devoting oneself to being happy.*
helioaeroterapia	**heliotherapy** *Treatment of disease with sunlight.*
helmintíase	**helminthiasis** *Being infected by a helminth.*
helminto	**helminth** *A fluke, tapeworm or nematode.*
hemaglutinina	**hemagglutinin** *An antibody that facilitates the agglutination of blood.*
hemangioma	**hemangioma** *A benign tumor composed of blood vessels.*
hemangioma cavernoso	**cavernous hemangioma** *A tumor composed of connective tissue with blood filled areas.*
hemartrose	**hemarthrosis** *Presence of intra-articular blood.*
hematêmese	**hematemesis** *Vomiting blood.*
hematina	**hematin** *The insoluble iron protoporphyrin component of hemoglobin.*
hematocele	**hematocele** *A mass or area of swelling caused by the accumulation of blood.*
hematoma	**hematoma** *A mass containing blood.*

Portuguese	English
hematoma epidural	**epidural hematoma** *Formation of a collection of blood outside the dural layer of the brain; usually caused by trauma.*
hematoma subdural	**subdural hematoma** *Formation of a blood clot between the dura mater and the arachnoid membrane.*
hematométria	**hematometra** *The accretion of blood in the uterus.*
hematomielia	**hematomyelia** *Accumulation of blood in the spinal cord.*
hematoporfirina	**hematoporphyrin** *A derivative of heme that does not contain iron.*
hematoquezia	**hematochezia** *Presence of blood in the excrement.*
hematossalpinge	**hematosalpinx** *Presence of blood in the fallopian tube.*
hematócrito	**hematocrit** *The measurement of the volume of red blood cells compared to the total volume of blood; recorded in percent.*
hematúria	**hematuria** *The presence of blood in the urine.*
heme	**heme** *A constituent of hemoglobin that is an insoluble iron protoporphyrin.*
hemeralopia	**hemeralopia** *Night blindness.*
hemianopsia bitemporal	**bitemporal hemianopsia** *A visual defect seen commonly in pituitary tumors in which the visual defect is in the temporal portion of each eye.*
hemianopsia quadrântica	**quadranic hemianopia** *Loss of a quarter of the visual field in one or both eyes. If bilateral, it may be further described as homonymous, heteronymous, binasal, bitemporal, or crossed.*
hemianopsia; hemianopia	**hemianopsia** *Blindness over half the field of vision.*
hemibalismo	**hemiballismus** *Severe motor restlessness unilaterally, usually from a subthalamic lesion.*
hemicolectomia	**hemicolectomy** *Surgical removal of part of the colon.*
hemicrânia	**hemicrania** *1. Pain on one side of the head. 2. Incomplete anencephaly.*
hemicrânia; enxaqueca	**migraine** *An episodic, unilateral headache accompanied by nausea.*
hemiparesia	**hemiparesis** *Unilateral muscle weakness (half the body).*
hemiplegia	**hemiplegia** *Paralysis of one side of the body.*
hemisfera	**hemisphere** *Referring to either the right or left portion of the cerebrum.*
hemizigoto	**hemizygote** *A cell with only one set of genes.*
hemocitômetro	**hemocytometer** *A device used for counting cells from a blood sample.*
hemoconcentração	**hemoconcentration** *Decrease in the total fluid content of the blood, leading at times to a falsely elevated hematocrit.*
hemocromatose	**hemochromatosis** *A hereditary condition exhibited by iron deposition in the tissue and leading to liver disease, bronze discoloration of the skin and diabetes.*
hemodiálise	**hemodialysis** *The process of filtering blood outside the body to remove toxins normally excreted by functioning kidneys.*
hemofilia	**hemophilia** *A hereditary bleeding disorder characterized by hemarthroses and deep tissue bleeding as a result of absence of a coagulation factor such as factor VIII.*
hemofílico	**hemophiliac** *A person with hemophilia.*
hemoftalmia	**hemophthalmia** *Bleeding within the eye.*
hemoglobina	**hemoglobin** *An iron containing protein used for the transport of oxygen in blood.*
hemoglobinúria	**hemoglobinuria** *Presence of free hemoglobin in the urine.*
hemolítico	**hemolytic** *Something that causes hemolysis.*
hemopericárdio	**hemopericardium** *Abnormal presence of blood in the pericardium.*

Portuguese	English
hemoperitôneo	**hemoperitoneum** *Abnormal presence of blood in the peritoneum.*
hemopneumotórax	**hemopneumothorax** *Accumulation of blood and air in the pleural space.*
hemopoiese	**hemopoiesis** *The production of blood cells from stem cells.*
hemopoiético	**hemopoietic** *Referring to a hormone secreted by the kidneys that stimulates the bone marrow to produce erythrocytes.*
hemoptise	**hemoptysis** *Expectoration of blood.*
hemorragia	**hemorrhage** *Bleeding from a damaged blood vessel.*
hemorroidectomia	**hemorrhoidectomy** *Surgical excision of a hemorrhoid.*
hemorróidas	**hemorrhoids** *Engorgement of the veins in the anus or rectum.*
hemostasia	**hemostasis** *The control of bleeding.*
hemotórax	**hemothrorax** *The abnormal presence of blood in the pleural cavity.*
hemólise	**hemolysis** *Breakdown of hemoglobin.*
heparina	**heparin** *A polysaccharide that occurs naturally in the liver and is used as a medication to induce a hypocoagulable state.*
hepatectomia	**hepatectomy** *Partial or complete surgical resection of the liver.*
hepatite	**hepatitis** *Inflammation of the liver.*
hepatite colestática	**cholestatic hepatitis** *Liver inflammation caused by obstruction of bile flow from the liver to the duodenum.*
hepatoma	**hepatoma** *A tumor of the liver.*
hepatomegalia	**hepatomegaly** *Enlargement of the liver.*
hepatosplenomegalia	**hepatosplenomegaly** *Enlargement of the spleen and the liver.*
hepatócito	**hepatocyte** *A liver cell.*
hepático	**hepatic** *Referring to the liver.*
hereditário	**hereditary** *That which is transmitted genetically*
hermafrodita	**hermaphrodite** *A person possessing gonadal characteristics of both sexes.*
herniação tronco cerebral	**brainstem herniation** *Movement of the brainstem into the incisura because of increased intracranial pressure.*
herniorrafia	**herniorrhaphy** *The surgical repair of a hernia.*
heroína	**heroin** *A morphine derivative that is highly addictive.*
herpangina	**herpangina** *An infectious disease caused by Coxsackie virus exhibited by vesicular lesion on the soft palate.*
herpes	**herpes** *A skin condition exhibited by formation of clustered vesicular lesions; herpes simplex is at times referred to, albeit incompletely, as herpes.*
herpes genital	**genital herpes** *A sexually transmitted infection caused by herpes simplex.*
herpes simples	**cold sore** *A perioral blister caused by herpes simplex.*
herpes zóster	**shingles** *A reactivation of herpes zoster.*
herpes zóster; zona	**herpes zoster; shingles** *A unilateral vesicular rash along one dermatome and caused by inflammation of a posterior nerve root by "the chicken pox virus".*
herpetiforme	**herpetiform** *Something that is characteristic of herpes.*
herpético	**herpetic** *Referring to herpes.*
heterogêneo	**heterogenous** *That which originates outside the organism.*
heterotopia	**heterotropia** *Synonym of strabismus.*
heterozigoto	**heterozygous** *Having different alleles concerning a certain trait.*
hélio	**helium** *An inert gas that is the lightest of the noble gases.*
hérnia encarcerada	**hernia, incarcerated** *An irreducible hernia.*

Portuguese	English
hérnia femoral	**hernia, femoral** *A bulge in the upper thigh/groin region because of bowel protruding through the muscle. Also called crural hernia.*
hérnia diafragmática	**diaphragmatic hernia** *Protrusion of visceral contents through the diaphragm.*
hérnia do hiato	**hiatus hernia** *Protrusion of part of the stomach through the esophageal hiatus of the diaphragm.*
hérnia inguinal	**hernia, inguinal** *Protrusion of abdominal-cavity contents through the inguinal canal.*
hérnia lombar	**hernia, lumbar** *Defect in the lumbar muscles or the posterior fascia, below the 12th rib and above the iliac crest.*
hérnia umbilical	**hernia, umbilical** *Protrusion of abdominal contents at the umbilicus.*
hialina	**hyaline** *Having a glassy, transparent appearance.*
hialóide	**hyaloid** *Transparent.*
hidatiforme	**hydatiform** *Referring to a hydatid cyst.*
hidradenite	**hidradenitis** *Inflammation of a sweat gland. When there is purulent discharge it is called hidradenitis suppurativa.*
hidrartrose	**hydrarthrosis** *An accumulation of water-like fluid in a joint cavity.*
hidratação	**hydration** *Used to describe fluid balance.*
hidrocefalia	**hydrocephalus** *The excessive accumulation of cerebral spinal fluid in the brain causing enlargement of the head.*
hidrocele	**hydrocele** *The accumulation of fluid in a body sac.*
hidrocele funicular	**scrotal hydrocele** *A benign collection of fluid in the scrotum.*
hidrocortisona	**hydrocortisone** *A natural steroid hormone secreted by the adrenal cortex and used in a synthetic formulation for treatment of various medical conditions.*
hidrofobia	**hydrophobia** *Abnormal fear of water.*
hidronefrose	**hydronephrosis** *Enlargement of a kidney due to interruption of outflow of urine from that kidney.*
hidropneumotórax	**hydropneumothorax** *Abnormal accumulation of fluid and air in the pleural space.*
hidropsia	**hydrops** *The abnormal collection of fluid in a cavity.*
hidropsia fetal	**hydrops fetalis** *The total body accumulation of fluid in a fetus; the result of a hemolytic reaction in a Rh neg mother.*
hidrose	**hidrosis** *The production and secretion of sweat.*
hidrossalpinge	**hydrosalpinx** *Collection of fluid in a fallopian tube.*
hidrotórax	**hydrothorax** *Accumulation of fluid within the thoracic cavity.*
hidrólise	**hydrolysis** *A reaction with water causing a compound to breakdown.*
hifema	**hyphema** *A blood collection in the front of the eye.*
higiene oral	**oral hygiene** *Cleansing of the mouth and associated structures.*
higroma	**hygroma** *A cyst or bursa filled with fluid.*
higroscópico	**hygroscopic** *The tendency to absorb moisture from the air.*
hilar	**hilar** *Referring to a hilus.*
hilo	**hilum or hilus** *A depression where blood vessels and nerve fibers enter an organ.*
himenotomia	**hymenotomy** *Surgically creating an opening in the hymen.*
hipcampo	**hippocampus** *The area at the base of the cerebral ventricles thought to be the center of memory and emotion.*
hiper-reflexia	**hyperreflexia** *Abnormally brisk and vigorous reflex.*
hiperalgesia	**hyperalgesia** *Greater than normal sensitivity to pain.*
hiperatividade	**hyperactivity** *Abnormal increase in activity.*

Portuguese	English
hiperácido	**hyperacidity** *An abnormally high acid level.*
hiperbárico	**hyperbaric** *Use of gas at a higher than normal pressure.*
hiperbilirrubinemia	**hyperbilirubinemia** *Higher than normal level of bilirubin in the blood.*
hipercalcemia	**hypercalcemia** *Higher than normal level of calcium in the blood.*
hipercalemia	**hyperkalemia** *Higher than normal level of potassium in the blood stream.*
hipercapnia	**hypercapnia** *Higher than normal level of carbon dioxide in the blood stream.*
hiperceratose	**hyperkeratosis** *Excessive thickening of the outer layer of skin.*
hipercinese	**hyperkinesis** *Excessive activity and inability to concentrate.*
hipercolesterolemia	**high cholesterol** *Elevated serum cholesterol.*
hipercolesterolemia	**hypercholesterolemia** *Higher than normal level of cholesterol in the blood.*
hipercromia	**hyperchromia** *An excessive level of hemoglobin in erythrocytes.*
hiperemia	**hyperemia** *An increase in blood for the area of concern.*
hiperesplenismo	**hypersplenism** *Excessive splenic activity resulting in decreased peripheral blood elements and sometimes splenomegaly.*
hiperestesia	**hyperesthesia** *Higher than normal skin sensitivity.*
hiperextensão	**hyperextension** *Extension of an articulation beyond the normal range.*
hiperfagia	**hyperphagia** *Excessive food ingestion.*
hiperflexão	**hyperflexion** *Flexion of an articulation beyond the normal range.*
hiperforia	**hyperphoria** *Upward deviation of the visual axis of the eye.*
hiperglicemia	**hyperglycemia** *Higher than normal level of glucose in the blood.*
hipergonadismo	**hypergonadism** *A condition of excessive gonadal activity and subsequently precocious sexual development.*
hiperidrose	**hyperhidrosis** *Excessive perspiration.*
hiperisotônico	**hypertonic** *Increased osmotic pressure.*
hiperlipemia	**hyperlipidemia** *Higher than normal level of lipids in the blood stream.*
hipermetropia	**hypermetropia** *Farsightedness.*
hipermiotonia	**hypermyotonia** *Excessive muscle tone.*
hipermnésia	**hypermnesia** *Unusually good memory.*
hipernatremia	**hypernatremia** *Elevated level of sodium in the blood.*
hipernefroma	**hypernephroma** *A renal tumor that mimic adrenal cortical tissue.*
hiperoníquia	**hyperonychia** *Hypertrophic nails.*
hiperopia	**hyperopia** *Farsightedness.*
hiperopia	**longsighted** *Synonym of hyperopia.*
hiperosmia	**hyperosmia** *Increased sense of smell.*
hiperparatireoidismo	**hyperparathyroidism** *Excessive level of parathyroid hormones in the blood stream causing weak bones and hypocalcemia.*
hiperpirexia	**hyperpyrexia** *Fever.*
hiperpituitarismo	**hyperpituitarism** *Excessive eosinophilic hormone resulting in acromegaly or excessive basophilic hormone resulting in pituitary compression and ultimately hypopituitarism.*
hiperplasia	**hyperplasia** *Excessive growth of normal cells.*
hiperpnéia	**hyperpnea** *Abnormal increase in rate and depth of respiration.*
hipersensibilidade	**hypersensitivity** *Abnormal increase in sensitivity.*

Portuguese	English
hipertemia	**hyperthermia** *Fever.*
hipertensão	**high blood pressure** *Elevated arterial blood pressure.*
hipertensão	**hypertension** *Higher than normal blood pressure.*
hipertensão maligna	**malignant hypertension** *Sudden, severe hypertension associated with neuroretinitis.*
hipertensão porta	**portal hypertension** *Hypertension in the portal system of the liver as seen in conditions causing obstruction to the portal vein.*
hipertireoidismo	**hyperthyroidism** *Increased thyroid activity resulting in exophthalmos and increased metabolic rate.*
hipertonia	**hypertonia** *Excessive tone or tension.*
hipertricose	**hypertrichosis** *Excessive hair growth.*
hipertrofia	**hypertrophy** *Pathologic organ enlargement.*
hiperuricemia	**hyperuricemia** *Elevated level of uric acid in the blood.*
hiperventilação	**hyperventilation** *Rapid and deep respirations.*
hipervolemia	**hypervolemia** *Abnormally large amount of fluid in the blood stream.*
hipnótico	**hypnotic** *Sleep inducing agent.*
hipocalcemia	**hypocalcemia** *Lower than normal level of calcium in the blood.*
hipocalemia	**hypokalemia** *Diminished level of potassium in the blood stream.*
hipocapnia	**hypocapnia** *A decreased level of carbon dioxide in the blood.*
hipocloridria	**hypochlorhydria** *A state of decreased secretion of hydrochloric acid in the stomach.*
hipocondria	**hypochondriac** *A person suffering from hypochondriasis.*
hipocondria	**hypochondriasis** *Abnormal increase in concern about one's own health.*
hipocôndrio	**hypochondrium** *The upper abdomen lateral to the epigastrium.*
hipocrômico	**hypochromic** *Referring to the abnormal decrease in hemoglobin content of erythrocytes.*
hipoestesia	**hypoesthesia** *Abnormally decreased skin sensitivity.*
hipofibrinogenemia	**hypofibrinogenemia** *Diminished blood fibrinogen level.*
hipofisectomia	**hypophysectomy** *Surgical removal of the pituitary gland.*
hipoforia	**hypophoria** *Downward deviation of the visual axis of the eye.*
hipofosfatasia	**hypophosphatasia** *A genetic defect of diminished alkaline phosphatase in the cells leading to bone demineralization.*
hipogastro	**hypogastrium** *The area of the central abdomen located below the stomach.*
hipogástrico	**hypogastric** *Referring to the hypogastrium.*
hipoglicemia	**hypoglycemia** *Abnormally low blood sugar.*
hipogonadismo	**hypogonadism** *Abnormal decrease in gonadal function with associated diminished growth and sexual development.*
hipomania	**hypomania** *A moderate form of mania.*
hiponatremia	**hyponatremia** *Diminished level of sodium in the blood stream.*
hipoparatireoidismo	**hypoparathyroidism** *Abnormal decrease in parathyroid function.*
hipopituitarismo	**hypopituitarism** *Diminished pituitary activity exhibited by obesity and persistence of adolescent characteristics.*
hipoplasia	**hypoplasia** *Incomplete development.*
hipospádia	**hypospadias** *Congenital condition exhibited by development of the urethral meatus on the inferior aspect of the penis.*
hipossalivação	**hyposalivation** *Secretion of saliva below the normal rate.*

Portuguese	English
hipotálamo	**hypothalamus** *Located inferior to the thalamus it controls visceral activities, water balance, temperature and sleep.*
hipotensão	**hypotension** *Abnormally low blood pressure.*
hipotensão postural; hipotensão ortostática	**postural hypotension** *A significant drop in blood pressure when going from the supine or sitting position to standing.*
hipotermia	**hypothermia** *Lower than normal temperature.*
hipotireoidismo	**hypothyroidism** *Reduced functioning of the thyroid.*
hipotonia	**hypotonia** *Reduced tone or activity.*
hipoxia	**hypoxia** *Diminished oxygen content.*
hipófise	**hypophysis** *Pituitary gland.*
hipópio	**hypopyon** *The presence of purulent fluid in the anterior chamber of the eye.*
hipóstase	**hypostasis** *The formation of a deposit.*
hirsutismo	**hirsutism** *Abnormal growth on hair on a person's face and body.*
hirsuto	**hairy** *A profuse amount of hair.*
histamina	**histamine** *A chemical responsible for the reaction exhibited when a person has an allergic reaction.*
histerectomia	**hysterectomy** *Surgical removal of the uterus.*
histeria	**hysteria** *A psychological condition exhibited by uncontrolled emotion or exaggerated manifestations.*
histerografia	**hysterography** *1. Recording of uterine contractions. 2. Roentgenography of the uterus after administration of contrast media.*
histeromiomectomia	**hysteromyomectomy** *Surgical removal of a uterine myoma.*
histeropexia	**hysteropexy** *Surgical fixation of the uterus by shortening of the round ligaments or by other means.*
histerossalpingografia	**hysterosalpingography** *Roentgenography of the uterus and fallopian tubes after instillation of contrast media.*
histerotomia	**hysterotomy** *Surgical opening of the uterus.*
histidina	**histidine** *An amino acid precursor to histamine.*
histioquímica	**histochemistry** *Study of intracellular distribution of chemicals, reaction sites and enzymes.*
histiócito	**histiocyte** *A phagocytic cell found in connective tissue.*
histologia	**histology** *The study of the structure and composition of minute structures.*
histoplasmose; doença de Darling	**histoplasmosis** *A fungal pulmonary infection from bat and bird excrement.*
híbrido	**hybrid** *An animal or plant produced from two different species.*
hímen	**hymen** *A membrane in the vagina.*
homem	**man** *Male human.*
homeopatia	**homeopathy** *A treatment of disease by use of minute doses of toxic substances that would normally be harmful.*
homeostase	**homeostasis** *The tendency of an organism to maintain a stable and uniform state.*
homicído	**homicide** *When one person kills another.*
homoenxerto	**homograft** *A graft of tissue from the same species as the recipient.*
homolateral	**homolateral** *Ipsilateral.*
homossexual	**homosexual** *A person sexually attracted to someone of the same gender.*
homozigoto	**homozygous** *Having identical alleles for a particular trait.*
homólogo	**homologous** *Referring to something derived from the same species but different genotype.*

Portuguese	English
hordéolo	**hordeolum** *Inflammation of the sebaceous gland of the eye.*
hormônio	**hormone** *A substance produced in the body that effects a specific organ.*
hormônio adrenocorticotrópico	**adrenocorticotrophic hormone (ACTH)** *A hormone that influences the cortex of the adrenal glands.*
hormônio antidiurético	**antidiuretic hormone** *Vasopressin.*
hormônio estimulante da tireóide	**thyroid stimulating hormone (TSH)** *A thyroid secreted by the pituitary that regulates the thyroid.*
hormônio folículo-estimulante	**follicle stimulating hormone (FSH)** *An anterior pituitary gland hormone responsible for production of sperm or ova.*
hormônio liberador	**releasing hormone** *Hormones that come from one gland such as the thalamus that cause release of hormones from another gland such as the pituitary.*
hormônio luteinizante	**luteinizing hormone (LH)** *A pituitary hormone that stimulates ovulation in females and androgen in males.*
hospital	**hospital** *Acute care medical/surgical facility.*
humano	**human** *Homo sapien.*
humor aquoso	**aqueous humor** *The fluid between the cornea and lens, anterior to the globe.*
humor aquoso	**humor, aqueous** *The gelatinous fluid circulating between the cornea and lens.*
humor vítreo	**humor, vitreous** *The fluid circulating between the lens and retina.*
iatrogênico	**iatrogenic** *A problem caused by medical treatment.*
icterícia	**icterus** *Yellowing of the skin and sclerae because of excess bilirubin.*
icterícia	**jaundice** *Yellowing of the sclerae and skin because of excessive bilirubin in the blood.*
icterícia do recém-nascido	**jaundice of the newborn** *A form of jaundice seen in newborns in the first two weeks of life; also called icterus neonatorum.*
icterícia nuclear	**kernicterus** *A condition associated with high bilirubin levels that causes yellow staining of cerebral tissues and subsequent neurologic dysfunction.*
ictiose	**ichthyosis** *A congenital anomaly exhibited by excessively dry, thick skin.*
id est	**i.e.** *A latin derived abbreviation for "that is to say"(In latin: id est)*
idade	**age** *Length of life.*
idiopático	**idiopathic** *Relating to a disease with an unknown cause.*
idosos	**elderly** *Advanced in years.*
igual	**equal** *The same or uniform.*
ileíte	**ileitis** *Inflammation of the ileum.*
ileocolite	**ileocolitis** *Inflammation of the ileum and cecum.*
ileocolostomia	**ileocolostomy** *Creating a surgical opening between the ileum and colon.*
ileoprotostomia	**ileoproctostomy** *Creating a surgical opening between the ileum and the rectum.*
ileostomia	**ileostomy** *Surgical creation of an opening in the ileum that is placed at the skin surface.*
ileterado	**illiterate** *Unable to read or write.*
ilhota	**islet** *Tissue that is structurally separate from adjacent tissues.*
iliococcígeo	**iliococcygeal** *Referring to the ilium and coccyx.*
imagem por ressonância magnética	**magnetic resonance imaging (MRI)** *Images are produced by evaluating the response of body tissue. nuclei to radio waves in a magnetic field.*

Portuguese	English
impactação cerúmen	**cerumen impaction** *External ear canal full of wax resulting in hearing loss until the impaction is removed.*
impactação dentária	**impaction, tooth** *A tooth that does not erupt because adjacent teeth prevent it.*
impactação fecal	**fecal impaction** *The presence of hard excrement in the rectum that requires manual removal.*
imperfurado	**imperforate** *Lack of an opening. An infant with an imperforate anus has a congenital defect with no anal opening.*
imperícia	**malpractice** *Negligent professional activity.*
impérvio	**impervious** *Not affected by.*
implante	**implant** *A device or prosthesis implanted in a person.*
implementação	**implementation** *The process of putting a plan into effect.*
impotência	**impotence** *Inability to act or inability to achieve a penile erection.*
impulso nervo	**nerve impulse** *A signal transmitted along a nerve fiber.*
imune	**immune** *Being resistant to an infection.*
imunização	**immunization** *A medication given to provide immunity.*
imunodeficiência	**immunodeficiency** *An inadequate immune response.*
imunoeletroforese	**immunoelectrophoresis** *A means of differentiating proteins and other compounds by comparing their mobility and antigenic specificities.*
imunoglobulina	**immunoglobulin** *Serum and cellular proteins of the immune system.*
imunoquímica	**immunochemistry** *The study of immune response and biochemistry.*
imunossupressão	**immunosuppression** *The inhibition of the immune response.*
inadaptação	**maladjustment** *Having the trait of being unable to cope normally.*
inalação	**inhalation** *The act of breathing in.*
inanição	**inanition** *Generalized weakness from lack of nutrition.*
inanição	**starvation** *Death related to starvation.*
inaplicável	**irrelevant** *Not pertinent.*
inarticulado	**inarticulate** *Indistinct speech.*
incapacidade	**disability** *Decreased or impaired mental or physical ability.*
incesto	**incest** *Sexual relations between related people.*
inchação	**puffiness** *Having a soft, swollen area.*
inchado	**bloated** *Sensation of having an abnormally large amount of air in the viscera.*
incipiente	**incipient** *Starting to happen.*
incisão	**incision** *An intentional surgical cut in the skin.*
incisivo	**incisor** *Sharp-edged tooth; humans have four incisors.*
incisura	**incisura** *A notch or indentation usually on the edge of a bone.*
incisura	**incisure** *A notch or incision.*
incisura jugular	**jugular notch** *The notch on the upper border of the sternum.*
inclinação	**learning** *The intentional acquisition of knowledge.*
incoerente	**incoherent** *Absence of intelligible speech.*
inconsciência	**unconsciousness** *Unable to respond to sensory stimuli.*
incontenência urinária	**urinary incontinence** *Involuntary micturition.*
incontinência	**incontinence** *Inability to control urination.*
incoordenação	**incoordination** *Absence of smooth, efficient body movement.*
incremento	**increment** *An increase on a fixed scale.*
incubador	**incubator** *A warming device for infants.*
indigestão	**indigestion** *Inadequate digestion for various reasons.*

Portuguese	English
indígeno	**indigenous** *Naturally occurring.*
indolente	**indolent** *1. Causing little pain. 2. Slow healing ulcer.*
induzir	**induce, to** *Facilitated. When referring to labor, it means medication was given to assist in delivery of the fetus.*
inebriação	**drunk** *Inebriated.*
inebriação	**inebriation** *Intoxication with drugs or alcohol.*
ineficaz	**ineffective** *Unsuccessful or inefficient.*
inervação	**innervation** *The presence of a nerve supply.*
inesperado	**unexpected** *Unforeseen.*
inevitável	**inevitable** *Not preventable.*
inércia	**inertia** *The tendency to remain unchanged.*
infantil	**infantile** *Referring to babies or young children.*
infartação	**infarction** *Dead tissue, for example, myocardial infarction.*
infartação lacunar	**lacunar infarction** *Small non-cortical cerebral infarcts.*
infartação miocárdico	**myocardial infarction** *The death of myocardial tissue as a result of an interruption in flow to the region supplied by a coronary vessel.*
infarto	**infarct** *Referring to dead tissue.*
infância	**childhood** *The time between infancy and puberty.*
infância	**infancy** *Early childhood.*
infeccionar	**fester, to** *To become infected.*
infeccioso	**infectious** *Contagious.*
infecção cruzada	**cross-infection** *Transfer of infection between individuals, each with a different organism.*
infecção nosocomial	**nosocomial infection** *An infection occurring after admission to a hospital.*
infecção orelha	**ear infection** *General term referring to otitis media or otitis externa.*
inferior	**inferior** *The lower aspect.*
infestação	**infestation** *The presence of large numbers, as in lice infestation.*
infestações por ácaros	**acariasis** *Mite infestation.*
inflamação	**inflammation** *Localized redness, excessive warmth and swelling.*
influenza aviária	**avian flu** *A viral disease found in birds and fowl that can be transmitted to humans; it is exhibited by respiratory and gastrointestinal symptoms but can lead to encephalitis.*
influenza; gripe	**influenza** *Viral infection causing fever, muscle aches and catarrh.*
infra-espinhoso	**infraspinous** *Below the scapular spine.*
infundíbulo	**infundibulum** *The connection between the hypothalamus and the posterior pituitary gland.*
infusão	**infusion** *The injection of fluid into tissue or a vein.*
infusão intravenoso	**intravenous infusion** *Administration of fluid into a vein.*
ingestão	**ingestion** *The intake of food or liquid orally.*
inguinal	**inguinal** *Referring to the groin.*
inhibidor da monoamina oxidase	**monoamine oxidase inhibitor (MAOI)** *A drug used to treat depression that allows accumulation of serotonin and norepinephrine.*
inibidor da enzima que converte a angiotensina	**angiotensin converting enzyme inhibitors (ACEI)** *A class of medicines that prevent conversion of angiotensin I to angiotensin II, a potent vasoconstrictor.*
injecção	**injection** *The act of a needle being inserted into a body.*
injeção hipodérmica	**hypodermic injection** *Subcutaneous injection.*

Portuguese	English
inoculação	**inoculation** *Injection with a vaccine to provide immunity.*
inofensivo	**harmless** *Safe or benign.*
inominada	**innominate** *Referring to the innominate artery.*
inorgânico	**inorganic** *Not coming from natural growth.*
insanidade	**insanity** *Referring to a serious mental illness.*
insano	**insane** *A term not used in formal medical evaluations that when used by a layperson means a serious mental illness.*
insensível	**insensible** *Unable to perceive a stimulus.*
inserção	**insertion** *The act of inserting something.*
inserção tubo nasogástrico	**nasogastric tube placement** *Insertion of a tube that is placed in the stomach via the nostril; it is used for administration of fluid or to suction gastric contents.*
insidioso	**insidious** *A slow, gradual and harmful advancement.*
insificiência cardíca congestiva	**congestive heart failure** *A diminished cardiac output leading to passive engorgement.*
insignificante	**meaningless** *Having no significance.*
insolação	**heat stroke** *A condition caused by excessive exposure to high ambient temperature; it is exhibited by dry skin, thirst, vertigo, muscle cramps and nausea. The three forms are heat exhaustion, heat cramps and sunstroke.*
insônia	**insomnia** *Sleeplessness.*
inspiração	**inspiration** *Drawing in a breath.*
inspissado	**inspissate, to** *To thicken or congeal.*
instável	**groggy** *Drowsy.*
insuficiência aórtica	**aortic insufficiency** *A dysfunction of the aortic valve allowing backflow of blood into the heart.*
insuficiência cardíaca congestiva	**cardiac failure** *Decreased cardiac output of the heart.*
insuficiência renal	**renal failure** *Diminution of kidney function.*
insuficiência vertebrobasilar	**vertebrobasilar insufficiency** *Diminished flow to the vertebral and basilar arteries causing posterior fossa symptoms.*
insulina	**insulin** *A hormone produced by the pancreas and synthetically to control blood glucose levels.*
insulinoma	**insulinoma** *An islet cell tumor that causes abnormally high insulin secretion and thus hypoglycemia.*
integumento	**integument** *Outer protective layer.*
intensivo	**intensive** *Very thorough or vigorous.*
interarticular	**interarticular** *Between the articular surfaces of a joint.*
intercelular	**intercellular** *Between cells.*
interior	**inside** *Inner part, center.*
intermitente	**intermittent** *Occurring at irregular intervals.*
interno	**internal** *Situated on the inside.*
interósseo	**interosseous** *Referring to something between bones, like the interosseous muscles of the hand.*
intersticial	**interstitial** *Referring to the interstices of tissue.*
intertrigo	**intertrigo** *Irritation present because adjacent surfaces rub together.*
intertrocantérica	**intertrochanteric** *Referring to the space within the trochanter.*
intervalo	**interval** *An intervening time.*
interventricular	**interventricular** *Between the ventricles.*
intestinal	**intestinal** *Referring to the intestines.*
intestino	**intestine** *A general term used for the section of bowel from the stomach to the anus.*

Portuguese	English
intolerância lactose	**lactose intolerance** *The inability of the small bowel to digest lactose.*
intossuscepção	**intussusception** *The inversion of one portion of the bowel into another.*
intoxicação alimentar	**food poisoning** *Poisoning where the active agent is in the food.*
intoxicação pelo iodo	**iodism** *A condition caused by excessive iodine intake resulting in diarrhea, weakness, and convulsions.*
intoxicação pelo monóxido de carbono	**carbon monoxide poisoning** *This tasteless, odorless gas causes constitutional symptoms but can lead to death upon inhalation.*
intoxicação por chumbo	**lead poisoning** *The ingestion of lead, exhibited in severe cases by paralysis, encephalopathy, purple gingiva, and colic.*
intra-abdominal	**intraabdominal** *Within the abdominal cavity.*
intra-articular	**intraarticular** *Within a joint space.*
intra-ósseo	**intraosseous** *Within a bone.*
intra-uterino	**intrauterine** *Within the uterus.*
intracelular	**intracellular** *Within a cell.*
intracerebral	**intracerebral** *Within the cerebrum.*
intracraniano	**intracranial** *Within the cranial vault.*
intradérmico	**intradermal** *Within the dermis.*
intradural	**intradural** *Within the dural space.*
intramedular	**intramedullary** *1. Within the medulla oblongata. 2. Within the bone marrow.*
intramuscular	**intramuscular** *Within a muscle.*
intraperitoneal	**intraperitoneal** *Within the peritoneal cavity.*
intratecal	**intrathecal** *Technically means within a sheath but this term is used when medication is instilled in the dura mater spinalis.*
intravenoso	**intravenous** *Within a vein.*
intubação	**intubation** *Placement of a tube; commonly used to refer to endotracheal intubation.*
inulina	**inulin** *A polysaccharide used in the testing of renal function.*
inunção	**inunction** *The application of lotion with friction.*
involucional	**involutional** *The shrinkage of an organ when it is not in use, as in the uterus after childbirth.*
invólucro	**involucrum** *A wrap or covering (referring to a sequestrum).*
iodo	**iodine** *A chemical used as an antiseptic and a deficiency of it can lead to goiter.*
ipsolateral	**ipsilateral** *On the same side.*
iridectomia	**iridectomy** *Surgical removal of part of the iris.*
iridociclite	**iridocyclitis** *Inflammation of the ciliary body and the iris.*
iridoplegia	**iridoplegia** *Paralysis of part of the iris with subsequent lack of contraction or dilation of the pupil.*
iridotomia	**iridotomy** *A surgical opening of the iris.*
irmão	**sibling** *A brother or sister.*
irradiação	**irradiation** *The process of being irradiated.*
isoanticorpo	**isoantibody** *A situation in which an antibody of person A reacts with an antigen of person B.*
isolamento	**isolation** *To be kept separate or apart.*
isótopo radioativo	**radioactive isotope** *An isotope with an unstable nucleus that is used in diagnostic imaging.*
isquemia	**ischemia** *Inadequate blood supply to a part of the body.*
istmo	**isthmus** *A narrow piece of tissue connecting two larger body parts.*

Portuguese	English
íleo	**ileum** *The portion of the small bowel from the jejunum to the cecum.*
íleo (obstrução mecânica)	**ileus** *A temporary obstruction in the intestine.*
íleo por verme	**verminous ileus** *Obstruction due to masses of intestinal parasites.*
índice de natalidade	**birth rate** *The number of live births per 1000 of a given population per year.*
íris	**iris** *The colored membrane posterior to the cornea.*
íris da heterocromia; síndrome de Eric	**heterochromia iridis or syndrome of Eric** *Congenital anomaly in which the iris of each eye is of a different color.*
ísquio	**ischium** *The inferoposterior portion of the pelvis.*
jarrete	**hamstrings** *Tendons of the posterior thigh.*
jato de água	**flush, to** *Term used to describe an irrigation procedure, as in flushing an NG tube.*
jejum	**fasting** *Absence of caloric intake for a specified period.*
jejunectomia	**jejunectomy** *Surgical removal of the jejunum.*
jejunostomia	**jejunostomy** *Surgical creation of an opening in the jejunum.*
joanete	**bunion** *Swelling of the bursa of the metatarsal head of the first metatarsal.*
joelho	**knee** *The joint at the distal femur and proximal tibia.*
joelho da dona-de-casa	**housemaid's knee** *Also referred to as prepatellar bursitis.*
joelho de Brodie	**Brodie's knee** *Also referred to as chronic hypertrophic synovitis of the knee.*
joelho travado	**unstable knee** *A condition with giving way of the knee due to ligamentous or cartilaginous dysfunction.*
joelho valgo	**genu valgum** *A condition exhibited by the knees turning inward, commonly referred to as knock-knee.*
joelho varo; perna arqueada	**genu varum** *A condition exhibited by the knees turning outward, commonly referred to as bowleg.*
jovem	**young** *Having lived for a short period.*
jugular	**jugular** *Referring to the neck, as in jugular vein.*
junção estreita	**tight junction** *An intercellular junction with an impermeable membrane.*
junta; articulação	**knuckle** *A metacarpophalagngeal joint or a finger joint when the fist is closed.*
juramento de Hipócrates	**Hippocratic oath** *An vow taken by doctors, indicating they will treat people properly.*
justarticular	**juxta-articular** *Positioned near a joint.*
kra-kra	**craw-craw** *A pruritic papular skin eruption sometimes caused by Onchocerca.*
labial	**labial** *Referring to the lip.*
labirintite	**labyrinthitis** *Inflammation of the labyrinth.*
labirinto	**labyrinth** *Inner ear structure concerned with balance.*
laboratório	**laboratory** *A room equipped to run blood, tissue and fluid samples.*
laceração	**laceration** *An injury that produced a cut in the skin or tissue such as a tear during childbirth.*
laceração	**tear** *Referring to a vaginal tear after childbirth.*
lacrimal	**lacrimal** *Referring to the secretion of tears.*
lacrimejamento	**lacrimation** *The secretion of tears.*
lactação	**lactation** *The secretion of milk from mammary glands.*
lactalbumina	**lactalbumin** *Proteins found in milk.*
lactase	**lactase** *An enzyme that facilitates the breakdown of lactose to glucose and galactose.*

Portuguese	English
lactente pósmaduro	**infant, post-term** *A neonate born after the normal gestation.*
lactente prematuro	**infant, pre-term** *A neonate born prior to normal gestation.*
lactente termo	**infant, term** *A neonate born at expected date.*
lactente; criança	**infant** *Newborn.*
lactose	**lactose** *A disaccharide present in milk.*
lacuna	**lacuna** *A small cavity or depression.*
lado	**side** *A position medial or lateral to center.*
lagoftalmia	**lagophthalmos** *Characterized by the inability to close the eyelid completely over the eye.*
laliofobia	**laliophobia** *Abnormal fear of speaking or stuttering.*
laloquezia	**lalochezia** *Relief of stress by uttering obscenities.*
lambdóide	**lambdoid** *The suture connecting the parietal bones with the occipital bone.*
lamela	**lamella** *A thin layer of bone.*
lamentação	**querulousness** *Whining or complaining.*
laminectomia	**laminectomy** *The surgical removal of part of a vertebrae.*
lanceta	**lancet** *A small sharp instrument used to obtain a drop of blood for testing.*
laparoscopia	**laparoscopy** *A procedure utilizing a laparoscope.*
laparoscópio	**laparoscope** *A fiber-optic instrument used to visualize the peritoneal contents.*
laparotomia	**laparotomy** *A surgical incision of the abdomen.*
laparotomia exploratório	**exploratory laparotomy** *Abdominal surgery with the intent of examining the abdominal contents.*
largura	**width** *Side to side measurement.*
laringe	**larynx** *A hollow muscular structure that contains the vocal cords.*
laringectomia	**laryngectomy** *Surgical removal of the larynx.*
laringismo estriduloso	**laryngismus stridulus** *Sudden, severe laryngeal spasm.*
laringite	**laryngitis** *Inflammation of the larynx.*
laringoestenose	**laryngostenosis** *Abnormal narrowing of the larynx.*
laringofaringe	**laryngopharynx** *The pharyngeal space between the superior aspect of the glottis and the opening of the larynx.*
laringologia	**laryngology** *The study of the larynx and related diseases.*
laringospasmo	**laryngospasm** *Sudden, involuntary muscle contraction of the larynx.*
laringotomia	**laryngotomy** *Surgical creation of an opening in the larynx.*
laríngeo	**laryngeal** *Referring to the larynx.*
lasca	**splinter** *A small, thin object; usually refers to the object being imbedded in the body.*
lateral; de lado	**lateral** *Referring to the side of the body.*
latirismo	**lathyrism** *A disease characterized by tremors, spastic paralysis and paresthesias caused by Lathyrus sativus.*
lavagem do estômago;	**gastric lavage** *Instillation and removal of large quantities of saline into the stomach in order to treat poisoning.*
lábil	**labile** *Easily altered; emotionally unstable.*
lábio	**labium** *Referring to any lip shaped structure.*
lábio	**labrum** *An edge or lip. The labrum acetabular is the fibrocartilagous rim attached to the acetabulum.*
lábio inferior	**lip, lower** *Labium inferius oris.*
lábio leporino; lábio fendido	**cleft lip** *A congenital abnormal opening of the lip.*
lábio pudendo menor	**labium minus (plural=labia minora)** *The folds of skin posterior to the labia majora.*

Portuguese	English
lábio, superior	**lip, upper** *Labium superius oris.*
láctico	**lactic** *Referring to milk.*
lágrima	**tear** *As in, to shed a tear.*
látero-desvio	**laterodeviation** *Pushed to the lateral aspect.*
lâmina	**slide** *A thin, rectangular piece of glass used for viewing specimen under a microscope.*
lecitina	**lecithin** *A compound widely used by tissues, derived from egg yolks and it consists of phospholipids linked to choline.*
leishmaniose	**leishmaniasis** *A condition caused by a flagellate protozoan parasite that is exhibited by visceral or dermatologic manifestations.*
leite de vaca	**cow's milk**
leito	**bed** *A mattress resting on a frame.*
leito de ungueal	**nail bed** *The area just beneath a finger or toenail.*
lente	**lens** *The transparent chamber between the posterior chamber and the vitreous body.*
lentes de contacto	**contact lens** *A lens that fits over the cornea to correct refractive errors.*
lenticular	**lenticular** *Referring to the lens of the eye.*
lentigo	**lentigo** *A benign condition exhibited by flat brown patches on the skin.*
lento	**slow** *Unhurried.*
leontíase óssea; doença de Virchow	**leontiasis ossea** *Bilateral hypertrophy of the bones of the face and cranium.*
lepra	**leprosy** *A contagious disease caused by Mycobacterium leprae that causes insensate papules and disfiguration.*
leproma	**leproma** *A superficial granulatomous papule that is seen in leprosy.*
leptomeningite	**leptomeningitis** *A general term used to describe meningitis of the pia and arachnoid of the brain.*
leptospirose	**leptospirosis** *A zoonosis caused by the spirochete Leptospira interrogans transmitted by rats and contaminated water.*
lesão	**injury** *A wound, abrasion or contusion.*
lesão cerebral por contragolpe	**injury, contrecoup of brain** *An injury to the brain on the side opposite of that which was struck.*
lesão da cabeça	**head trauma** *Any injury to the brain.*
lesão de desluvamento	**injury, degloving** *Trauma that involves the ripping of skin and subcutaneous tissue from the underlying tissue.*
lesão de pele	**skin lesion** *An abnormal but not necessarily cancerous lesion.*
lesão de punção-agulha	**needle-stick injury** *The inadvertent self-puncture with a needle that had been used previously to inject a patient.*
lesão de rajada	**blast injury** *Trauma from a wave of air pressure.*
lesão de virilha	**groin pull** *A muscle strain in the inguinal region.*
lesão fechada da cabeça	**injury, closed head** *Brain trauma not associated with damage to the dura or skull.*
lesão por hiperextensão e hiperflexão	**injury, hyperextension-hyperflexion** *An injury, usually to the cervical spine, that involves rapid deceleration, causing pronounced extension and flexion.*
letal	**lethal** *Deadly.*
letargia	**lethargy** *Absence of energy.*
leucemia	**leukemia** *A malignant disease causing an increase in the number of abnormal and immature leukocytes.*
leucemia linfocítico	**lymphocytic leukemia** *Chronic accumulation of functionally incompetent lymphocytes.*

Portuguese	English
leucina	**leukine (or leucine)** *An amino acid obtained from hydrolysis of some proteins.*
leucocitemia	**leukocythemia** *Synonym of leukemia.*
leucocitose	**leukocytosis** *An increase in the number of leukocytes.*
leucocitólise	**leukocytolysis** *Destruction of white blood cells.*
leucodermia	**leukodermia** *A localized loss of skin pigment.*
leuconíquia	**leukonychia** *A whitish discoloration of the fingernails and toenails.*
leucopenia	**leukopenia** *A decreased number of leukocytes in the blood.*
leucopoiese	**leukopoiesis** *Production of white blood cells.*
leucorréia	**leukorrhea** *Thick white vaginal discharge.*
leucócito	**leukocyte** *A white blood cell.*
levantar	**raise, to** *To lift or bring up.*
leve	**light** *Not heavy.*
levedura	**yeast** *A unicellular fungus.*
levulose	**levulose** *Synonym for fructose.*
lésbica	**lesbian** *A woman with same gender preference.*
liberdade	**loose** *Not tight.*
libido	**libido** *Sexual desire.*
lidar com	**cope, to** *To deal with a difficult situation.*
ligado a	**related to** *Causally connected.*
ligadura	**ligature** *A thread used to tie a vessel.*
ligamento	**ligament** *A band of fibrous connective tissue that connects two bones or cartilage.*
ligamento bifurcado	**bifurcate ligament** *A ligament on the dorsum of the foot that includes the calcaneonavicular and calcaneocuboid ligaments.*
ligamento largo	**broad ligament of uterus** *Supports the uterus on both sides.*
ligamento pectíneo	**pectineal ligament** *A continuation of the lacunar ligament along the pectineal line in the pubis.*
ligamento redondo do útero	**round ligament of the uterus** *The supporting structure of the uterus.*
limbo	**limbus** *The margin of a structure, for example, of the cornea and sclera.*
linctura	**lincture** *A medicine mixed with a sweet substance.*
linfa	**lymph** *A transparent and sometimes opalescent fluid that flows in the lymph channels.*
linfadenite	**lymphadenitis** *Inflammation of a lymph node.*
linfangiectasia	**lymphangiectasis** *Distention of the lymph channels.*
linfangioma	**lymphangioma** *A mass composed of newly formed lymph tissue.*
linfangite	**lymphangitis** *Inflammation of the lymph vessels.*
linfático	**lymphatic** *Referring to the lymph system.*
linfocitemia	**lymphocythemia** *Abnormally high number of lymphocytes in the blood.*
linfocitopenia	**lymphocytopenia** *Decrease in the usual number of lymphocytes in the blood.*
linfocitose	**lymphocytosis** *The organization of cysts containing lymph.*
linfoma	**lymphoma** *A malignant disease of the lymph system, Hodgkin's lymphoma for example.*
linfonodo	**lymph node** *An area of organized lymphatic tissue.*
linfossarcoma	**lymphosarcoma** *A malignant disease of the lymph system that does not include Hodgkin's lymphoma.*
linfócito	**lymphocyte** *A white blood cell produced by the lymph tissue.*

Portuguese	English
linfóide	**lymphoid** *Similar to lymph.*
linha branca	**linea alba** *The tendinous portion of the anterior abdomen between the two rectus muscles.*
linha do meio	**midline** *A median line of bilateral separation.*
linha negra	**lingua nigra** *A condition characterized by a dark fur-like covering on the dorsum of the tongue.*
lipase	**lipase** *A pancreatic enzyme that facilitates the breakdown of fats.*
lipemia	**lipemia** *Abnormally high fat content in the blood.*
lipídeo	**lipid** *A compound that is a fatty acid which is insoluble in water but soluble in organic solvents.*
lipoatrofia	**lipoatrophy** *Fatty tissue atrophy.*
lipodistrofia	**lipodystrophy** *Abnormal fat metabolism.*
lipoidose	**lipoidosis** *Abnormal lipid metabolism.*
lipoma	**lipoma** *A benign tumor consisting of fat cells.*
lipoproteína	**lipoprotein** *A soluble protein used to transport fat or lipids.*
lipócito	**lipocyte** *A fat cell.*
lipóide	**lipoid** *Referring to fat.*
lise	**lysis** *The rupture of a cell wall or membrane.*
lisina	**lysine** *An amino acid found in most proteins.*
lisossoma	**lysosome** *An organelle contained in the cytoplasm of eukaryotic cells.*
lisossoma; muramidase	**lysozyme** *An enzyme in tears that facilitates destruction of certain bacterial cell walls.*
listeriose	**listeriosis** *A disease caused by Listeria monocytogenes that occurs in the pregnant and immunocompromised.*
litmo	**litmus** *A dye that turns red with low pH and blue with high pH.*
litolapaxia	**litholapaxy** *The crushing and then removal of a calculus.*
litotomia	**lithotomy** *Surgical removal of a calculus.*
litotriptor	**lithotriptor** *An instrument used to crush a calculus.*
lividez pós-morte	**post-mortem lividity** *The purplish discoloration occurring 30-120 minutes after death in dependent body parts.*
livre	**free** *Lacking or absent.*
língua	**tongue** *The fleshy muscular organ of the mouth.*
língua de framboesa	**strawberry tongue** *A characteristic discoloration of the tongue seen in an early phase of scarlet fever.*
língua pilosa	**hairy tongue** *Lingua villosa, a benign condition associated with antibiotic used caused by candida albicans infection.*
líquen	**lichen** *A term used to describe a variety of papular skin diseases. Lichen planus is a shiny, flat, violaceous eruption of the mucous membranes, skin and genitalia.*
lítico	**lytic** *Referring to lysis.*
lobar	**lobar** *Referring to a lobe.*
lobectomia	**lobectomy** *Surgical removal of a lobe (generally lung or liver).*
lobo	**lobe** *A body part divided by a fissure.*
lobotomia	**lobotomy** *Surgical incision into the prefrontal lobe; historically a treatment of mental illness.*
localização	**localization** *Establishment of a site of a disease process.*
localizado	**localized** *Toward one point or area.*
loculação	**loculated** *Divided into small cavities.*
lodo	**sludge** *A viscous fluid.*
loíasis	**loiasis** *A disease caused by the filarial nematode Loa loa.*

Portuguese	English
lombar	**lumbar** *Referring to the spinal region inferior to the thoracic spine.*
longevidade	**longevity** *Long life.*
lordose	**lordosis** *An abnormal depth of the inward curvature of the spine.*
loucura	**madness** *Common term for insanity.*
lóbulo	**lobule** *A small lobe.*
lóbulo da oelha	**earlobe** *The soft, fleshy inferior portion of the pinna.*
lóquios	**lochia** *Vaginal secretions noted within two weeks of childbirth.*
lubrificante	**lubricant** *Emollient.*
luteotrópico	**luteotropic** *Synonym of prolactin.*
luto	**mourning** *A period of grieving.*
luva	**glove** *A covering for hand protection.*
luz	**light** *Illumination, bright.*
lúcido	**clear** *Lucid.*
lúnula	**lunula** *The pale area at the base of a fingernail.*
lúpus eriematoso	**lupus erythematosous** *An autoimmune inflammatory disease exhibited by a butterfly shaped rash on the face along with visceral and connective tissue abnormalities.*
maconha	**marijuana** *Cannabis.*
macrocitose	**macrocytosis** *Referring to the status of an increased number of large erythrocytes as seen in Vitamin B12 deficiency.*
macrodactilia	**macrodactyly** *Abnormally large digits.*
macroencefalia	**macroencephaly** *Having an abnormally large head.*
macroglobulina	**macroglobulinemia** *A condition exhibited by an increase number of macroglobulins in the blood.*
macroglossia	**macroglossia** *Abnormally large tongue.*
macromastia	**macromastia** *Abnormally large breasts.*
macromelia	**macromelia** *Abnormally large head or extremity.*
macroquilia	**macrocheilia** *Abnormally large lips.*
macrostomia	**macrostomia** *Abnormal increase in the width of the mouth.*
macrócito	**macrocyte** *A large red blood cell.*
macrófago	**macrophage** *A phagocytic cell that originates in the tissues.*
maculopápula	**maculopapule** *A skin lesion that is similar to both a macule and a papule.*
madatário	**mandatory** *Obligatory.*
magneto	**magnet** *A piece of iron with atoms ordered to make it magnetic.*
magnético	**magnetic** *Having the properties of a magnet.*
mais velho	**older** *Being around more than compared with another.*
mal-alinhamento	**malalignment (dental)** *Displacement of the teeth from their normal position.*
mal-estar	**malaise** *A vague feeling of discomfort or unease.*
malacia	**malacia** *The abnormal softening of a body part or tissue.*
malaxação	**petrissage** *Massage using a kneading action.*
malária	**malaria** *A condition caused by a protozoan of the genus Plasmodium. It is transmitted by mosquitos and is exhibited by fever, chills, headache. In the severe form it can lead to convulsions, increased ICP and death.*
malária cerebral	**cerebral malaria** *A severe form of malaria manifested by seizures and a decreased level of consciousness.*
maléolo	**malleolus** *A bony protrusion on medial and lateral aspect of each ankle.*
maléolo lateral	**malleolus, lateral** *The lateral aspect of the distal fibula.*

Portuguese	English
maléolo medial	**malleolus, medial** *The medial aspect of the distal portion of the tibia.*
malformação arteriovenoso	**arteriovenous malformation** *A sac like structure created by the abnormal communication of an adjacent artery and vein.*
maligno	**detrimental** *Harmful.*
maligno	**malignant** *Tendency of a tumor to invade normal tissue.*
maltose	**maltose** *A disaccharide hydrolyzed by amylase.*
mamário	**mammary** *Referring to the breast.*
mamilar	**mammillary** *Referring to a nipple.*
mamilo	**nipple** *The small projection on the breast thru which milk is secreted.*
mamografia	**mammography** *Roentgenography of the breasts, used as a screening test for cancer.*
mamona	**castor bean** *A bean that can yield the poisonous compound ricin.*
mamoplastia	**mammaplasty** *Plastic surgery of the breast.*
mancha algodonosas	**cotton wool spots** *Condition characterized by blue or white discoloration on the retina related to nerve ischemia.*
manchas de Koplik	**Koplik's spots** *Red buccal macules with a blue center; seen in measles.*
mandíbula	**jaw** *Mandible.*
mandíbula	**mandible** *The lower jaw.*
maneuver de Mcdonald	**Mcdonald's maneuver** *A measurement of the uterus in centimeters that corresponds to gestational age in weeks.*
manguito rotador do ombro; manguito musculotendinoso	**rotator cuff** *The structure around the capsule of the shoulder joint formed by the infraspinatus, supraspinatus, teres minor and subscapularis muscles.*
mania	**mania** *A mental disorder exhibited by hyperexcitability, delusions and euphoria.*
manobra de Adson	**Adson maneuver** *A test used to screen for thoracic outlet syndrome.*
manobra de Bill	**Bill maneuver** *During childbirth, use of forceps at midpelvis to help extract the head.*
manobra de Bracht	**Bracht maneuver** *Delivery of a fetus in a breech position.*
manobra de Buzzard	**Buzzard maneuver** *Testing of the patellar reflex while the client firmly touches the floor with their toes in a sitting position.*
manobra de Credé	**Credé's maneuver** *Manual pressure over the bladder to assist in expression of urine in an atonic bladder.*
manobra de Hampton	**Hampton maneuver** *Rolling a patient during gastrointestinal fluoroscopy in order to obtain an air contrast of the antrum and duodenum.*
manobra de Heimlich	**Heimlich maneuver** *A forceful upward thrust to the diaphragm to dislodge an airway obstruction.*
manobra de Hillis-Müller	**Hillis-Müller maneuver** *A procedure to determine the descent of the head during active labor.*
manobra de Hueter	**Hueter's maneuver** *The application of downward and forward pressure on the tongue while passing an gastric tube.*
manobra de Jendrassik	**Jendrassik's maneuver** *A method of distracting a patient while checking the patellar reflex.*
manobra de Leopold	**Leopold's maneuver** *Used to determine fetal position.*
manobra de Ritgen	**Ritgen's maneuver** *A procedure that controls the rate of delivery of the infant's head during childbirth.*

Portuguese	English
manobra de Valsalva	**Valsalva's maneuver** *A technique in which one attempts to exhale with the mouth and nose closed; this equalizes pressure in the ears.*
manômetro	**manometer** *Device used for pressure monitoring.*
manúbrio esternal	**manubrium sterni** *The superior segment of the sternum which articulates with the clavicle and first rib.*
mapeamento	**mapping** *A collection of data points showing spatial distribution.*
marasmo	**marasmus** *Progressive weight loss and emaciation.*
marca de vinho do Porto; nevo flâmeo	**port-wine mark** *Also called nevus flammeus, it is a vascular anomaly characterized by purplish skin discoloration.*
marca-passo cardíaco	**pacemaker** *An electrical device used to stimulate the heart used for bradyarrhythmias.*
marcha em passos altos	**drop foot gait** *A gait characterized by dragging the foot, as there is no ankle dorsiflexion; usually associated with steppage gait.*
marcha festinante	**festinating gait** *Walking with increased speed involuntarily; often seen in Parkinson's disease.*
marcha gingada	**waddling gait** *Walking in short steps in a swaying fashion.*
marcha; andadura	**gait** *The way one walks.*
margem	**border** *Margin.*
marisco	**shellfish** *An aquatic shelled crustacean or mollusk.*
marsupialização	**marsupialization** *Creation of a surgical pouch.*
martelo	**malleus** *Small bone in the inner ear that articulates with the incus.*
massa	**mass** *Tumor.*
mastalgia	**mastodynia** *Breast pain.*
mastectomia	**mastectomy** *Surgical resection of one or both breasts.*
mastigação	**mastication** *Chewing.*
mastigar	**chew, to** *Masticate.*
mastite	**mastitis** *Inflammation of the breast.*
mastoidectomia	**mastoidectomy** *Surgical removal of the mastoid.*
mastoidite	**mastoiditis** *Inflammation of the mastoid process.*
mastóide	**mastoid** *Referring to the mastoid process.*
matéria	**content** *What something is made up of.*
maxilar	**maxilla** *The upper jaw that also forms the inferior portion of the orbit and part of the nose.*
maxilofacial	**maxillofacial** *Referring to the maxilla and the face.*
mazamorra	**mazamorra** *Dermatitis caused by hookworm larvae indigenous to Puerto Rico.*
má união	**malunion** *The union of a fracture in a faulty position.*
mácula	**macula** *1. The area of the eye of greatest visual acuity that surrounds the fovea. 2. A small flat discoloration of the skin (synonym for macule).*
máculas amareladas	**macula solaris** *Formal medical term describing a freckle.*
máquina coração-pulmão	**heart lung machine** *Device used during cardiac surgery to replace the function of the heart and lungs while surgery is performed.*
máscara de Hutchinson	**Hutchinson's mask** *The sensation the face is covered in cobwebs, associated with tabes dorsalis.*
máscara de não-reinalação	**non-rebreather mask** *A type of oxygen mask used to deliver a higher oxygen concentration.*
mão	**hand** *The upper extremity distal to the wrist.*

Portuguese	English
mão em garra	**clawhand** *A hand deformity caused by ulnar nerve palsy exhibited by the hyperextension of the metacarpophalangeal joints and flexion of the interphalangeal articulations.*
meato	**meatus** *Opening to the body, such as urethral meatus.*
mecônico	**meconium** *The first newborn feces which are green.*
medial	**medial** *Situated toward the midline.*
mediastino	**mediastinum** *The thoracic area between the lungs.*
mediastinoscopia	**medianstinoscopy** *Visual inspection of the mediastinum with a scope.*
medicação; medicamento (P)	**medication** *A substance used for medical treatment.*
medicamento para cálculo	**lithagogue** *A treatment of a calculus.*
medicamento por hiperlipemia	**lipid-lowering agent** *A medication used to treat hyperlipidemia.*
medicamento; estudo de doenças	**medicine** *A substance used for medical treatment or the art and science of healing patients.*
medicina nuclear	**nuclear medicine** *The branch of medicine associated with the use of radioactive material in the evaluation and treatment of disease.*
medicocirúrgico	**medicosurgical** *Referring to medicine and surgery.*
medida de cintura	**abdominal girth** *Waist circumference.*
medo	**fear** *Fright or trepidation.*
medo mórbido de fadiga	**kopophobia** *A morbid fear of fatigue.*
medula óssea	**bone marrow** *The soft material filling the cavity of bones.*
medula da glândula supra-renal	**adrenal medulla** *The innermost part of the adrenal gland.*
medula oblonga	**medulla oblongata** *The inferior portion of the brainstem.*
medular	**medullary** *1. The inner part of an organ. 2. Referring to the medulla oblongata.*
meduloblastoma	**medulloblastoma** *A malignant tumor of the cerebellum found mostly in children.*
megacariócito	**megakaryocyte** *A cell found in the bone marrow that is a source of platelet production.*
megacefalia	**megacephaly** *Having a larger than normal cranial capacity.*
megacólon	**megacolon** *Abnormal enlargement and dilatation of the colon.*
megaloblasto	**megaloblast** *A large red blood cell noted primarily in pernicious anemia.*
megalomania	**megalomania** *A mental disorder characterized by abnormal feelings of self-importance.*
meia-vida	**half-life** *The time a drug decreases its effect in half over time.*
meias	**socks** *Worn on the feet before one puts on shoes.*
meio cultura	**culture broth** *A medium used to grow bacteria.*
meio-dia	**noon** *The 12 o'clock mid-day hour.*
meiose	**meiosis** *Cell division creating two daughter cells each with half the number of cells as the parent cell.*
melancolia	**melancholia** *Profound sadness.*
melanina	**melanin** *A dark pigment found on the skin, hair or iris.*
melanoma	**melanoma** *Malignant cancer, typically found in the skin.*
melena	**black stools** *Common term for melena.*
melena	**melena** *The passage of black, tarry stools indicative of upper gastrointestinal bleeding.*
melhor	**best** *Optimal or ideal.*
melhoria	**amelioration** *The act of making something better or improvement.*
melissofobia	**melissophobia** *Also called apiphobia, a fear of bees.*

Portuguese	English
melite	**melitis** *Inflammation of the cheek.*
membrana celular	**cell membrane** *The semipermeable structure surrounding the cytoplasm of a cell.*
membrana timpânico	**tympanic membrane** *The membrane between the external and middle ear.*
membro	**limb** *An extremity or branch.*
membro	**member** *Referring to an extremity (arm or leg).*
membro superior	**upper limb** *Referring to either arm.*
memória	**memory** *Ability to remember.*
menarca	**menarche** *The time of the initial menstrual period.*
mencionar	**mention, to** *Refer to or allude to.*
meningioma	**meningioma** *A tumor of the meningeal tissue; generally benign.*
meningismo	**meningism** *Signs and symptoms of meningitis without infection of the meninges.*
meningite	**meningitis** *Inflammation of the meninges exhibited by fever, photophobia, nuchal rigidity and in severe cases coma and convulsions.*
meningite criptocócica	**cryptococcal meningitis** *A meningeal infection associated with AIDS.*
meningocele	**meningocele** *A congenital defect exhibited by protrusion of the meninges through a defect in the spinal column.*
meningococcemia	**meningococcemia** *Presence of N. meningitidis in the blood.*
meniscectomia	**meniscectomy** *Surgical excision of a meniscus.*
menisco	**meniscus** *A thin cartilage between joint surfaces.*
meníngeo	**meningeal** *Referring to the dura mater, arachnoid and the pia mater.*
menopausa	**menopause** *The time when menstruation ceases.*
menorragia	**menorrhagia** *Abnormally large amount of menstrual blood.*
menos	**less** *A smaller amount.*
menstruação	**menses** *The blood and other material expelled from the uterus during menstruation.*
menstruação	**menstruation** *Synonym of menses.*
mento; queixo	**chin** *Mentum; the anterior projection of the lower jaw.*
mentual	**mental** *Cognitive or psychological.*
mergulhador	**diver** *A person who swims in deep water.*
mesarterite	**mesarteritis** *Inflammation of the middle layer of an artery.*
mesencéfalo	**mesencephalon** *Midbrain.*
mesentério	**mesentery** *The fold of peritoneum that connects the small bowel, pancreas and spleen to the posterior portion of the abdominal wall.*
mesênquima	**mesenchyme** *Organized mesodermal cells that produce connective tissue, lymphatics and bone.*
mesoapêndice	**mesoappendix** *The portion of the mesentery vermiform appendix.*
mesocólon	**mesocolon** *The mesentery connecting the colon to the posterior abdominal wall.*
mesoderma	**mesoderm** *The middle germ layer in an embryo that is the source of bone, muscle and skin.*
mesonefroma	**mesonephroma** *Usually a tumor of the female genital tract that is thought to stem from the mesonephros.*
mesossalpinge	**mesosalpinx** *A portion of the broad ligament supporting the fallopian tubes.*
mesotelioma	**mesothelioma** *A tumor that stems from mesothelial tissue; a known cause is asbestos exposure.*

Portuguese	English
mesovário	**mesovarium** *The portion of the mesentery connecting the ovary with the abdominal wall.*
metabólico	**metabolic** *Referring to the physical and chemical reactions involved with keeping an organism functioning.*
metacarpiano	**metacarpal** *The name for any of the five hand bones.*
metacarpofalangiano	**metacarpophalangeal** *Referring to the metacarpus and the phalanges.*
metade	**half** *Divided in two.*
metaplasia	**metaplasia** *Abnormal change in the nature or character of tissue.*
metatarsalgia	**metatarsalgia** *Foot pain.*
metatársico	**metatarsal** *Any of the bones of the foot.*
metáfise	**metaphysis** *The region between the diaphysis and the epiphysis.*
metemoblobina	**methemoglobin** *A substance formed with the oxidation of hemoglobin.*
metencéfalo	**hindbrain** *The brainstem which includes the pons, medulla oblongata and cerebellum.*
metionina	**methionine** *A sulfur-containing amino acid used in the biosynthesis of cysteine.*
metro	**meter** *Unit if measurement. (instrument for measurement)*
metrorragia	**metrorrhagia** *Uterine bleeding in normal amounts but at irregular intervals.*
médico	**physician** *Medical practitioner.*
médico antecedente de família	**family history** *A review of past medical history of related persons.*
médico especialista em dietas	**dietitian** *A professional who works with diet and nutrition.*
médico legista	**coroner** *A person who investigates sudden or suspicious deaths.*
método de Ziehl-Neelsen	**Ziehl-Neelsen carbolfuchsin stain** *A stain used to detect acid-fast bacilli that appear red on the methylene blue background.*
mialgia	**myalgia** *Muscle pain.*
miastenia grave	**myasthenia gravis** *An autoimmune disease characterized by fluctuating weakness of the ocular, limb and respiratory muscles.*
micação	**voiding** *The act of urinating.*
micção	**micturition** *Synonym of urination.*
micetoma	**mycetoma** *Persistent inflammation of the tissues caused by an infection.*
micose	**mycosis** *A disease caused by a fungal infection.*
micose do pé	**athlete's foot** *Common term for tinea pedis.*
micotoxina	**mycotoxin** *A substance toxic to fungus.*
microbiologia	**microbiology** *The study of microorganisms.*
microcefálico	**microcephalic** *A congenital deformity exhibited by an abnormally small head.*
microftalmia	**microphthalmos** *A congenital condition characterized by smallness of the eyes.*
micrognatia	**micrognathia** *Abnormally small maxilla or mandible.*
micrograma	**microgram** *One millionth of one gram.*
microrganismo	**microorganism** *An organism only seen with a microscope.*
microscópio	**microscope** *A instrument used to magnify and view small objects.*
microscópio eletrônico	**electron microscope** *A device that uses electron beams and lenses to give high magnification.*
micróbio	**microbe** *A microorganism.*

Portuguese	English
micrócito	**microcyte** *An unusually small erythrocyte associated with anemias, such as iron deficiency anemia.*
micrômetro	**micrometer** *One millionth of one meter.*
midríase	**mydriasis** *Pupillary dilation.*
mielina	**myelin** *The substance that forms a sheath around some nerve fibers.*
mielite	**myelitis** *Inflammation of the spinal cord.*
mielocele	**myelocele** *Protrusion of the spinal cord through a defect in the bony structure.*
mielograma	**myelogram** *CT scan or roentgenography of the spinal canal after injection of contrast media.*
mieloma	**myeloma** *Malignant tumor of the bone marrow.*
mielomatose	**myelomatosis** *A leukemic disease in which there is an abnormally high amount of myeloblasts in the blood.*
mielomeningocele	**myelomeningocele** *A protrusion of the spinal cord and its meninges through a defect in the vertebral canal.*
mielopatia	**myelopathy** *A condition of the spinal cord.*
mielóide	**myeloid** *Referring to the bone marrow or spinal cord.*
miliária	**miliary** *Referring to a disease that is exhibited by small seed-like lesions (millet), such as miliary tuberculosis.*
miligrama	**milligram** *A unit of weight, 1/1000 of a gram.*
mililitro	**milliliter** *A unit of volume, 1/1000 of a liter.*
milímetro	**millimeter** *A unit of measurement, 1/1000 of a meter.*
minuto	**minute** *A unit of time.*
minúsculo	**minute** *Something very small.*
miocardite	**myocarditis** *An inflammation of the heart.*
miocárdio	**myocardial** *Referring to the muscular tissue of the heart.*
miocárdio	**myocardium** *The middle layer of the heart wall.*
mioclonia	**myoclonus** *Contraction or spasm of a group of muscles.*
mioclonia palatal	**palatal myoclonus** *An involuntary, persistent, rapid regular tremor of the soft palate and face.*
mioglobina	**myoglobin** *A protein within muscle that carries and stores oxygen.*
mioma	**myoma** *A benign neoplasm of muscular tissue.*
miomectomia	**myomectomy** *Surgical resection of a myoma.*
miométrio	**myometrium** *The smooth muscle layer of the uterus.*
miopatia	**myopathy** *Muscle disease.*
miopia; visão curta	**myopia** *Nearsightedness.*
miosina	**myosin** *A protein that when coupled with actin form the contractile complex of a muscle cells.*
miosite	**myositis** *Inflammation of muscle tissue.*
miossarcoma	**myosarcoma** *A mass with myoma and sarcoma characteristics.*
miostie ossificante	**myositis ossificans** *Inflammation of muscle tissue with presence of bony deposits.*
miotomia	**myotomy** *The surgical removal of muscle tissue.*
miriachite	**miryachit** *A disease of Siberia characterized by an exaggerated startle response; also referred to as jumping disease.*
miringite	**myringitis** *Inflammation of the tympanic membrane.*
miringoplastia	**myringoplasty** *Surgical repair of tympanic membrane defects.*
miringotomia	**myringotomy** *Surgical opening of the tympanic membrane.*
misantropia	**misanthropy** *A severe dislike of homo sapiens.*
misofobia	**mysophobia** *Severe fear of dirt or contamination from common objects.*

Portuguese	English
mitocôndria	**mitochondria** *Organelle found in cells responsible for energy production.*
mitose	**mitosis** *Cell division in which two daughter cells are formed that have the same number of chromosomes as the parent cell.*
mitral	**mitral** *Referring to the mitral valve.*
mixedema	**myxedema** *Diffuse edema with a wax-like appearance of the skin; this condition is associated with hypothyroidism.*
mixoma	**myxoma** *A tumor composed of mucous tissue.*
mixossarcoma	**myxosarcoma** *A sarcoma that also has mucous tissue.*
mocidade	**youth** *The time between childhood and being an adult.*
modíolo	**modiolus** *A column located in the cochlea.*
modo	**mood** *A temporary state of mind or feeling.*
molalidade	**molality** *The number of moles of a solution per kilogram of pure solvent.*
molde de gesso	**cast; plaster cast** *Use of plaster of paris to immobilize an extremity.*
molde gessado	**plaster cast** *Use of gypsum impregnated gauze to immobilize fractured extremities.*
molde gessado por ambulação	**walking cast** *A cast used for simple fractures of the lower leg.*
molécula	**molecule** *A combination of at least two atoms.*
monitor	**monitor** *A person that observes a process or a monitoring device.*
monitor fetal	**fetal monitor** *Device used to monitor fetal heart rate and rhythm.*
monitorar ECG ambulatorial	**ambulatory electrocardiographic monitoring** *A continuous recording of the electrocardiogram used to detect occult dysrhythmias.*
monocitose	**monocytosis** *An abnormal increase in the number of monocytes in the blood.*
monoclonal	**monoclonal** *Asexual formation of a clone from a single cell.*
monofosfato de adenosina	**adenosine monophosphate** *A nucleotide, it is produced when ATP is converted to ADP.*
monomania	**monomania** *A psychotic obsession about a single subject.*
mononeurite	**mononeuritis** *Inflammation of a single nerve.*
mononeuropatia cranial III	**cranial mononeuropathy III** *Dysfunction of the third cranial nerve causes double vision and eyelid drooping.*
mononeuropatia cranial VI	**cranial mononeuropathy VI** *A disorder of the sixth cranial nerve causes double vision.*
mononuclear	**mononuclear** *A cell having only one nucleus.*
mononucleose	**mononucleosis** *An infectious disease exhibited by malaise and lymphadenopathy.*
monoplegia	**monoplegia** *Paralysis of a single limb.*
monócito	**monocyte** *A leukocyte with an oval nucleus and grey cytoplasm.*
monte pubiano	**mons pubis** *The fleshy protuberance over the symphysis pubis.*
morbidade	**morbidity** *The state of disease.*
mordedura por carrapato	**tick bite**
morféia	**morphea** *A condition exhibited by an elevated or depressed patch of pink skin with a purple border.*
morfina	**morphine** *An opioid analgesic.*
morfologia	**morphology** *The study of living organisms and the correlation between their structure.*
morgue; necrotério	**morgue** *A room where deceased patients are housed until sent to a funeral home.*
moribundo	**moribund** *Near death.*

Portuguese	English
morrer	**die, to** *To stop living, to expire.*
morte	**death** *The action of dying.*
morte cerebral	**brain death** *Cessation of cerebral functioning.*
morto	**dead** *Deceased.*
mosca preto	**black fly** *From the family Simuliidae, a gnat that can cause disease in humans; also called buffalo fly.*
mosqueamento	**mottled** *An irregular arrangement of patches of color.*
motor	**motor** *Referring to muscles.*
movimento fetal	**fetal movements** *Sensations by the mother of fetal activity.*
movimento rápido dos olhos	**REM (rapid eye movement) sleep** *This period of sleep is associated with irregular respirations and heart rate, involuntary movements and dreaming.*
movimentos oculares rápidos (MOR)	**Rapid Eye Movement** *The movement of a person's eyes during this period of sleep.*
mórbido	**morbid** *Indicative of disease.*
mórula	**morula** *A solid mass created by the splitting of an ovum.*
mucilagem	**mucilage** *1. A viscous bodily fluid. 2. A polysaccharide used in medicines and glue.*
mucina	**mucin** *A glycoprotein that is the primary constituent in mucous.*
muco	**mucus** *A substance secreted by mucous membranes.*
mucocele	**mucocele** *An accumulation of mucous in a dilated cavity.*
mucolítico	**mucolytic** *A substance that breaks down mucous.*
mucopolissacaridose do tipo ; síndrome de Morquio	**mucopolysaccharidosis type IV** *Also referred to as Morquio syndrome, persons do not produce galactosamine-6-sulfatase or in some cases beta-galactosidase. Symptoms include hypermobile joints, macrocephaly, short stature and wide spaced teeth.*
mucopolissacaridose do tipo I; síndrome de Hurler	**mucopolysaccharidosis type I** *Also referred to as Hurler syndrome, persons cannot make lysosomal alpha-L-iduronidase which breaks down glycosaminoglycans.*
mucopolissacaridose do tipo II; síndrome de Hunter	**mucopolysaccharidosis type II** *Also referred to as Hunter syndrome, persons with this inherited condition cannot produce iduronate sulfatase. There are mild to severe forms but all forms have deafness, coarse facial features, hypertrichosis and macrocephaly.*
mucopolissacaridose do tipo III; síndrome de Sanfilippo	**mucopolysaccharidosis type III** *Also referred to as Sanfilippo syndrome, persons cannot catabolize the heparan sulfate sugar chain. Symptoms include stiff joints, thick eyebrows, coarse facial features and developmental delays.*
mucopolissacaridose do tipo IS; síndrome de Scheie	**mucopolysaccharidosis type Is** *Also referred to as Scheie syndrome, persons cannot produce lysosomal alpha-L-iduronidase. Symptoms include cloudy cornea, hirsutism, prognathism and stiff joints.*
mucopolissacaridose do tipo VI; síndrome de Marotaeux-Lamy	**mucopolysaccharidosis type VI** *Also referred to as Maroteaux-Lamy syndrome. It is characterized by hydrocephalus, macroglossia and coarse facial features but normal intelligence.*
mucopurulento	**mucopurulent** *That which contains both mucous and pus.*
mucosa	**mucosa** *A mucous membrane like the buccal mucosa.*
mucóide	**mucoid** *Referring to mucous.*
mudo	**mute** *Refraining from or being speechless.*
muitos	**lots of** *An abundance of.*
muleta	**crutch** *Long metal or wooden stick used for support while walking.*
muleta de antebraço	**forearm crutch** *A long stick with a place for a hand-grip to aid in ambulation when there is lower extremity weakness.*

Portuguese	English
multigrávida	**multigravida** *A woman who has been pregnant more than once.*
multilocular	**multilocular** *The presence of more than one cell within a cavity.*
multípara	**multipara** *A woman with more than one live births.*
muscular	**muscular** *Referring to muscles.*
mutação	**mutation** *A gene alteration that can be passed to the next generation.*
mutismo	**mutism** *Inability to speak.*
músculo	**muscle** *A band if fibrous tissue that can contract.*
músculo abdutor curto do polegar	**abductor pollicis brevis** *Abducts the thumb.*
músculo abdutor longo do polegar	**abductor pollicis longus** *Abducts and flexes the thumb.*
músculo bucinador	**buccinator muscle** *Pulls the mouth posteriorly.*
músculo estapédio	**stapedius muscle** *Located in the tympanic interior, it reduces stapedial movement.*
músculo glúteo	**gluteal or gluteus muscle** *A paired set of three muscles, the gluteus maximus, medius and minimus, that all have origins in the ilium and insertions in the femur. (buttocks)*
músculo occipitofrontal	**occipitofrontal muscle** *Raises the eyebrows.*
músculo reto abdominal	**rectus abdominis muscle** *The pair of long, flat muscles that connect the sternum with the pubis.*
músculo sartório	**sartorius muscle** *The thigh muscle that runs from the pelvis to the proximal, medial aspect of the tibia.*
músculo solear	**soleus muscle** *Assists with ankle plantar flexion.*
músculo trapézio	**trapezius muscle** *The muscle with an origin of occipital bone and seventh cervical vertebra, insertion of clavicle and scapula, and it draws the scapula backward.*
myatonia	**amyotonia** *A condition associated with the lack of muscle tone.*
narcisismo	**narcissism** *Abnormally excessive self-interest.*
narcolepsia	**narcolepsy** *A condition exhibited by a strong desire to sleep and by sudden onset of sleep at increased intervals.*
narcose	**narcosis** *A reversible medication-induced condition of excessive drowsiness or unconsciousness.*
narcótico	**narcotic** *A medication that produces narcosis.*
narimorto	**stillborn** *Refers to a newborn that died in utero.*
narinas	**nostril** *One of two openings in the nose used for air passage.*
nariz	**nose** *The midface protuberance used for smelling and breathing.*
nariz sangrante	**nosebleed** *Common term for epistaxis.*
nasal; rinal	**nasal** *Referring to the nose.*
nascer	**born, to be** *Being present as a result of birth.*
nasofaringe	**nasopharynx** *The part of the pharynx which lies superior to the soft palate.*
nasofaríngeo	**nasopharyngeal** *Referring to the nose and pharynx.*
nasolacrimal	**nasolacrimal** *Referring to the nose and tear apparatus.*
navicular	**navicular** *1. boat shaped 2. Referring to the navicular bone of the hand or foot.*
nádegas	**buttocks** *The bilateral region covering the gluteal muscles.*
náusea	**nausea** *A feeling that one wants to vomit.*
náusea das alturas; doença de Acosta; doença das montanhas	**altitude sickness** *A general term used for an illness that occurs at high altitude.*
não ressuscitar	**DNR Do not resuscitate.** *The term used to indicate a person should not have life sustaining measures taken if they were to have cardiopulmonary arrest.*

Portuguese	English
nebulizador	**nebulizer** *A device used for transforming a liquid into a fine mist for inhalation as in nebulized albuterol for an acute exacerbation of asthma.*
nebuloso	**hazy** *Cloudy.*
necroscopia	**necropsy** *Synonym of autopsy.*
necrose	**necrosis** *The death of most of the cells of the affected part.*
necrose avascular	**avascular necrosis** *Bone death caused by poor blood supply.*
necrótico	**necrotic** *Referring to necrosis.*
nefrectomia	**nephrectomy** *Surgical removal of a kidney.*
nefrite	**nephritis** *A general term meaning inflammation of a kidney that is further categorized depending on the associated pathology.*
nefroblastoma	**nephroblastoma** *Congenital tumor of the kidney, also called Wilms' tumor.*
nefrocalcinose	**nephrocalcinosis** *A condition exhibited by calcium phosphate deposition in the renal tubules; a cause of renal insufficiency.*
nefrolitíase	**nephrolithiasis** *A calculus in the kidney.*
nefrolitotomia	**nephrolithotomy** *Surgical removal of a renal calculus.*
nefroma	**nephroma** *A renal tumor.*
nefropatia	**nephropathy** *Renal disease.*
nefropexia	**nephropexy** *The surgical fixation of a kidney that was previously floating.*
nefroptose	**nephroptosis** *Inferior displacement of the kidney.*
nefrosclerose	**nephrosclerosis** *Hardening of the kidney.*
nefrose	**nephrosis** *A kidney disease exhibited by edema and proteinuria; also called nephrotic syndrome.*
nefrostomia	**nephrostomy** *Surgical creation of an opening between the renal pelvis and an opening in the skin.*
nefrotomia	**nephrotomy** *Surgical incision of the kidney.*
nefrótico	**nephrotic** *Referring to nephrosis.*
negar	**deny, to** *To reject or repudiate.*
negar	**withhold, to** *To refuse to give something.*
negativo	**negative** *Contrary or opposing.*
nematódeo	**nematode** *An endoparasite belonging to the class of the Nemathelminthes including roundworms and threadworms.*
neonado	**neonate** *The term for a newborn infant for the first four weeks.*
neonatal	**neonatal** *Referring to the first four weeks after birth.*
neoplasma	**neoplasm** *A new and abnormal growth.*
nervo	**nerve** *A fibrous band made up of axons and dendrites that connects the nervous systems with other organs.*
nervo acessório, nervo espinhal	**accessory nerve (XI)** *Supplies motor innervation to the sternocleidomastoid and trapezius.*
nervo circunflexo	**circumflex nerve** *The axillary nerve that has an origin in the posterior branch of the brachial plexus.*
nervo espinhal	**spinal nerve** *The term for each of the thirty pairs of nerves that originate in the spine and traverse between the vertebrae. There are eight cervical, twelve thoracic, five lumbar, five sacral and one coccygeal nerve pairs.*
nervo esplâncnico	**splanchnic nerves** *The nerves supplying the abdominal viscera and blood vessels.*
nervo facial (VII)	**facial nerve** *Cranial nerve VII that supplies the face and tongue.*
nervo femoral	**femoral nerve** *Supplies the motor function of the quadriceps and the sensation over the anterior and medial thigh.*
nervo hipoglosso	**hypoglossal nerve** *Twelfth cranial nerve pair.*

Portuguese	English
nervo motor ocular externo (P) nervo abducente (B)	**abducens nerve** *A motor nerve (6th cranial nerve) that controls the lateral rectus muscle of the eye.)*
nervo oculomotor	**oculomotor nerve** *Referring to cranial nerve III which is one of the nerves responsible for extraocular movements.*
nervo sensitivo	**sensory nerve** *A nerve that receives input from various receptors.*
nervo trigêmeo	**trigeminal nerve** *The fifth cranial nerve which supplies the motor function of mastication and has three sensory branches, the ophthalmic, maxillary and mandibular.*
nervo troclear	**trochlear nerve** *The fourth cranial nerve that supplies the superior oblique muscle of the eyeball.*
nervo ulnar; nervo cubital	**ulnar nerve** *Arises from the C8-T1 nerves and supplies the hand. (Injury to the ulnar nerve causes loss of flexion of the metacarpophalangeal joints and extension at the interphalangeal joints, thus the common term, claw hand.)*
nervo vago	**vagus nerve** *The tenth cranial nerve that supplies the heart, lungs visceral organs; its function is tested by assessment of elevation of the uvula.*
neural	**neural** *Referring to a nerve or nerve impulse.*
neuralgia geniculada	**geniculate neuralgia** *Severe intermittent pain in the external ear and deep in the ear.*
neuralgia trigêmeo	**trigeminal neuralgia** *Pain in the region of one or more branches of the fifth cranial nerve sensory branches.*
neuralgia; neurodinia	**neuralgia** *Severe pain along the course of a nerve.*
neurapraxia	**neurapraxia** *Paralysis from nerve injury but no degeneration of the nerve.*
neurastenia	**neurasthenia** *A psychoneurosis exhibited by severe fatigue.*
neurectomia	**neurectomy** *Excision of a section of a nerve.*
neurite	**neuritis** *Inflammation of a nerve.*
neurite retrobulbar	**retrobulbar optic neuritis** *An inflammatory, demyelinating condition in the retrobulbar region.*
neuroblastoma	**neuroblastoma** *A nervous system malignant tumor composed of neuroblasts.*
neurocirurgia	**neurosurgery** *Surgery of the brain or spinal cord.*
neurodermatite	**neurodermatitis** *A pruritic, thickened eruption in the axillary and inguinal thought to be exacerbated by emotions.*
neuroepitélio	**neuroepithelium** *Cells specialized to serve as sensory cells such as cells of the cochlea and tongue.*
neurofibroma	**neurofibroma** *A tumor formed by excessive growth of perineurium and endoneurium.*
neurofibromatose	**neurofibromatosis** *A hereditary condition exhibited by formation of multiple soft tumors scattered throughout the skin surface. Also known as von Recklinghausen disease.*
neurolema	**neurilemma** *The membrane covering a myelinated nerve fiber or the axon of an unmyelinated nerve fiber.*
neuroléptico	**neuroleptic** *A drug that causes neurologic symptoms.*
neurologia	**neurology** *The study of the nervous system.*
neurologista	**neurologist** *A physician who specializes in the study of the nervous system.*
neuroma	**neuroma** *A mass composed of nerve cells and fibers.*
neuroma acústico	**acoustic neuroma** *A nonmalignant tumor that can cause deafness, tinnitus and vertigo.*
neuropatia	**neuropathy** *Structural of pathologic changes of the peripheral nervous system.*
neuropatia de encarceramento	**entrapment neuropathy** *Weakness or numbness caused by compression of a peripheral nerve.*

Portuguese	English
neuropatia diabético	**diabetic neuropathy** *Pain and burning initially in the feet, associated with diabetes mellitus.*
neuropatia em bulbo de cebola; neuropatia intersticial hipertrófica	**onion bulb neuropathy** *Also known as hypertrophic interstitial neuropathy which is a sensorimotor polyneuropathy.*
neuropatia óptica isquêmica	**ischemic optic neuropathy** *A general category of a cause of blindness with several subcategories.*
neuropatia plexo braquial	**brachial plexus neuropathy** *Characterized by acute arm or shoulder pain followed by focal muscle weakness.*
neuropatia por vitamina B12; degeneração subaguda combinada da medula espinhal	**vitamin B12 neuropathy** *Abnormal sensation related to a chronic deficiency of cyanocobalamin;also called subacute combined degeneration of the spinal cord or Putnam-Dana syndrome.*
neuropático	**neuropathic** *Referring to neuropathy.*
neurose	**neurosis** *A mental disorder.*
neurossífilis	**neurosyphilis** *Infection of the central nervous system with Treponema pallidum.*
neurotmese	**neurotmesis** *The severing of a nerve.*
neurotomia	**neurotomy** *Surgical incision into a nerve.*
neurotransmissor	**neurotransmitter** *A substance released at the end of a nerve fiber that facilitates transmission of an impulse.*
neuróglia	**neuroglia** *A type of connective tissue of the nervous system.*
neurônio	**neuron** *A nerve cell.*
neutropenia	**neutropenia** *Diminished number of neutrophils in the blood.*
neutrófilo	**neutrophil** *A polymorphonuclear leukocyte.*
nevo arâneo	**spider nevus** *A papule with telangiectases radiating from the center.*
nevo capilar	**capillary nevus** *A growth of skin that involves the capillaries.*
nevo; espiloma	**nevus** *A benign, well-circumscribed growth of tissue of congenital origin.*
nébula	**nebula** *An opaque spot on the cornea causing impaired vision.*
néfron	**nephron** *A functional unit of the kidney that consists of the glomerulus, the proximal and distal convoluted tubules, the loop of Henle and the collecting tubule.*
nistagmo	**nystagmus** *Rapid involuntary movement of the eyes; it can be horizontal, vertical or rotary.*
nistagmo pendular	**oscillating nystagmus** *Abnormal movement of the eyes in a wave-like pattern.*
nitrato de prata	**silver nitrate stick** *A medical device used to treat hypergranulation tissue.*
nitrogênio	**nitrogen** *A colorless, odorless gas used as a coolant in the liquid form.*
nocivo	**noxious** *Harmful or poisonous.*
noctúria	**nocturia** *Urination at night.*
nodo	**node** *A swelling or prominence.*
nodo sinoatrial	**sinoatrial node** *A mass of cardiac tissue that acts as the pacemaker.*
nodos de Herberden	**Heberden's node** *Hard nodules formed at the distal interphalangeal joints in osteoarthritis.*
nome	**name** *A word by which a person is known.*
nome de solteira	**maiden name** *The surname a woman uses prior to being married.*
norepinefrina	**norepinephrine** *A hormone secreted by the adrenal medulla and a synthetic drug used as a pressor agent.*
normoblasto	**normoblast** *A precursor cell for erythrocytes.*

Portuguese	English
normócito	**normocyte** *A normal erythrocyte.*
nosofobia	**nosophobia** *Unwarranted, excessive fear of any disease.*
nosologia	**nosology** *The medical science of disease classification.*
noturno	**nocturnal** *Referring to events that happen at night.*
nó	**knot** *A fastening made by tying a suture, for instance.*
nó sincicial	**syncytial knot** *Aggregation of syncytiotrophoblastic nuclei in the villi of the placenta during early pregnancy.*
nódulo	**nodule** *A small node in the skin of up to 1cm and in the lung up to 3cm.*
nódulo da Irmã Joseph	**Sister Mary Joseph nodule** *A nodule at the umbilicus associated with metastatic abdominal cancer.*
nódulo de Schmorl	**Schmorl's nodule** *Protrusion of the nucleus pulposus through the vertebral body endplate into the adjacent vertebra.*
nódulos de Caplan	**Caplan nodules** *These are pulmonary nodules noted in people with rheumatoid arthritis who were exposed to coal dust.*
nuclear	**nuclear** *Referring to a nucleus.*
nucleoproteína	**nucleoprotein** *A substance composed of a nucleic acid and a protein.*
nuligrávida	**nulligravida** *A woman who has never been pregnant.*
nulípara	**nullipara** *A woman who has never given birth.*
numulação	**nummulation** *Formed as round, flat discs.*
nutação	**nutation** *Referring to nodding of the head.*
nutrição	**nutrition** *The process of supplying food needed for growth.*
nutrição entérico	**enteral feeding** *Nutrition supplied via the alimentary canal.*
nutrição magro	**low-fat foods** *Nutrients with lower than normal fat content.*
nutriente	**nutrient** *A substance that provides essential nourishment.*
núcleo	**core** *Central part of a structure.*
núcleo arqueado	**arcuate nucleus** *Small masses of gray matter found on the medulla oblongata.*
núcleo vermelho	**red nucleus** *A collection of gray matter near the subthalamus that receives data from the superior cerebellar peduncle.*
obesidade	**obesity** *Having a body mass index over 30kilograms/meters squared.*
obsessão	**obsession** *A pathologic preoccupation.*
obsoleto	**obsolete** *No longer in use; antiquated.*
obstetra	**obstetrician** *A physician who specializes in the management of pregnancy, labor and the peuperium.*
obstetrícia	**midwifery** *The occupation of assisting in childbirth.*
obstétrico	**obstetric** *Referring to The management of pregnancy, labor and the peuperium.*
obstrução	**obstructed** *To be blocked or halted.*
obstrução intestinal	**intestinal obstruction** *Blockage of the intestine by mass or volvulus.*
obturador	**obturator** *A device used to close an artificial or natural opening.*
obtuso	**obtuse** *Rather insensitive or hard to understand.*
occipital	**occipital** *Referring to the back part of the head.*
oclusão	**occlusion** *A pathway that is blocked or obstructed.*
oclusão coronaria	**coronary occlusion** *A blockage in a coronary artery.*
ocular	**ocular** *Referring to the eye.*
oculogírico	**oculogyric** *Referring to movement of the eye around the anteroposterior axis.*
odinofagia	**odynophagia** *Pain associated with swallowing.*

Portuguese	English
odinofonia	**odynophonia** *Pain associated with speaking.*
odontalgia	**odontalgia** *Tooth pain.*
odontalgia	**toothache** *Dental pain.*
odontologia	**odontology** *Synonym of dentistry.*
odontóide	**odontoid** *A prominence on the second cervical vertebra on which the first cervical vertebra pivots.*
odor; cheiro	**odor** *A smell that is given off someone or something.*
odorífero	**odiferous** *Having an unpleasant or distinctive smell.*
oftalmia	**ophthalmia** *Profound inflammation of the eye or its structures.*
oftalmia gonorréica	**gonorrheal ophthalmia** *An acute purulent conjunctivitis that can occur in neonates within 2-5 days of birth.*
oftalmologia	**ophthalmology** *The study of diseases of the eye.*
oftalmologista	**ophthalmologist** *A physician specializing in diseases of the eye.*
oftalmoplegia	**ophthalmoplegia** *Paralysis of the eye muscles.*
oftalmoplegia supranuclear	**supranuclear ophthalmoplegia** *A disorder that effects the extraocular movements especially limiting the upward movement of the eyes.*
oftalmoscópio	**ophthalmoscope** *A device used to visually inspect the interior eye.*
oftálmico	**ophthalmic** *Referring to the eye.*
ofuscamento	**glare** *An angry stare.*
olecrânio; olécrano	**olecranon** *The bony protrusion at the proximal ulna at the elbow.*
olfatório	**olfactory** *Referring to the sense of smell.*
oligodactilia	**oligodactyly** *Presence of fewer than 5 digits on a hand or foot.*
oligodendria	**oligodendroglia** *The ectodermal cells forming part of the central nervous system.*
oligoidrâmnios	**oligohydramnios** *Inadequate amount of amniotic fluid.*
oligomenorréia	**oligomenorrhea** *Infrequent menstruation or low volume menstrual flow.*
oligoptialismo	**oligoptyalism** *Insufficient secretion of saliva; also oligosialia.*
oligospermia	**oligospermia** *Abnormally low sperm count.*
oligotrofia	**oligotrophia or hypotrichosis** *Less than normal amount of head/body hair.*
oligúria	**oliguria** *Abnormally low urine output.*
ombro (ombro direito, ombro esquerdo)	**shoulder** *The joint were the scapula joins the clavicle and humerus. (right shoulder, left shoulder)*
ombro congelado; capsulite adesiva	**frozen shoulder** *Common term for adhesive capsulitis.*
ombrofobia	**ombrophobia** *An abnormal fear of rain.*
omento	**omentum** *A fold of peritoneum fastening the stomach to other organs in the viscera.*
omentocele	**omentocele** *A herniated protrusion of omentum.*
omentopexia	**omentopexy** *Surgically fastening the omentum to an adjacent tissue it was not previously attached to.*
oncologia	**oncology** *The study of cancer.*
oncologista	**oncologist** *A physician specializing in the treatment of cancer.*
onda alfa	**alpha wave** *Electroencephalographic waves with a frequency of 8-13 per second.*
onfalite	**omphalitis** *Inflammation of the umbilicus.*
onfalocele	**omphalocele** *A large congenital, umbilical hernia with only a thin membranous covering.*
ONG ouvido, nariz, e garganta	**ENT** *Abbreviation for ears, nose and throat.*

Portuguese	English
onicocriptose	**onychocryptosis** *Ingrown toenail.*
onicocriptose; unha encravada	**ingrown nail** *Also referred to as onychocryptosis.*
onicofagia	**onychophagia** *Habitually chewing on one's fingernails.*
onicogrifose	**onychogryphosis** *A deformed nail that is incurved or hooked.*
onicomicose	**onychomycosis** *Fungal disease of the toenails or fingernails.*
oniquia	**onychia** *Inflammation of the toenail or fingernail matrix.*
oniquia seca	**onychia sicca** *Brittle fingernails or toenails.*
ooforectomia	**oophorectomy** *Surgical removal of an ovary.*
ooforite	**oophoritis** *Inflammation of an ovary.*
ooforossalpingectomia	**oophorosalpingectomy** *Surgical removal of an ovary and fallopian tube.*
oogênese	**oogenesis** *The initiation and development of an ovum.*
oócito	**oocyte** *An ovarian cell that needs to undergo meiotic division to become an ovum.*
oóforo	**oophoron** *Synonym for ovary.*
operação	**operation** *A surgical procedure.*
opiáceo	**opiate** *Referring to opium.*
opióide	**opioid** *A substance similar to opium that binds to at least one of the opium receptors in the body.*
opistótono	**opisthotonos** *A profound spasm in which the head/neck is hyperextended, the feet are touching the bed and with the patient supine the body arched upward.*
oponente	**opponens** *Synonym for opponent muscle.*
opsonina	**opsonin** *An antibody used to facilitate phagocytosis of a bacterium.*
optometria	**optometry** *The profession of examination of the eyes for disease (not a medical doctor).*
optometrista	**optometrist** *A person who practices optometry.*
oral	**oral** *Relating to the mouth.*
oralmente	**orally** *By mouth.*
orbicular	**orbicular** *Rounded or circular.*
orbitário	**orbital** *Referring to the orbit.*
orelha; ouvido	**ear** *The organ of hearing and balance.*
Organização Mundial de Saúde (da ONU em Geneva)	**World Health Organization (WHO)**
organomegalia	**organomegaly** *Enlargement of an organ, typically referring to an intraabdominal organ.*
orifício	**orifice** *Synonym of foramen.*
ornitose	**ornithosis** *A viral infection transmitted by birds that is manifested by chills, headache, photophobia, fever, nausea and vomiting.*
orofaringe	**oropharynx** *The portion of the pharynx between the soft palate and the superior aspect of the epiglottis.*
orquialgia	**orchialgia** *Testicular pain.*
orquidectomia	**orchidectomy** *Synonym of orchiectomy; removal of one or both testes.*
orquiepididimite	**orchiepididymitis** *Inflammation of the testis and epididymis.*
orquiopexia	**orchidopexy** *Surgical repair of an undescended testis.*
orquite	**orchitis** *Inflammation of one or both testes.*
ortodôntica	**orthodontics** *A subspecialty of dentistry concerned with treatment of dental irregularities and malocclusion, including the use of braces.*
ortografia errada	**misspelling** *Incorrect spelling of a word.*

Portuguese	English
ortopedia	**orthopedics** *A surgical specialty concerned with treatment of skeletal problems.*
ortopnéia	**orthopnea** *The inability to breath comfortably except in the upright position.*
ortose	**orthosis** *Straightening of a malaligned part with the use of braces and other supportive devices.*
ortostático	**orthostatic** *Referring to the standing position. Orthostatic hypotension is low blood pressure in the standing position.*
oscilante	**unsteady** *Unstable or wobbly.*
osmol	**osmole** *The recognized unit of osmotic pressure.*
osmolalidade	**osmolality** *The concentration expressed in total number of solute particles per kilogram.*
osmose	**osmosis** *The movement of a solvent from a solution of greater concentration to one of lower concentration through a semi-permeable membrane until the two solutions have equal concentration.*
osmótico	**osmotic** *Referring to osmosis.*
ossificação	**ossification** *The formation of bone.*
ossículo	**ossicle** *A small bone. (auditory ossicle)*
osso	**bone** *Skeletal tissue formed by osteoblasts.*
osso capitato	**capitate bone** *The bone at the base of the palm that articulates with the third metacarpal.*
osso escafóide	**scaphoid bone** *The most lateral of the carpal bones; it articulates with the radius.*
osso etmóide	**ethmoid bone** *A bone at the root of the nose which has perforations for the olfactory nerves to transit.*
osso hamato; unciforme	**unciforme bone** *Hamate bone. The bone on the ulnar side of the distal row of the carpus. It articulates withe the 4th and 5th metacarpal, triquetral, lunate and capitate.*
osso hióde	**hyoid bone** *A horseshoe shaped bone located between the chin and thyroid cartilage.*
osso ilíaco	**ilium** *The large bone at the superior aspect of the pelvis which is present bilaterally.*
osso intermédio	**lunate bone; os lunatum** *A carpal bone that articulates with the wrist.*
osso navicular de mão	**navicular bone** *The most lateral bone in the proximal row of carpal bones.*
osso trapezóide	**trapezoid bone** *A bone that articulates with the second metacarpal, trapezium, capitate and scaphoid.*
osso zigomático	**zygomatic bone** *The triangular cheek bone.*
ossos turbinadso	**turbinate bones** *The three curved shelves in the nasal cavity.*
osteíte	**osteitis** *Inflammation of the bone.*
ostensivamente	**ostensibly** *Synonym of apparently and seemingly.*
osteoartrite	**osteoarthritis** *A long term, progressive degenerative joint disease.*
osteoartrose	**osteoarthrosis** *Arthritis without inflammation.*
osteoblasto	**osteoblast** *A cell that matures from a fibroblast and produces bone.*
osteoclasia	**osteoclasis** *The surgical fracture of a bone usually in order to restore proper alignment.*
osteoclasto	**osteoclast** *A large bone cell that is associated with bone reabsorption and removal.*
osteoclastoma	**osteoclastoma** *A tumor composed of giant cells or osteoclasts.*
osteocondrite	**osteochondritis** *Inflammation of bone and cartilage.*

Portuguese	English
osteocondroma	**osteochondroma** *A tumor with bony and cartilaginous characteristics.*
osteocondroso	**osteochondral** *Referring to bone and cartilage.*
osteodistrofia	**osteodystrophy** *Abnormal bone formation.*
osteofonia	**osteophony** *The sound conduction of bone.*
osteogênese	**osteogenesis** *Development of new bones.*
osteogênese imperfeita	**ostogenesis imperfecta** *A connective tissue disorder characterized by bone fragility, skeletal deformity, blue sclerae, ligament laxity, and hearing loss.*
osteolítico	**osteolytic** *Referring to the removal or loss of calcium from the bone.*
osteomalacia	**osteomalacia** *Softening of the bones because of a deficiency of vitamin D, calcium or phosphorus.*
osteomielite	**osteomyelitis** *Inflammation of the bone or bone marrow because of a microorganism.*
osteopatia	**osteopathy** *1. Any disease of the bone. 2. Medical practice concerning treatment of disease by manipulation and massage of bones, joints, and muscles.*
osteopetrose; doença de Albers-Schönberg	**osteopetrosis** *Increased bone density with no change in modeling.*
osteoporose	**osteoporosis** *Loss of bone substance because the osteoblasts fail to produce bone matrix.*
osteosclerose	**osteosclerosis** *Abnormal hardening of bone.*
osteossarcoma	**osteosarcoma** *A tumor composed of a sarcoma and osseous material.*
osteotomia	**osteotomy** *Creation of a surgical opening in bone.*
osteócito	**osteocyte** *An osteoblast within the bone matrix.*
osteófito	**osteophyte** *Abnormal growth of a bone protuberance.*
otalgia	**earache** *Pain associated with the ear.*
otalgia	**otalgia** *Ear pain.*
otitie	**otitis** *Inflammation of the ear. (otitis media or otitis externa)*
otolaringologista	**otolaryngologist** *Surgical specialist concerned with organs of the ears, nose and throat.*
otologia	**otology** *Study of conditions and anatomy of the ear.*
otomicose	**otomycosis** *Fungal infection of the ear.*
otosclerose	**otosclerosis** *A hereditary condition exhibited by progressive hearing loss because of bone overgrowth in the inner ear.*
otoscópio	**otoscope** *A device used for inspection of the tympanic membrane.*
ototóxico	**ototoxic** *A substance harmful to the ear or its nerve supply.*
otólito	**otolith** *A calcium based calculus in the inner ear.*
ouro	**gold** *Precious metal with atomic number of 79.*
ouvido externo	**ear, external** *Auris externa.*
ouvido externo	**external ear canal** *Auditory canal.*
ouvido interno	**ear, inner** *Auris interna.*
ouvido interno	**inner ear** *Made up of the cochlea and semicircular canals.*
ouvido médio	**ear, middle** *Auris media.*
ouvido médio	**middle ear** *The portion of the ear containing the stapes, incus and malleus.*
ovarite	**ovaritis** *Synonym for oophoritis.*
oviduto	**oviduct** *The channel which an ovum passes from the ovary.*
ovo	**egg**
ovulação	**ovulation** *The release of an ova from the ovary.*

Portuguese	English
oxalúria	**oxaluria** *Existence of oxalates in the urine.*
oxicefalia	**oxycephaly** *The deformation of the skull so that it appears pointed.*
oxidação	**oxidation** *The process of a chemical combining with oxygen.*
oxigenação	**oxygenation** *Saturated with oxygen.*
oxigenoterapia	**oxygen therapy** *Utilization of supplemental oxygen.*
oxigênio	**oxygen** *A colorless, odorless gas with atomic number 8.*
oxitocina	**oxytocin** *A natural hormone released by the pituitary or a synthetic hormone that facilitates uterine contraction.*
oxitócico	**oxytocic** *Referring to rapid parturition.*
oxiúro	**pinworm** *Common term for Enterobius vermincularis; a nematode worm that is a parasite.*
oxímetro	**oximeter** *A medical device used to measure the percent of oxygen that is saturated in the blood (oxygen saturation).*
oxyemoglobina	**oxyhemoglobin** *The combination of oxygen and hemoglobin using a covalent bond.*
ozena	**ozena** *Various nasal conditions, all of which include fetid discharge.*
ozônio	**ozone** *A toxic chemical that has profound oxidizing properties. It has three atoms in its molecule compared with oxygen which has two.*
óculos	**eyeglasses** *Eye wear used for cosmetic or prescription purposes.*
óculos de proteção	**goggles** *Close fitting, protective eyeglasses.*
ópio	**opium** *An addictive drug derived from opium poppy; synthetic versions are used as analgesics.*
óptico	**optic** *Referring to the eye.*
óptico	**optician** *A person who makes eyeglasses.*
órbita	**orbit** *The bony structure enclosing the eyeball.*
órgão	**organ** *A part of the body that is self contained and serves a vital function.*
órgão terminal	**end organ** *The encapsulated end of a sensory nerve.*
ósseo	**osseous** *Possessing the quality of bone.*
óstio	**ostium** *A vessel or body cavity opening.*
óvulo	**ovule** *An immature ovum.*
óxido nitroso	**nitrous oxide** *An inhalant gas used as an anesthetic agent.*
paciente	**patient** *The client being treated for a medical or surgical condition.*
pagofagia	**pagophagia** *Compulsive need to eat ice which is usually associated with iron deficiency anemia.*
paladar tardio	**after-taste** *The sensation of a prolonged savor following eating/drinking.*
palato	**palate** *The roof of the mouth.*
palatoplegia; estafiloplegia	**palatoplegia** *Paralysis of the palate.*
paliativo	**palliative** *A treatment used to reduce pain when cure is not possible.*
palidectomia	**pallidectomy** *Surgical resection of all or part of the palate.*
palidez	**pallor** *Unusually pale appearance.*
palma da mão	**palm** *The anterior aspect of the hand.*
palmar	**palmar** *Referring to the palm.*
palmo	**span** *A distance between two objects.*
palpação	**palpation** *The assessment of the body with the use of one's hands.*

Portuguese	English
palpitação	**palpitation** *Sensation of a forceful, rapid, irregular heartbeat present after exercise or with anxiety.*
paludismo	**paludism** *Synonym of malaria.*
pan-artrite	**panarthritis** *Inflammation of the joints.*
pan-cardite	**pancarditis** *Inflammation of pericardium, myocardium and endocardium.*
pan-hipopituitarismo	**panhypopituitarism** *Insufficiency of the anterior pituitary.*
pan-oftalmite	**panophthalmia** *Inflammation of the eye and all its structures.*
pan-otite	**panotitis** *Inflammation of each part of a bone.*
pancreatectomia	**pancreatectomy** *Surgical excision of part or all of the pancreas.*
pancreatite	**pancreatitis** *Inflammation of the pancreas.*
pancreozimina	**pancreozymin** *A duodenal mucosal enzyme that facilitates the secretion of amylase and other enzymes from the pancreas.*
pandêmico	**pandemic** *When a disease is present over an entire region.*
paniculite	**panniculitis** *Inflammation of a section of subcutaneous tissue containing large amounts of fat.*
panturrilha; barriga da perna	**calf** *Muscles of the posterior portion of the lower leg.*
papiledema	**papilledema** *Swelling of the optic disc.*
papilite	**papillitits** *Swelling of a papilla.*
papiloma	**papilloma** *A benign, lobulated tumor coming from epithelium.*
paquidermia	**pachydermia** *An abnormally thick skin.*
paquileptomeningite	**pachymeningitis** *Inflammation of the dura mater.*
paracentese	**nyxis** *Paracentesis or a puncture.*
paracentese	**paracentesis** *A procedure involving aspiration of fluid from the abdominal cavity.*
paracusia	**paracusia** *Any abnormality in the sense of hearing.*
parada cardíaca	**cardiac arrest** *Cessation of function of the heart.*
parafimose	**paraphimosis** *A condition in which the foreskin is retracted but cannot be replace because of a restricted foreskin.*
paralisia	**palsy** *Paralysis that is usually associated with tremors.*
paralisia bulbar	**bulbar palsy** *Paralysis due to changes in the motor center of the medulla oblongata.*
paralisia cerebral	**cerebral palsy** *A condition exhibited by motor incoordination and speech changes that is the result of brain injury occurring ante-, intra- or post- partum.*
paralisia com agitação	**paralysis agitans** *Synonym of Parkinson's disease.*
paralisia de Bell	**Bell's palsy** *Unilateral facial paralysis related to dysfunction of the seventh cranial nerve.*
paralisia facial	**facial paralysis** *Lack of movement or sensation in the distribution of the facial nerve.*
paralisia ocular	**ocular paralysis**. *Paralysis of intraocular and extraocular muscles.*
paralisia periódica	**periodic paralysis** *A familial muscle disorder exhibited by recurrent episodes flaccid paralysis without change in level of consciousness.*
paralisia periódica hiperpotassêmica	**hypokalemic periodic paralysis** *An inherited disorder that leads to muscle weakness related to a low serum potassium level.*
paralisia pseudobulbar	**pseudobulbar palsy** *Sudden outbursts of laughter or tearfulness sometimes seen in amyotrophic lateral sclerosis.*
paralítico	**paralytic** *1. Referring to paralysis. 2. A person who is paralyzed.*
paramediano	**paramedian** *Situated toward the middle of the body.*

Portuguese	English
parametrite	**parametritis** *Inflammation of the parametrium.*
paramédico	**paramedical** *Hospital support staff excluding physicians.*
paramétrio	**parametrium** *The connective tissue and smooth muscle between the broad ligament serous layers.*
paramimia	**paramnesia** *A condition exhibited by a person's belief they have memory for an event that never happened.*
paranasal	**paranasal** *Situated adjacent to the nose.*
paranóia	**paranoia** *A mental condition exhibited by delusions of persecution.*
paranóide	**paranoid** *Having the symptom of paranoia.*
parapleglia	**paraplegia** *Paralysis of the lower extremities.*
parapraxia	**parapraxis** *1. Unable to perform purposeful movements. 1. Irrational behavior.*
pararretal	**pararectal** *Adjacent to the rectum.*
parasita	**parasite** *An organism that lives on or within another organism without benefit to the latter.*
parassimpático	**parasympathetic** *Part of the autonomic nervous system that opposes sympathetic stimulation.*
paratireóide	**parathyroid** *Positioned adjacent to the thyroid.*
paratormônio	**parathormone** *Synonym for parathyroid hormone.*
paravertebral	**paravertebral** *Positioned adjacent to the vertebra.*
parede celular	**cell wall** *The peripheral border of the cell.*
parede torácica	**chest wall** *Thoracic wall.*
parenteral	**parenteral** *Other than the alimentary canal.*
parentesco	**relation** *1. A person who has a blood or marriage connection.*
paresia	**paresis** *Incomplete paralysis.*
parestesia	**paresthesia** *An abnormal sensation usually described as pins and needles.*
parênquima	**parenchyma** *The functional elements of an organ.*
parietal	**parietal** *Referring to the wall of a part or cavity.*
paroníquia	**paronychia** *Inflammation of the tissue bordering a fingernail*
paroníquia	**whitlow** *An abscess occurring on the palmar surface of the fingertips.*
parosmia	**parosmia** *An alteration in the sense of smell.*
parotidite	**parotiditis** *Inflammation of the parotid gland.*
paroxismos de taquicardia ventricular	**torsade de pointe** *Ventricular cardiac rhythm disturbance.*
paroxístico	**paroxysmal** *Occurring in sudden attacks.*
parótida	**parotid** *A gland near the ear.*
parte cardial do estômago, que circunda a junção esofagogástrica	**cardia** *The superior aspect of the stomach at the opening of the esophagus.*
parteiro	**midwife** *A person trained to assist in childbirth.*
partenogênese	**parthenogenesis** *Reproduction that occurs without an egg being fertilized by sperm.*
partida	**parting** *Separating.*
parto	**childbirth** *Parturition; the process of labor and delivery of an infant.*
parto nádegas	**breech birth** *Delivery with the feet or buttocks coming first.*
parto pósmaduro	**post-term birth** *An infant born after the normal length of pregnancy.*
parto; nascimento	**birth** *The process of bearing offspring from the uterus.*
parto; nascimento	**delivery** *The process of giving birth.*
parturição	**parturition** *The process of giving birth.*

Portuguese	English
parúlide	**gumboil** *Swelling noted on the gingiva over a dental abscess.*
passagem de uma vela	**bougienage** *Passage of a bougie through a body orifice with the goal of increasing the diameter of the orifice.*
passivo	**passive** *Not achieved through active effort.*
passo	**pace** *Consistent and continuous movement.*
passo	**stride** *Walk with long definitive steps.*
pasta de documentos	**file** *Patient record or folder.*
patela	**kneecap** *Common term for patella.*
patelectomia	**patellectomy** *Surgical excision of the patella.*
patogênese	**pathogenesis** *The course of a disease.*
patogênico	**pathogenic** *Referring to an organism that can cause disease.*
patognomônico	**pathognomonic** *Characteristic of something.*
patologia	**pathology** *1. The branch of medicine dealing with the study of tissues and the forensic application. 2. Referring to a condition that is abnormal.*
patológico	**pathological** *Referring to pathology.*
pavio; fio	**wick** *A drain using a thin piece of cloth or tubing.*
pálpebra	**eyelid** *Palpebra.*
pálpebra	**palpebra, palpebrae** *Eyelid, eyelids.*
pápula	**papule** *A small, well-circumscribed elevation of the skin.*
pápula; placa de urticária	**wheal** *A circumscribed urticarial lesion.*
páreas secundinas	**afterbirth** *The tissue expelled after the birth of a child that includes the placenta and allied membranes.*
pâncreas	**pancreas** *A gland that secretes digestive enzymes into the duodenum and insulin and glucagon into the blood.*
pecilocitose	**poikilocytosis** *The presence of abnormally shaped erythrocytes.*
pecilotermia	**poikilothermy** *A condition of cold-blooded animals in which their temperature varies based on the ambient temperature.*
pectorilóquia	**pectoriloquy** *The examiner's voice is clearly audible when the patient speaks as when the examiner listens to an area of consolidation in the lungs of the speaker.*
pectorilóquia sussurrada	**whispered pectoriloquy** *The sound heard through the stethoscope when listening to a person's lungs. The sound resonates as it would when listening over a bronchus if there is an area of consolidation.*
pedaço	**lump** *A protuberance.*
pediatra	**pediatrician** *Physician who is a specialist in pediatrics.*
pediatria	**pediatrics** *Medical specialty concerned with the treatment and prevention of childhood disease.*
pediculado	**pediculate** *Referring to pedicle.*
pediculose	**pediculosis** *Lice infestation.*
pedículo	**pedicle** *Part of a skin/tissue graft temporarily left connected to the original site.*
pedúnculo	**peduncle** *1. A stalk-like protrusion. 2. A bundle of nerve fibers connecting two parts of the brain.*
pedúnculo cerebelar superior	**brachium cerebelli** *Synonym of pedunculus cerebellaris superior (upper portion the cerebellum).*
pegar faringite (B); apanhar uma constipação (P)	**catch a cold** *To come down with a viral upper respiratory tract infection.*
peidar	**fart, to** *Slang term for releasing flatus.*
peito do pé	**instep** *The medial aspect of the foot between the ankle and the ball of the foot.*
peito; mama	**breast** *Mammary tissue including the areola.*
peitoral	**pectoral** *Referring to the pectoral muscle.*

Portuguese	English
peixe; pescado	**fish** *A cold-blooded vertebrate with gills and fins.*
pelagra infantil	**kwashiorkor** *A form of malnutrition from inadequate protein intake.*
pelagra; coceira de Santo Inácio	**pellagra** *A deficiency in nicotinic acid exhibited by diarrhea and dermatitis.*
pele	**dermis** *The "true skin" that lies beneath the epidermis.*
pele	**skin** *Flesh.*
pele de ganso	**goose bumps** *Cutis anserina.*
pelve	**pelvis** *The bony structure at the base of the spine.*
pelve andróide	**android pelvis** *A pelvis shaped like a man's.*
pelve renal	**renal pelvis** *The kidney collecting system.*
pelvimetria	**pelvimetry** *Measurement of the dimensions of the pelvis to determine whether a patient is capable of natural childbirth.*
penetração	**penetration** *The process of making a way through something.*
penfigóide bulhosa	**bullous pemphigoid** *A benign disease of the aged characterized by large bullae forming on the torso and extremities.*
penicilina	**penicillin** *A synthetic antibiotic originally produced from blue mold.*
pentosúria	**pentosuria** *The presence of pentose in the urine (a monosaccharide with five carbon atoms in the molecule).*
pepsina	**pepsin** *A proteolytic gastric enzyme.*
peptído	**peptide** *A compound with low molecular weight and containing two or more amino acids.*
percevejo	**bedbug Cimex lectularius.** *A small insect that is parasitic and hides in clothing or bedding.*
percussão	**percussion** *A manual procedure involving tapping a body part to determine the size or density (liquid or air) of a part.*
perfuração	**perforation** *Presence of a hole.*
periartrite	**periarthritis** *Inflammation of the tissues around a joint.*
pericardite	**pericarditis** *Inflammation of the pericardium.*
pericardíaco	**pericardial** *Referring to around the heart.*
pericárdio	**pericardium** *The structure enclosing the heart which contains a fibrous outer layer and serous inner layer.*
pericolite	**pericolitis** *Inflammation of the membrane covering the colon.*
pericondrite	**perichondritis** *Inflammation of the perichondrium.*
pericôndrio	**perichondrium** *The membrane that encloses a cartilage.*
periférico	**peripheral** *Referring to an outward part or surface.*
perilinfa	**perilymph** *The fluid separating the membranous and osseous labyrinth.*
perinatologia	**perinatology** *The study of disease in the period just before and right after birth.*
perineorrafia	**perineorrhaphy** *Surgical repair of the perineum.*
perinéfrico	**perinephric** *Around the kidney.*
periostite	**periostitis** *Inflammation of the periosteum.*
periósteo	**periosteum** *A layer of connective tissue covering the bones.*
perióstico	**periosteal** *Referring to the periosteum.*
periproctite	**periproctitis** *Inflammation of the tissue encircling the anus and rectum.*
peristaltismo	**peristalsis** *The contraction of the longitudinal and circular muscle fibers of the alimentary canal so food is propelled.*
peritomia	**peritomy** *Surgically creating an opening of the periosteum.*
peritoneal	**peritoneal** *Referring to the peritoneum.*

Portuguese	English
peritonite	**peritonitis** *Inflammation of the peritoneum.*
peritonsilar	**peritonsillar** *Surrounding the tonsils.*
peritônio	**peritoneum** *The serous membrane covering the abdominal organs and lining the abdominal walls.*
periuretral	**periurethral** *Surrounding the urethra.*
perineal	**perineal** *Referring to the perineum.*
perineo	**perineum** *The area between the anus and scrotum or anus and vulva.*
período de gestação	**full-term** *A normal length pregnancy.*
perna	**leg** *One of two lower extremities.*
perna de leite ou branca; flegmasia trombótica	**phlegmasia alba dolens** *Phlebitis of the femoral vein that can occur after pregnancy or typhoid fever.*
perniciose	**pernicious** *1. Having a detrimental effect. 2. Pernicious anemia is a reduced red blood cell count due to Vitamin B12 deficiency.*
peroneiro	**peroneal** *Referring to the fibula or the outer part of the leg.*
personalidade	**personality** *Qualities that form a person's unique character.*
perspiração	**perspiration** *The process of sweating.*
pesadelo	**nightmare** *An unpleasant or frightening dream.*
pescoço	**neck** *The part of the body that connects the body to the head.*
pescotapa; semelhente à chicotada	**whiplash** *Common term for cervical strain following a sudden deceleration.*
peso (corpo)	**body weight** *Relative mass as measured in kilograms or pounds.*
pessário	**pessary** *A supportive device placed in the rectum or vagina.*
pessoa	**heavy** *Possessing great weight.*
pessoa	**soft** *Easy to mold or compress.*
peste bubônica	**bubonic plague** *A form of plague exhibited by the formation of buboes.*
petéquias	**petechia** *A small red or purple macule on the skin caused by bleeding.*
petroso	**petrous** *Possessing a density of a stone.*
pé	**foot** *The lower extremity distal to the ankle.*
pé caído	**foot drop** *Caused by palsy of the nerve controlling foot dorsiflexion.*
pé cavo	**pes cavus** *Excessive height of the longitudinal arch of the foot.*
pé chato	**flatfoot** *Common term for pes planus.*
pé em gota; pé caído	**drop foot** *The symptom in a person with a nerve injury causing impaired ankle dorsiflexion.*
pé plano	**pes planus** *Medical term for flat foot.*
pé valgo	**pes valgus** *Abnormal longitudinal arch- it is flat.*
pélvico	**pelvic** *Referring to the pelvis.*
péptico	**peptic** *Referring to pepsin or concerning digestion.*
pênfigo	**pemphigus** *A skin disorder with large bullous lesions.*
pênis	**penis** *Male genital organ used for the transfer of sperm and elimination of urine.*
pia-máter	**pia mater** *The first layer of three covering the brain and spinal cord.*
pica	**pica** *A desire for unusual substances as occurs in pregnancy and some psychological conditions.*
picada	**sting** *A small puncture as in a bee sting.*
picada de abelha	**bee sting** *A piercing from a bee.*
picnose	**pyknosis** *The degeneration of a cell with the nucleus shrinking.*
pielite	**pyelitis** *Renal pelvis inflammation.*

Portuguese	English
pielografia	**pyelography** *Use of a contrast agent to radiologically study the kidney, ureters and bladder.*
pielolitotomia	**pyelolithotomy** *Surgical excision of a calculus from the renal pelvis.*
pielonefrite	**pyelonephritis** *Inflammation of the renal parenchyma usually due to bacterial infection.*
pielonefrose	**pyelonephrosis** *Term, rarely used anymore, used to describe disease of the renal pelvis.*
piemia	**pyemia** *Sepsis characterized by the presence of secondary abscesses.*
pigmento biliar	**bile pigments** *The golden brown or green-yellow color associated with bile.*
piloro	**pylorus** *The opening at the distal stomach that opens into the duodenum.*
piloroplastia	**pyloroplasty** *Surgical enlargement of a pylorus that previously was stenotic.*
pilórico	**pyloric** *Referring to the pylorus.*
pinguécula	**pinguecula** *The yellow tissue on the bulbar conjunctiva adjacent to the sclerocorneal junction.*
pino intramedular	**pin, intramedullary** *Hardware used for fracture management or during joint replacement.*
pinocitose	**pinocytosis** *The absorption of fluid into a cell by the formation of vesicles on the cell membrane.*
piodermatite	**pyoderma** *A purulent skin infection.*
piogênico	**pyogenic** *Referring to the formation of pus.*
piolho caranguejo; piolho pubiano	**crab louse** *Phthirus pubis is formal name for a louse that infests pubic hair and causes intense itching.*
piolhos	**lice** *Plural for louse, a small parasite that lives on the skin. Pediculus humanus capitis is a head louse.*
pionefrose	**pyonephrosis** *Injury to the renal parenchyma due to pus.*
piorar	**worsen, to** *To deteriorate.*
piorréia	**pyorrhea** *Emission of pus.*
piossalpinge	**pyosalpinx** *Purulent material in the oviduct.*
pipeta	**pipet** *A slender tube with a bulb used for transferring liquids.*
piramidal	**pyramidal** *A term that is used to describe various spinal tracts that originate in the cerebral cortex.*
pirexia	**pyrexia** *Fever.*
piridixina	**pyridoxine** *Synonym for vitamin B6.*
pirogênio	**pyrogen** *A fever producing substance released by bacteria.*
pirose	**pyrosis** *Synonym for heartburn.*
piscar	**blinking** *To open and close the eyelid rapidly.*
pitiríase rósea	**pityriasis rosea** *A skin disease characterized by dry pink oval papulosquamous eruptions.*
pícnico	**pyknic** *Possessing a short, stocky physique.*
piúria	**pyuria** *Presence of purulent material in the urine.*
pílula	**pill** *A medicated tablet or capsule.*
placa terminal	**motor end plate** *The expansions on a motor nerve where the branches terminate on muscle fiber.*
placenta	**placenta** *The vascular tissue that nourishes a fetus through an umbilical cord.*
placenta prévia	**placenta praevia** *A condition in which the placenta covers the cervical os.*
placentário	**placental** *Referring to the placenta.*

Portuguese	English
plagiocefalia	**plagiocephaly** *A condition characterized by an asymmetric skull because the cranial sutures do not close normally.*
plantar	**plantar** *Referring to the bottom of the foot.*
plaqueta	**platelet** *An oval cell without a nucleus used in coagulation; also called a thrombocyte.*
plasmacitose	**plasmacytosis** *The existence of plasma cells in the blood.*
plasmaferese	**plasmapheresis** *A method of removing blood and reinfusing it after the elimination of antibodies.*
plesiomorfismo	**pleomorphism** *The ability of an organism or substance to attain distinct forms.*
pletismógrafo	**plethysmograph** *A device used to measure the amount of blood flowing through a body part; impedance plethysmography is used to check for deep venous thrombosis.*
pletora	**plethora** *An excess of something.*
pleura	**pleura** *The serous membrane lining each lung.*
pleura cervical; cúpula da pleura	**cervical pleura** *The dome-like cap of the pleura.*
pleurisia	**pleurisy** *Inflammation of the pleura.*
plexo braquial	**brachial plexus** *A cluster of nerves coming off the last four cervical and first thoracic spinal nerves form the nerve supply the the chest and arms.*
plexo solar	**solar plexus** *A cluster of ganglia and nerves, located at the base of the sternum, that surround the celiac trunk.*
plural de cilium	**cilia** *The hairs growing on the eyelid or a motile extension of a cell surface.*
pneumatocele	**pneumatocele** *1. A hernia-like protrusion of lung tissue. 2. A collection of gas in a sac such as the scrotum.*
pneumatúria	**pneumaturia** *Presence of air or gas in the urine.*
pneumococos	**pneumococcus** *A bacterium causing pneumonia and meningitis. A common type is Streptococcus pneumoniae.*
pneumoconiose	**pneumoconiosis** *Fibrosis of the lung due to dust inhalation.*
pneumonectomia	**pneumonectomy** *Surgical excision of all or part of a lung.*
pneumonia	**pneumonia** *Inflammation of the lung due to an infection caused by a virus or bacterium.*
pneumonia pneumocística jiroveci	**pneumocystis jiroveci pneumonia**. *A pulmonary infection associated with AIDS. Formerly called pneumocystis carinii pneumonia*
pneumonia por aspiração	**aspiration pneumonia** *Taking air or matter into the lungs.*
pneumotórax	**pneumothorax** *Abnormal presence of air between the lung and chest wall.*
polegar	**thumb** *The first digit of each hand.*
poliarterite nodosa	**polyarteritis nodosa** *A systemic necrotizing vasculitis that effects medium sized arteries.*
policitemia	**polycythemia** *Excess in the number of erythrocytes in the blood.*
policitemia rubra	**polycythemia vera** *Condition characterized by increase in erythrocytes, thrombocytes and leukocytes, as well as, splenomegaly.*
policístico	**polycystic** *Possessing more than one cyst.*
policondrite	**polychondritis** *Inflammation of the cartilage at more than one site.*
polidactilia	**polydactyly** *Congenital anomaly exhibited by more than 5 digits on the hands and/or feet.*
polidipsia	**polydipsia** *Profound thirst.*
polimenorréia	**polymenorrhea** *Increase in the frequency of menstruation.*
polimiosite	**polymyositis** *Inflammation of several muscle groups at once.*

Portuguese	English
polineurite	**polyneuritis** *Inflammation of more than one nerve.*
polineuropatia	**polyneuropathy** *A condition involving more than one nerve.*
polioencefalite	**polioencephalitis** *Polio infection of the brain.*
poliomielite	**poliomyelitis** *An infectious viral disease exhibited by constitutional symptoms that can lead to quadriplegia.*
poliopia	**polyopia** *A condition in which one object is seen abnormally as two or more.*
polipo	**polypus** *Synonym of polyp (a prominent growth from a mucous membrane).*
polipose	**polyposis** *The formation of multiple polyps.*
poliptialismo	**polysialia** *Abnormal increase in saliva.*
polissacarídeo	**polysaccharide** *A carbohydrate that upon hydrolysis forms more than ten monosaccharides.*
politraumatiso	**polytrauma** *A condition exhibited by multiple injuries from blunt or penetrating trauma.*
poliúria	**polyuria** *Abnormal increase in volume of urine excreted.*
polpa	**pulp** *The tissue filling the root canals of a tooth.*
polvilho	**powder** *Fine dry particles.*
Pomo-de-Adão	**Adam's apple** *A prominence on the anterior neck caused by the thyroid cartilage of the larynx.*
poncionar lombar	**lumbar puncture** *Insertion of a needle into the spinal canal in the region of L3-4 to obtain a sample of CSF.*
poncionar medula óssea	**bone marrow puncture** *The aspiration of marrow to look for pressure of disease.*
ponfólige	**pompholyx** *A condition exhibited by interdigital vesicles of the hands and feet.*
ponte	**pons** *The part of the brainstem that connects the medulla oblongata with the thalamus.*
pontilhado	**stippling** *Having numerous small specks or spots.*
pontino	**pontine** *Referring to the pons.*
ponto do dedo	**fingertip** *Distal aspect of a finger.*
ponto terminal	**end point** *The last stage of a process.*
poplíteo	**popliteal** *Referring to the posterior aspect of the knee.*
por toda a vida	**lifetime** *Duration of a person's life.*
porfiria	**porphyria** *A hereditary condition currently classified based on the specific enzyme deficiency. The most common form is porphyria cutanea tarda that causes blistering lesions.*
porfirina	**porphyrin** *A class of pigments that contain a flat ring of four heterocyclic groups.*
porta-agulha	**needle holder** *A surgical instrument used to grasp a needle during suturing.*
portal	**portal** *Referring to an entrance such as porta hepatis.*
posição de litotomia	**lithotomy position** *Buttocks positioned at the end of the OR table, the hips and knees flexed and the feet strapped in. Dorsosacral position.*
posição fetal	**fetal position** *Refers to how the fetus lies within the uterus.*
posição genocubital	**knee elbow position** *Knees and elbows are on the table and the chest is in the air.*
posição varo	**varus position** *Refers to a joint being abnormally angulated toward the midline of the body.*
positivo	**positive** *Indicating the presence of something.*
pospor	**postpone, to** *To delay.*
posterior	**posterior** *Further back in position; opposite of anterior.*
postural	**postural** *Referring to position or posture.*

Portuguese	English
potássio	**potassium** *A chemical of the alkali metal group.*
potencial evocado	**evoked potential** *Electrical impulses that can be noted after stimulation of sensory organs.*
potential de ação	**action potential** *The alteration in electrical potential associated with the movement along a nerve cell.*
potência	**potency** *Strength or power.*
pouco visível	**blind spot** *An area of insensitivity to light located at the point of entry of the optic nerve on the retina.*
pó	**dust** *Dry earthen particles found on the ground and surfaces.*
pós-carga	**after-load** *Referring to the amount of pressure the heart needs to pump against. If one has left heart failure it is beneficial to reduce after-load.*
pós-descarga	**discharge, postpartum vaginal** *The secretions noted after delivery.*
pós-íctico	**postictal** *The period of time after a seizure.*
pós-maduro	**postmaturity** *Generally referring to a pregnancy that goes beyond the due date.*
prata	**silver** *A precious metal with atomic number 47.*
precipitina	**precipitin** *An antibody-antigen reaction producing a precipitate.*
preconceituoso	**biased** *Prejudiced.*
precordialgia	**precordialgia** *Pain in the precordium.*
preço	**cost** *The fee or penalty.*
precórdio	**precordium** *The area occupying the epigastrium and lower sternum.*
prega	**plica** *A fold, as in a fold in the peritoneum.*
prematuro; pré-madura	**premature** *Occurring earlier than expected.*
preocupar	**worry, to** *To fret or have unease.*
prepúcio	**foreskin** *Also called prepuce, the skin that naturally covers the glans but can be rolled back.*
presbiacusia	**presbyacusia** *An age related, progressive hearing loss.*
presbiopia	**presbyopia** *Farsightedness associated with aging.*
prescrição; receita (P)	**prescription** *The action of prescribing a medication or treatment.*
presença de ar na cavidade peritoneal	**pneumoperitoneum** *Abnormal or induced presence of air or gas in the peritoneum.*
preservativo	**condom** *A covering for the penis or the vagina (female condom) used during sexual intercourse that is meant to reduce the chance of pregnancy or infection.*
pressão arterial	**blood pressure** *Written as the measurement in mmHg at the time of systole of the left ventricle over the time of diastole.*
preto	**black** *Referring to the color, as in the color of coal.*
prevenir	**prevent, to** *To stave off or hinder.*
pré-auricular	**preauricular** *Anterior to the ear.*
pré-canceroso	**precancerous** *Referring to an early stage in cancer development.*
pré-eclâmpsia	**preeclampsia** *Hypertension with proteinuria and/or edema in the setting of pregnancy.*
pré-menstrual	**premenstrual** *Occurring prior to the onset of menstruation.*
pré-natal	**prenatal** *Referring to the time prior to birth.*
pré-systólico	**presystolic** *The time just before systole.*
priapismo	**priapism** *A painful and abnormally prolonged erection.*
primeiros socorros	**first aid** *The initial treatment after an injury.*
primípara	**primipara** *A woman giving birth for the first time.*

Portuguese	English
privação	**deprivation** *The lack of a necessity.*
probabilidade	**likelihood** *The probability or feasibility.*
problema	**problem** *Difficulty or complaint.*
processo mastóide	**mastoid process** *The posterior part of the temporal bone bordered by the parietal bone superiorly and the occipital bone posteriorly.*
processo xifóide	**xiphoid process** *The inferior segment of the sternum.*
proctalgia	**proctalgia** *A chronic high, dull rectal pain worse with sitting position.*
proctectomia	**proctectomy** *Surgical excision of the rectum.*
proctite	**proctitis** *Inflammation of the rectum.*
proctocele	**proctocele** *A hernia-type protrusion of the rectum into the vagina.*
proctoscopia	**proctoscopy** *Inspection of the rectum with a scope.*
proeminência hipotenar	**hypothenar eminence** *The prominence on the palm at the base of the fingers adjacent to the ulna.*
profilaxia	**prophylaxis** *That which is done to prevent disease.*
profundo	**deep** *Having significant depth.*
progeria	**progeria** *A childhood disorder exhibited by signs of aging including gray hair, wrinkled skin and short height.*
progestogênio	**progesterone** *A steroid hormone that prepares the uterus for pregnancy.*
proglote	**proglottis** *Any segment of a tapeworm.*
prognatismo	**prognathism** *Protrusion of the mandible which can cause malocclusion.*
prognóstico	**prognosis** *The likely course of a disease.*
progressivo	**progressive** *Developing gradually.*
prolactina	**prolactin** *A pituitary hormone that facilitates milk production.*
prolapso	**prolapse** *The slipping downward of a body part, such as rectal prolapse.*
prolapso do cordão umbilical	**cord presentation** *The presence of the umbilical cord at the cervix during active labor.*
prolapso do cordão umbilical	**prolapse of the umbilical cord** *Refers to the umbilical cord protruding from the cervix during active labor.*
prolapso uterino	**prolapse of the uterus** *Eversion of the uterus through the vagina.*
prolapso uterino	**uterine prolapse** *Protrusion of the uterus out the vagina.*
promonócito	**promonocyte** *An intermediate cell stage between monocyte and monoblast.*
promontório	**promontory** *A protruding eminence.*
pronação	**pronation** *Turning posteriorly. When the hand is pronated, it is turned medially until the palm is facing posteriorly (when the body was initially in the anatomic position).*
prono	**prone** *Lying with the abdomen and face downward.*
pronunciar indistintamente	**slurring** *Indistinct yet comprehensible speech.*
proprioceptor	**proprioceptor** *A receptor that responds to sensory input including position sense.*
proptose do olho	**proptosis oculi** *Synonym of exophthalmos; bulging of the eye.*
prostaciclina	**prostacyclin** *A prostaglandin that functions as an anticoagulant and vasodilator.*
prostaglandina	**prostaglandin** *A compound first found in semen (thus "prosta" in the name from prostate) with many effects including uterine contraction.*
prostatectomia	**prostatectomy** *Surgical excision of the prostate.*

Portuguese	English
prostração	**prostration** *Profound exhaustion.*
proteinúria	**proteinuria** *The presence of protein in the urine.*
proteína	**protein** *A class of nitrogenous organic compound.*
proteólise	**proteolysis** *Enzyme action on proteins to form amino acids.*
protoplasma	**protoplasm** *The cytoplasm, organelles and nucleus of a living cell.*
Protozoa	**Protozoa** *A single celled microscopic organism including amoebas among others.*
protrombina	**prothrombin** *A compound converted to thrombin during coagulation of blood.*
prova antiglobulina	**antiglobulin test (Coombs' test)** *Test used to detect erythroblastosis fetalis.*
prova da fixação de complemento	**complement fixation test** *A laboratory test for the presence of an antibody in the serum that involves inactivation of the complement in the serum.*
prova da fragilidade capilar	**capillary fragility test** *Application of a blood pressure cuff high enough to restrict venous return and after five minutes count the number or petechiae produced.*
prova de tolerância à glícose	**glucose tolerance test** *The oral administration of a carbohydrate load and then evaluation of the blood sugar at timed intervals.*
provocar	**provoke, to** *To evoke or elicit.*
proximal	**proximal** *Situated closer to the center of the body (opposed to that which is farther away, as in distal).*
próstata	**prostate** *A gland found in men that surrounds the neck of the urethra and bladder.*
prótese	**prosthesis** *An artificial body part. (above the knee) [below the knee]*
próximo	**near** *In close proximity.*
prudente	**wise** *Possessing much knowledge.*
prurida da copra	**copra itch** *A pruritus noted in people working with copra (dried kernel from a coconut).*
prurido	**itch** *A sensation that makes one want to scratch.*
prurido	**pruritus** *A general term for conditions exhibited by itching.*
prurido da palha	**straw itch** *Pruritus associated with exposure to straw that is infested with the mite Pyemotes ventricosus. Also referred to as dermatitis pediculoides ventricosus.*
prurido de inverno	**frost itch** *A pruritus noted when exposed to cold weather.*
prurido de Santo Inácio; pelagra	**Saint Ignatius' itch** *Pruritus noted with a cluster of symptoms related to niacin deficiency. Generally referred to as pellagra.*
prurido do axo	**azo itch** *A pruritus noted in people who use azo dyes.*
prurido do barbeiro	**barber's itch** *Ringworm that is transmitted by contaminated shaving equipment.*
prurido do nadador	**swimmer's itch** *Pruritus caused by exposure to schistosomes.*
prurido do solo	**ground itch** *Marked pruritus caused by a hookworm larvae, known otherwise as cutaneous larva migrans.*
prurido do verão;	**summer itch** *Pruritus noted upon exposure to hot weather, also known as pruritus aestivalis.*
prurigo	**prurigo** *A chronic, pruritic papular skin eruption.*
pseudartrose	**pseudarthrosis** *Deossification of weight bearing long bones.*
pseudomnésia	**pseudomnesia** *Sensing the memory of an event that has never happened.*
psicoastenia	**psychasthenia** *Essentially any non-hysterical neuroses.*
psicologia	**psychology** *The study of the human mind and emotions.*

Portuguese	English
psiconeurose	**psychoneurosis** *A mental disorder that could include depression or anxiety but does not include hallucinations.*
psicopatologia	**psychopathology** *Scientific examination of mental disease.*
psicose	**psychosis** *A profound mental disorder that can include delusions and hallucinations.*
psicose pós-parto	**postpartum psychosis** *A episode of abnormal thought or hallucinations following delivery.*
psicossomático	**psychosomatic** *Physical ailments arising from mental disease.*
psicoterapia	**psychotherapy** *Treatment of mental disease with cognitive-behavioral approaches.*
psicólogo	**psychologist** *A professional specializing in psychology.*
psiquiatria	**psychiatry** *A branch of medicine specializing in the treatment of mental disorders.*
psitacose	**psittacosis** *A chlamydial pneumonia that is transmitted by birds.*
psoríase	**psoriasis** *A chronic papulosquamous dermatosis characterized by silver plaques.*
pterígo	**pterygium** *A membrane in the interpalpebral fissure present from the conjunctiva to the cornea.*
ptialina	**ptyalin** *An enzyme found in saliva.*
ptose	**ptosis** *Drooping of the upper eyelid usually due to paralysis of the third cranial nerve.*
puberdade	**puberty** *The time when adolescents become capable of sexual reproduction.*
pudendo	**pudendal** *Referring to the female genitalia*
pudendo; os genitais externos	**pudendum** *The mons, pubis, labia majora, labia minora and the vagina.*
puerpério	**puerperium** *The six week period after childbirth.*
puérpera	**puerpera** *A woman who just gave birth.*
pulga	**flea** *A small wingless insect that feeds on blood of mammals.*
pulite	**pulpitis** *Dental pulp inflammation.*
pulmão	**lung** *One of a pair of respiratory organs.*
pulmão dos fazendeiros	**farmer's lung** *Coined because farmers are susceptible to this disease by inhaling fungi from hay; also called Aspergillosis.*
pulmonar	**pulmonary** *Referring to the lungs.*
pulsátil	**pulsatile** *Relating to pulsation.*
pulsação	**pulsation** *The action of expanding and contracting.*
pulsar	**throb, to** *The beat with strong regular rhythm.*
pulso	**pulse** *The rhythmic throbbing of arteries felt at major vessels.*
pulso alternante	**pulsus alternans** *A regular alternation of weak and strong beats of the pulse.*
puncionar	**tap** *A puncture with the intent of draining fluid as in spinal tap.*
punção cisternal	**cisternal puncture** *A trans-occipitoatlantoid ligament puncture of the cisterna magna so CSF can be obtained.*
punho	**fist** *When a person has their fingers clenched tightly to the palm.*
punho caído	**wrist drop** *The inability to hyperextend the wrist due to radial nerve injury.*
punho; pulso	**wrist** *The articulation of the hand and radius/ulna.*
pupila	**pupil** *The opening at the center of the iris.*
pupila amaurótica	**amaurotic pupil** *A pupil that will not respond to light when directly exposed but will respond when the other eye is exposed to light.*

Portuguese	English
pupila de Adie	**Adie's pupil** *Characterized by a weak light reaction and a strong but slow near response.*
pupila de Bumke	**Bumke's pupil** *Dilation of the pupil in response to anxiety.*
pupila de gato	**cat's eye pupil** *A pupil in the shape of an oval.*
pupila de Hutchinson	**Hutchinson's pupil** *Dilation of a pupil related to third nerve palsy on the side of the lesion as seen in herniation.*
pupila paradoxal	**paradoxical pupil** *Constriction of the pupil when exposed to darkness.*
purulento	**purulent** *Referring to pus.*
pus	**pus** *Thick yellow or green opaque liquid as seen with infection.*
putrefação	**putrefaction** *The rotting or decaying of organic matter.*
puxar	**pull, to** *To exert force on something.*
púbis	**pubis** *The anterior inferior part of the hip bone on each side that articulates at the pubic symphysis.*
púrpura	**purpura** *The presence of patches of ecchymosis or petechiae.*
púrpura de Henoch	**Henoch purpura** *Exhibited by vomiting, diarrhea, abdominal pain and hematuria; a non-thrombocytopenic purpura.*
pústula	**pox** *A general term for fluid filled papules that upon rupturing leave pockmarks.*
quadril	**hip** *The lateral eminence of the pelvis from the waist to the thigh; it is formed by the iliac crest and greater trochanter.*
quadriplegia	**quadriplegia** *Paralysis of all four extremities.*
quadríceps	**quadriceps** *The anterior thigh muscle composed of four muscles.*
qualificar	**qualify** *To become eligible by fulfilling a necessary standard.*
quarentena	**quarantine** *A place of isolation for infectious persons until it can be certain it is safe to let them mingle.*
queimadura	**burn** *An injury caused by exposure to heat.*
queixa	**complaint** *Grievance.*
quelação	**chelation** *The process used to bind a compound with metal typically used in the treatment of poisoning.*
quelóide	**keloid** *Hypertrophic scar tissue that forms after a minor cut or surgical procedure.*
quente	**hot** *Very warm.*
quiasma	**chiasma** *The optic chiasma is the area inferior to the hypothalamus where the optic nerves cross.*
quiescente	**quiescent** *A time of inactivity.*
quilite	**cheilitis** *Inflammation of the lip.*
quilo	**chyle** *A combination of lymph fluid and fat that enters the blood via the thoracic duct.*
quilomícron	**chylomicron** *A one micron particle of emulsified fat.*
quiloníquia	**koilonychia** *Thin and concave fingernails.*
quiloso	**chylous** *Referring to chyle.*
quimera	**chimera** *A mixture of genetically distinct tissues.*
quimiorrecptor	**chemoreceptor** *A sense organ that responds to stimuli.*
quimiotaxia	**chemotaxis** *The response of an organism to chemical agents.*
quimioterapia	**chemotherapy** *Use of medication (chemical agents) in the treatment of disease. This term is commonly used to refer to the treatment of cancer patients with medication.*
quimo	**chyme** *The gruel produced by gastric digestion.*
quinta doença	**Fifth disease** *Erythema infectiosum is a viral disease caused by parovirus B19.*
quiropodista	**chiropodist** *A doctor trained in the treatment of feet.*

Portuguese	English
quiroprástica	**chiropractor** *A medical practitioner who is involved with the treatment of disease by manipulating malaligned joints.*
quiroprástico	**chiropractic** *Referring to the medical practice of adjusting malaligned joints.*
quociente de inteligência	**intelligence quotient (IQ)** *A number representing a person's ability to problem solve compared to a matched-control.*
rabdomiólose	**rhabdomyolysis** *A acute destruction of muscle documented by myoglobinemia and myoglobinuria.*
racemoso	**racemose** *A gland having the form of a cluster.*
radiação	**radiation** *1. The emission of energy in the form of electromagnetic waves. 2. Divergence from a common point.*
radiação ionizante	**ionizing radiation** *High energy radiation that produces ion pairs in matter.*
radial	**radial** *Referring to the radius.*
radiculite	**radiculitis** *Inflammation of a spinal nerve root.*
radioativo	**radioactive** *Referring to the emission of ionizing particles or radiation.*
radiobiologia	**radiobiology** *The study of the effects of radiation on organisms.*
radioepitelite	**radioepithelitis** *The injury to epithelial cells due to effects of radiation.*
radiografia	**radiography** *The department where images are produced on sensitive film by x-rays.*
radiografia de tórax	**chest x-ray** *Roentography of the thorax.*
radiologia	**radiology** *The branch of medicine concerned with roentgenography and other high-energy radiation.*
radiologista	**radiologist** *A physician specializing in radiology.*
radionuclídeo	**radionuclide** *A radioactive nuclide.*
radiossensibilidade	**radiosensitivity** *The susceptibility of the skin to radiation.*
radioterapia	**radiotherapy** *Treatment of cancer with radiation.*
radônio-219	**actinon** *A radioactive element, radon-219; short lived isotope of radon.*
raio-X (P)	**x-ray**
raios gama	**gamma ray** *A type of electromagnetic radiation.*
raios ultravioleta	**ultraviolet rays** *Electromagnetic radiation with wavelength longer than x rays.*
raiva	**rage** *Uncontrollable anger.*
raiz	**root** *An embedded part of an organ or structure.*
raiz anterior	**anterior root** *A motor nerve root that is in the anterior part of the spinal cord between the anterior and lateral funiculi.*
raiz dorsal	**dorsal root** *A description of the site of ganglion found on the dorsal root of each spinal nerve.*
raiz quadrada	**square root** *The result noted when a number is multiplied by itself.*
ramo	**ramus** *A branch; a term used to describe a smaller vessel branching off from a larger one.*
raquitismo	**rickets** *A condition exhibited by softening and bowing of the long bones; caused by Vitamin D deficiency.*
raspado	**scrape** *An injury caused by having a body part rubbed against a rough surface.*
rábico	**rabies** *An infectious viral disease transmitted through the bite of a mammal. Symptoms include hydrophobia, pharyngeal spasms and hyperactivity.*
rágades	**rhagade** *Fissures in the skin, particularly adjacent to body orifices.*
rápido	**brisk** *Rapid or fast.*

Portuguese	English
rânula	**ranula** *A retention cyst formed because of obstruction of a salivary gland in the floor of the mouth.*
rã	**frog** *A tailless amphibian that is short with long hind legs for jumping.*
reactivo	**reactive** *A response to a stimulus.*
reação	**reaction** *A response to an action.*
reação cruzada	**cross-matching (blood)** *Evaluation of blood to determine compatibility between the donor and recipient prior to transfusion.*
reação de conversão	**conversion reaction** *When referring to a psychiatric condition it is the exhibition of physical symptoms as a manifestation of mental disease.*
reação despertar	**arousal reaction** *The change in brain wave patterns upon awakening.*
reação dopa	**dopa reaction** *A dopa-oxidase reaction, changing dopa into melanin.*
reação por drogas	**drug reaction** *Typically refers to an adverse effect of medication.*
realizar	**achieve, to** *To complete something one was striving for.*
receptor	**receptor** *A cell or organ that accepts stimuli and transmits data to a sensory nerve.*
recessivo	**recessive** *This refers to genetic controlled traits that are only inherited when code from both parents is the same.*
recordação	**recollection** *Memory.*
recorrência	**relapse** *The return to a prior state of ill health.*
recúbito	**recumbent** *Lying down.*
rede mosquito	**mosquito net** *A fine mesh fabric hung over a bed as a mosquito repellent.*
redução	**reduction** *Return of a dislocated joint or fractured bone to its proper position.*
redução aberta (de fraturas)	**open reduction (of fractures)** *The realignment of a fractured bone using a surgical approach.*
redução fechada (de fraturas)	**closed reduction** *The realignment of a fracture without use of surgery.*
refexo glúteo	**gluteal reflex** *After the skin of the buttocks are stimulated the gluteal muscles contract.*
reflexo bicipital	**biceps reflex** *The biceps brachii tendon is hit with a reflex hammer and results in flexion of the forearm as a normal response. This assesses the C5-C6 region.*
reflexo bulbocavernoso	**bulbocavernosus reflex** *Brisk contraction of the ischiocavernosus and bulbocavernosus muscles when the glans penis is compressed.*
reflexo conjuntiva	**conjunctival reflex** *Closure of the eyes in response to irritation of the conjunctiva.*
reflexo corneano	**corneal reflex** *Closure of the eyelids when the cornea is touched lightly with a soft material. Also called the lid reflex.*
reflexo cremastérico	**cremasteric reflex** *Retraction of the testicle and scrotum upon stroking of the ipsilateral inner thigh.*
reflexo da apreensão	**grasp reflex** *Flexion of the fingers or toes when stimulated.*
reflexo de ânisia	**gag reflex** *Contraction of the pharynx muscles when the back of the pharynx is stimulated by touch.*
reflexo de Babinski; reflexo cutâneo-plantar	**Babinski's sign** *A reflex that occurs when the plantar surface of the foot is stimulated. The great toe turns upward- normal in infancy but when it turns upward in an adult it means there is central nervous system injury.*

Portuguese	English
reflexo de Bainbridge	**Bainbridge reflex** *Increase in heart rate due to increased pressure in the right atrium.*
reflexo de Bechterew-Mendel	**Bechterew-Mendel reflex** *Plantar flexion of the toes when the examiner percusses the dorsum of the foot; seen with pyramidal lesion.*
reflexo de Bezold-Jarisch	**Bezold-Jarisch reflex** *A reflex in the vagus, originating in the heart, resulting in sinus bradycardia, hypotension & peripheral vasodilation.*
reflexo de Oppenheim	**Oppenheim reflex** *Extension of the toes elicited by scratching of the medial leg; present when the patient has cerebral irritation.*
reflexo de Rossolimo	**Rossolimo reflex** *Flexion of the toes when the tips of the toes are flicked. This abnormal response is present in pyramidal tract lesions.*
reflexo de Strümpell	**Strümpell reflex** *Flexion of the leg and adduction of the foot elicited by stroking of the thigh or abdomen.*
reflexo do polegar	**finger-thumb reflex** *Opposition and adduction of the thumb with flexion at the MCP joint and extension at the interphalangeal joint when there is flexion of the 3rd, 4th, and 5th finger. This is present normally and absent with with pyramidal lesions.*
reflexo do quadríceps	**quadriceps jerk (reflex)** *Also referred to as the patellar reflex.*
reflexo do seio carótico	**carotid sinus reflex** *Bradycardia as a result of pressure on the carotid sinus.*
reflexo do tendão	**tendon reflex** *A deep reflex elicited by gently tapping the tendon.*
reflexo do tendão de Aquiles; reflexo aquiliano	**Achilles tendon reflex** *The normal response to tapping the achilles tendon with a reflex hammer is the plantar flexion of the foot.*
reflexo do tríceps	**triceps reflex** *A tendon reflex causing extension of the arm when the triceps tendon is gently tapped.*
reflexo espinhal	**spinal reflex** *A reflex that has an arc passing through the spine.*
reflexo facial	**facial reflex or bulbomimic reflex** *Pressure on the eyeballs causes contraction of facial muscles on the side contralateral to the side of the lesion in the patient in a coma. In coma from a metabolic problem the reflex is present bilaterally.*
reflexo gastrocólico	**gastrocolic reflex** *Peristalsis of the colon produced by food entering the stomach.*
reflexo luminoso consensual	**consensual light reflex** *Constriction of the pupil of one eye in sync with the other pupil upon exposure to light.*
reflexo mandibular	**jaw reflex** *Contraction of the temporal muscles when a relaxed mandible is given a downward tap. Also, masseter reflex or jaw jerk.*
reflexo patelar; reflexo de contração do joelho	**knee jerk reflex** *Contraction of the quadriceps, yielding leg extension when the quadriceps tendon is tapped.*
reflexo plantar	**extensor plantar response** *Great toe extension indicating a positive Babinski sign.*
reflexo profundo tendinoso	**deep tendon reflex** *Reflexes exhibited by the stretching of a tendon.*
reflexos abdominais	**abdominal reflexes** *Elicited by stroking the abdomen lightly from mid-axillary line to umbilicus. A normal response is contraction of the umbilicus toward the stimulated side.*
refluxo hepatojugular	**hepatojugular reflex** *The presence of jugular venous distension with compression of the abdomen for at least 10 seconds.*
registro médico	**medical record** *The electronic or paper report on a patient.*
registro médico	**patient chart** *The file containing the client's medical record.*

Portuguese	English
registro operatório	**operative note** *A detailed description of a surgical procedure performed on a specific patient.*
regurgitação	**regurgitation** *1. Backflow of blood in the heart. 2. Movement of gastric contents into the mouth.*
regurgitação mitral	**mitral regurgitation** *Backflow of blood from the left ventricle to the left atrium because of dysfunctional valve.*
relações sexuais	**sexual intercourse** *The act of copulation.*
relaxante	**relaxant** *Term generally used to refer to a muscle relaxant.*
relaxina	**relaxin** *A hormone secreted by the placenta which dilates the cervix.*
remissão	**remission** *A decrease in severity or a temporary resolution.*
remoção	**removal** *The act of removing something.*
renal; néfrico	**renal** *Referring to the kidney.*
renina	**renin** *A renal enzyme that facilitates the production of angiotensin.*
repouso	**rest** *Relaxation or respite.*
repouso no leito	**bed rest** *A medical order requiring one to stay in bed.*
resina	**resin** *An organic substance that is insoluble in water. There are many types. Cholestyramine resin is used for hypercholesterolemia.*
resmungar	**mumble, to** *To speak quietly and indistinctly.*
respiração de Cheyne-Stokes	**Cheyne-Stokes respirations** *A breathing pattern characterized by alternating apnea with hyperpnea.*
respiração de Kussmaul	**Kussmaul respiration** *The slow, deep breathing noted in patients with acidosis.*
respiração; fôlego	**breath** *One respiration.*
respirador	**respirator** *A device used to artificially ventilate a patient.*
respiratório	**respiratory** *Referring to respiration or the organs of respiration.*
resposta imune	**immune response** *The body's reaction to what is perceived as a foreign substance.*
ressalto	**rebound** *A term used to describe a type of tenderness found with peritonitis.*
ressecção	**resection** *The removal of tissue.*
ressonância magnética nuclear (RMN)	**nuclear magnetic resonance (NMR)** *A type a diagnostic body imaging utilizing electromagnetic radiation in a magnetic field.*
ressuscitação boca-a-boca	**mouth to mouth resuscitation** *A form of emergency management of respiratory failure.*
ressuscitação cardiopulmonar	**cardiopulmonary resuscitation** *Use of artificial means to support respiration and circulation.*
resultado	**disease outcome** *The response obtained from treatment.*
resultado laboratório	**lab result** *The data obtained from a laboratory test.*
retal	**rectal** *Referring to the rectum.*
reticular	**reticular** *Referring to a matrix of membranous tubules inside the cytoplasm of a eukaryotic cells.*
reticuloendotelial	**reticulo-endothelial** *Referring to the system of phagocytes involved in the immune system.*
reticulócite	**reticulocytosis** *An abnormal increase in circulating reticulocytes.*
reticulócito	**reticulocyte** *A red blood cell without a nucleus.*
retina	**retina** *The innermost of three layers of the eyeball; it surrounds the vitreous body and is continuous with the optic nerve.*
retina descolada	**retinal detachment** *A tear or hole in the retina caused by vitreous traction.*

Portuguese	English
retinite	**retinitis** *Inflammation of the retina.*
retinoblastoma	**retinoblastoma** *A tumor consisting of retinal germ cells.*
retinopatia	**retinopathy** *Any one of a number of retinal inflammatory conditions.*
retículo endoplasmático	**endoplasmic reticulum** *A framework of tubules within the cytoplasm of eukaryotic cells.*
retocele	**rectocele** *A herniation of the wall between the rectum and vagina.*
retoscopia	**rectoscopy** *Visualization of the rectum with a scope.*
retossigmóidectomia	**rectosigmoidectomy** *Surgical resection of the rectum and sigmoid colon.*
retração	**retraction** *Being drawn back.*
retrator	**retractor** *A device for pulling back tissue during surgery.*
retrofaríngeo	**retropharyngeal** *Referring to the area posterior to the pharynx.*
retroperitônio	**retroperitoneal** *Situated or referring to the area posterior to the peritoneum.*
retrógrado	**retrograde** *Referring to backward movement.*
reumatismo	**rheumatism** *Any condition exhibited by inflammation and pain in the joints and muscles.*
reumático	**rheumatic** *Referring to rheumatism.*
riboflavina	**riboflavin** *Also called vitamin B2, this essential vitamin is present in food such as eggs and is synthesized in the small bowel.*
rickettsia	**rickettsia** *A genus of bacteria transmitted by ticks or fleas; Rocky Mountain Spotted fever is one of many diseases caused by this bacterium.*
rigidez cadavérica	**rigor mortis** *The normal stiffening of the muscles and joints that occurs a few hours after death.*
rigidez descerebrada	**decerebrate rigidity** *Rigid extension of the arms which is an abnormal posture associated with increased intracranial pressure.*
rigidez em roda dentada	**cogwheel rigidity** *As in cogwheel rigidity which is a jerky passive movement after there was increased tone.*
rijo	**stiff** *Not easily bent.*
rim	**kidney** *One of two glandular organs that form urine.*
rim em ferradura	**horseshoe kidney** *Anomalous renal development.*
rima pudenda; fenda urogenital	**vulval cleft** *The area between the labia majora where the vagina and urethra rest.*
rinite	**rhinitis** *A viral infection or allergic reaction exhibited by nasal mucosal inflammation.*
rinoplastia	**rhinoplasty** *Plastic surgery performed on the nose.*
rinorréia	**rhinorrhea** *Abundant nasal mucosal drainage.*
rinoscopia	**rhinoscopy** *Examination of the nasal passages.*
riso sardônico	**risus sardonicus** *A spasm of the facial muscles causing what appears to be a smile on one's face.*
ritmo	**rhythm** *The pattern or cadence.*
ritmo circadiano	**circadian rhythm** *Naturally recurring fluctuations in a 24 hour period.*
ritmo de galope	**cantering rhythm** *Gallop rhythm.*
rizotomia	**rhizotomy** *Interruption of the spinal nerve roots within the spinal canal.*
rodopsina	**rhodopsin** *A reddish purple light sensitive pigment in the human retina.*
roedor	**rodent** *A gnawing mammal that includes rats and mice.*

Portuguese	English
roentgen	**Roentgen** *One unit of ionizing radiation named after the German physicist Wilhelm Conrad Röntgen.*
rombóide	**rhomboid** *A back muscle that elevates, retracts and adducts the scapula.*
roncar	**snore, to** *To snore or grunt while breathing during sleep.*
ronco	**rhonchus** *A coarse, dry sound heard on auscultation of the lungs.*
rosa; erisipila	**erysipelas** *An acute infection caused by Streptococcus pyogenes that causes fever along with swelling and inflammation. The infection frequently effects the face or one leg.*
rosácea	**acne rosacea** *A chronic disease characterized by the presence of flushing of the skin of the nose, forehead and cheeks.*
rosácea	**rosacea** *Erythema of the cheeks and nose caused by chronic vascular and follicular dilation.*
rotação	**rotation** *Movement around an axis.*
rotúla condromalacia	**chondromalacia of the patella** *Softening of the articular cartilage of the patella.*
rouco	**hoarse** *A rough, harsh sounding voice.*
roupa de cama	**sheet (bed)** *A rectangular fabric covering a bed.*
rouquidão	**frog in the throat, to have** *An expression describing hoarseness.*
rótula; patela	**patella** *The bone situated in the anterior portion of the knee.*
rubefaciente	**rubefacient** *A substance that reddens the skin.*
rubéola; sarampo alemão	**rubella** *Also called German measles, it is characterized by a rash, fever, headache.*
rubor	**blush, to** *To have an increased volume of blood flow to one's face causing a red tint to the skin.*
rubor	**flushing** *Transient erythema due to heat, stress or disease.*
rubor climatérico	**hot flash** *A symptom of menopause manifested as a sudden sensation of fever.*
rude	**rude** *Ill-mannered.*
rugina	**rugine** *A surgical instrument that resembles a rasp.*
ruído	**bruit** *An abnormal sound heard through a stethoscope indicating turbulent blood flow.*
ruído carótido	**carotid bruit** *An abnormal noise heard over the carotid artery that may be a sign of stenosis or aortic valvular disease.*
ruptura	**rupture** *An instance of bursting suddenly.*
ruptura prolongamento de membrano placentário	**prolonged rupture of the membranes** *Rupture of the membranes more than 24 hours before delivery.*
rúpia	**rupia** *A sign of tertiary syphilis in which there are bullae or vesicles formed on the skin that erupt and form crusts.*
sabão	**soap** *A compound made with fats/oils and an alkali; it is used for washing.*
sabido	**known** *Recognized or familiar.*
sabor; gosto	**taste** *Sensation of flavor perceived in one's mouth.*
sacral	**sacral** *Referring to the sacrum.*
sacralização	**sacralization** *The fusion of the fifth lumbar vertebra to the sacrum.*
sacro	**sacrum** *The bone formed by five fused vertebrae that is situated between the two hip bones.*
sacudir	**shake, to** *To tremble uncontrollably.*
sadio	**healthy** *In good health.*
safena	**saphena** *Referring to either of the two superficial saphenous veins.*

Portuguese	English
sais biliares	**bile salts** *Normally occurring salts of bile acids.*
sal	**salt** *Typically referring to sodium chloride.*
sala	**room** *A division in a building surrounded by walls.*
sala de emergência	**emergency room** *A ward used for initial treatment of critical patients.*
sala de parto	**labor room** *The hospital room used while a woman is in labor.*
sala de recuperação	**recovery room** *The immediate post-operative room where patients are stabilized prior to going to a general ward.*
salino	**saline** *A solution of sodium chloride.*
saliva	**saliva** *The watery liquid secreted by the salivary glands.*
saliva	**spit** *A term used to describe saliva that is ejected from the mouth.*
salivação	**salivation** *The process of secreting saliva.*
salpingectomia	**salpingectomy** *Surgical resection of the fallopian tubes.*
salpingite	**salpingitis** *Inflammation of the fallopian tubes.*
salpingografia	**salpingography** *Roentgenography of the fallopian tubes after administration of contrast media.*
salpingostomia	**salpingostomy** *A surgical procedure involving cutting the fallopian tube.*
salurético	**saluretic** *An agent that promotes excretion of sodium and chloride in the urine.*
sangramento uterino	**uterine bleeding** *Bleeding that emanates from the uterus.*
sangria	**bleeding** *Loss of blood.*
sangue	**blood** *Plasma containing erythrocytes, leukocytes and platelets.*
sangue oculto	**occult blood** *Presence of blood from an unknown source.*
sanguessuga	**leech** *An annelid used in some tropical regions for drawing out blood; they have an anticoagulant effect locally and have been attached to digits of persons with acute peripheral ischemia.*
sapato	**shoe** *Article of clothing worn on each foot.*
saponificar	**saponify,to** *The creation of soap from oil using an alkali.*
saprófita	**saprophyte** *Any organism living on dead organic material.*
sarampo	**measles** *A childhood viral, infectious disease exhibited by rash and fever.*
sarampo alemão	**German measles** *(rubella) A contagious viral infection.*
sarampo; rubéola	**Rubeola** *Another term for measles, an acute exanthematous disease.*
sarcoidose	**sarcoidosis** *A chronic disease characterized by lymphadenopathy and widespread granulomas.*
sarcolema	**sarcolemme** *The sheath that covers skeletal muscle fibers.*
sarcoma	**sarcoma** *A non-epithelial malignant tumor.*
sarcoma de Kaposi	**Kaposi sarcoma** *Typically seen in AIDS patients, it is characterized by cutaneous reddish-purple macules and plaques.Also called multiple idiopathic hemorrhagic sarcoma.*
sarcóide	**sarcoid** *Referring to sarcoidosis.*
saturação	**saturation** *An amount, expressed in a percentage, that expresses the degree something is absorbed versus the maximal absorption possible.*
saúde	**health** *The state of being free of illness.*
sebáceo	**sebaceous** *Referring to a sebaceous gland or what it secretes.*
seborréia	**seborrhea** *Abnormal amount of sebum production.*
seco	**dry** *Absence of moisture.*
secreção	**secretion** *The discharge of substances from cells or glands.*
secreção do estômago	**gastric secretions** *Fluids secreted from gastric mucosa.*

Portuguese	English
secretina	**secretin** *A hormone that increases secretion from the pancreas and liver.*
sedativo	**sedative** *A medication used to facilitate sleep or calm a person.*
sede	**thirst** *The desire to drink.*
sedimento urinário	**urinary sediments** *The debris that settles in a urine sample when left undisturbed.*
seguinte	**next** *The following or upcoming.*
seio cavernoso	**cavernous sinus** *Large venous sinus located adjacent to the sphenoid bone and posterior to the petrosal sinuses.*
seio esfenoidal	**sphenoidal sinus** *Part of the sphenoid bone; it communicates with the most superior aspect of the nasal meatus.*
seio frontal	**frontal sinus** *A paranasal sinus on both sides of the lower part of the frontal bone.*
seios paranasais	**paranasal sinuses** *Any of the sinuses (ethmoidal, frontal, maxillary or sphenoidal) that communicate with the nasal cavity.*
seleção	**choice** *Selection or decision.*
selo	**seal** *A device or substance used to bind two things together.*
sem dentes	**toothless** *Edentulous.*
sem responder a	**lost to follow-up** *This describes a situation in which a patient has a chronic medical problem but has not been seen regularly.*
semanalemente	**weekly** *That which occurs every seven days.*
seminoma	**seminoma** *A malignant tumor of the testis.*
senescência	**senescence** *The normal process of deterioration with age.*
senil	**senile** *Generally referring to mental deterioration associated with aging.*
senilidade	**senility** *The process of being senile.*
sensação	**sensation** *A perception when one is touched.*
sensibilidade	**sensibility** *Ability to feel or perceive.*
sensibilização	**sensitization** *The change in an organ by a hormone so it will respond to another stimulus.*
sensibilizar	**sensitized** *Being abnormally sensitive to a substance.*
sensível	**sensible** *When referring to a choice, chosen with wisdom.*
sentido horário	**clockwise** *Movement in the same direction as a normal clock.*
sentir	**feel, to** *To perceive or discern.*
sentir-se melhor	**feel better, to** *To have improved health symptomatically.*
septicopiemia	**septicemia** *A systemic disease in which microorganisms or their toxins are in the blood stream.*
septo	**septum** *A wall separating two chambers, the nasal septum for example.*
septo desviado	**deviated septum** *Characterized by deviation of the nasal septum.*
septo retovesical	**rectovesical septum** *The wall between the rectum and the urinary bladder.*
seqüela	**sequela** *A medical problem related to an initial injury or disease.(late sequelae)*
seqüestro	**sequestrum** *Necrotic bone present in an injured or diseased bone.*
ser surdo	**hard of hearing** *Decreased sense of hearing.*
seringa	**syringe** *A device used for administering medication through various routes.*
seringa de gavagem	**gavage syringe** *A syringe used for irrigation.*
seroso	**serous** *Referring to serum or similar to serum.*
serotonina	**serotonin** *A neurotransmitter that constricts blood vessels.*

Portuguese	English
serpiginoso	**serpiginous** *A skin lesion having wavy margin.*
serra	**saw** *A hand or power-driven tool used for cutting.*
severo	**severe** *Intense or very great.*
sexo	**sex** *Gender.*
sépsis	**sepsis** *A condition exhibited by overwhelming inflammation due to infection.*
séptico	**septic** *Referring to a state of sepsis.*
séssil	**sessile** *Having a broad base with no stalk.*
sialoadenite	**sialadenitis** *Inflammation of a salivary gland.*
sialogogo	**sialogogue** *A substance that increase salivary flow.*
sialólito	**sialolith** *A calculus in a salivary duct.*
sibilos devido a respiração ofegante (P), respirar com dificuldade (B)	**wheezing** *A whistling or musical sound made by air passing through a narrowed airway.*
sicose	**sycosis** *A bacterial infection affecting the hair follicles on a person's face.*
SIDA (P), AIDS (B)	**AIDS** *Acquired Immunodeficiency Syndrome*
siderose	**siderosis** *Discoloration of a part due to iron deposition.*
sigmoidectomia	**sigmoidoscopy** *Visualization of the sigmoid colon with a scope.*
sigmoidoscopia	**sigmoidostomy** *Formation of an opening in the sigmoid colon that communicates with the outside of the body.*
sigmóide	**sigmoid** *Referring to the portion of the colon that leads into the rectum.*
silencioso	**silent** *Absence of noise or no indication of something.*
silicose	**silicosis** *Grinders's disease; fibrotic lung disease caused by inhalation of silica.*
simbiose	**symbiosis** *The living together of two organisms.*
simetria	**symmetry** *Being equally bilaterally.*
simpatectomia	**sympathectomy** *The surgical resection of a sympathetic nerve to reduce undesired effects.*
simulador	**malingerer** *A person who feigns illness.*
simultâneo	**simultaneous** *Occurring at the same time.*
sinais de vida	**quickening** *Signs of life noted by a mother as the fetus moves.*
sinais vitais	**vital signs** *The designation for blood pressure, pulse, respirations and temperature.*
sinal da cimitarra	**scimitar sign** *An abnormal radiologic finding associated with anomalous pulmonary venous drainage.*
sinal de Brudzinski	**Brudzinski sign** *Involuntary flexion of the knees and hips after flexion of the neck while supine; seen in meningitis.*
sinal de Graefe	**Graefe's sign** *Also called lid lag, a sign characterized by the upper eyelid not closing over the globe. This is seen commonly in exophthalmic goiter.*
sinapse	**synapse** *The intersection of two nerve cells.*
sinartrose	**synarthrosis** *Adjacent bones connected by a joint but the joint is fixed.*
sincondrose	**synchondrosis** *A joint with little motion that uses cartilage such as the vertebral bodies.*
sindrome de Asperger	**Asperger's syndrome** *A condition characterized by disturbed social interaction; if was named after the Austrian scientist who first described it.*
sinéquia	**synechia** *The adhesion of two body parts, such as synechia vulvae in which the labia minora are congenitally adherent.*
sinistrocardia	**sinistrocardia** *Location of the heart toward the left (more than normally seen).*

Portuguese	English
sinoatrial	**sinoatrial** *Referring to the cardiac node of the same name.*
sinovectomia	**synovectomy** *Surgical resection of a synovial membrane.*
sinovite	**synovitis** *Inflammation of the synovium.*
sinstrotorção	**sinistrotorsion** *Distorsion toward the left; in reference to the eye generally.*
sintoma	**symptom** *A physical feature that is characteristic of disease.*
sintoma Argyll Robertson	**Argyll Robertson symptom** *Presence of small pupils that do not react to light but will constrict when the person focuses on a near object.*
sintoma apresentado	**presenting symptom** *The initial subjective complaint that initiated a visit.*
sinusite	**sinusitis** *Inflammation of the sinuses.*
sinusóide	**sinusoid** *An irregular vessel having almost no adventitia that is found in the liver, heart, parathyroid, spleen and pancreas.*
siringomielia	**syringomelia** *A condition exhibited by fluid-filled cavities in the spinal cord.*
sistema do grupo sanguíneo ABO	**ABO system** *The system using human blood antigens to determine blood type.*
sistema métrico	**metric system**
sistema nervoso autônomo	**autonomic nervous system** *Responsible for regulation of cardiac muscle, smooth muscle and glandular activity.*
sistema nervoso central (SNC)	**central nervous system (CNS)** *The brain and spinal cord.*
sistema nervoso simpático	**sympathetic nervous system** *The nerves responsible for the flight or fight response.*
sistólico	**systolic** *Referring to systole or that which occurs during systole.*
sífilis	**syphilis** *A infectious disease caused by Treponema pallidum that causes a painless penile ulcer in the primary stage but can lead to irreversible brain damage in the untreated tertiary stage.*
sífilis congênito	**congenital syphilis** *Passed to the child in utero, the child may have failure to thrive, fever and a flattened bridge of the nose.*
síncope	**syncope** *Sudden loss of consciousness.*
síncope do seio carótico	**carotid sinus syncope** *Dizziness and syncope that results from hyperactivity of the carotid sinus reflex.*
síndrome alcoólica fetal	**fetal alcohol syndrome** *A condition caused by alcohol use by the mother during pregnancy and exhibited by poor intrauterine growth, decreased muscle tone, delayed development and widened palpebral fissures.*
síndrome da alça aferente	**afferent loop syndrome** *The obstruction of the duodenum or jejunum after gastrojejunostomy, resulting in duodenal distention.*
síndrome da alça cega	**blind loop syndrome** *A condition in which there is a non-functional section of the bowel that is thought to be responsible for malabsorption and Vitamin B12 deficiency.*
síndrome da angústia respiratório	**respiratory distress syndrome** *A disease in infants that is caused by a surfactant deficiency.*
síndrome da cauda eqüina	**cauda equina syndrome** *Neurologic condition manifested by pain, paresthesia and weakness but no bowel/bladder dysfunction.*
síndrome da imunodeficiência adquirida (SIDA)	**Acquired Immunodeficiency Syndrome (AIDS)** *Presence of an AIDS defining illness or having a CD4 of less than 200/mm3.*
síndrome da morte súbita do lactente	**sudden infant death syndrome** *A leading cause of death of infants from one month to one year; the etiology is unknown.*
síndrome das pernas inquietas	**restless legs** *Associated with a syndrome exhibited by continuous movement of the legs from uncertain etiology.*

Portuguese	English
síndrome de Adam-Stokes; doença de Adam-Stokes	**Adams-Stokes Syndrome** *Characterized by bradycardia, syncope and convulsions.*
síndrome de Aicardi	**Aicardi syndrome** *A rare genetic anomaly in which the corpus callosum is absent or insufficient. It is characterized by seizures, microphthalmos, coloboma and developmental delays.*
síndrome de Bartter	**Bartter's syndrome** *An autosomal recessive renal disorder with a defect in chloride reabsorption and secondary hyperaldosteronism.*
síndrome de Behçet	**Behçet syndrome** *Characterized by recurrent oral and genital ulcers, uveitis, iridocyclitis and frequently arthritis.*
síndrome de Boerhaave	**Boerhaave Syndrome** *Rupture of the esophagus from vigorous vomiting, with resultant mediastinitis.*
síndrome de Brown-Séquard	**Brown-Séquard syndrome** *Unilateral spinal cord lesions, proprioception loss and weakness occur ipsilateral to the lesion, while pain and temperature loss occur contralateral.*
síndrome de Budd-Chiari	**Budd-Chiari syndrome** *Hepatomegaly, severe portal hypertension and ascites related to thrombosis of the hepatic vein.*
síndrome de Cushing	**Cushing's syndrome** *Characterized by truncal obesity, moon face, acne, abdominal striae, hypertension, decreased carbohydrate tolerance, protein catabolism, psychiatric disturbances, and osteoporosis.*
síndrome de Down	**Down's syndrome** *A congenital chromosomal defect (trisomy 21) that causes diminished intellectual function, short stature and a broad face.*
síndrome de esmagamento	**crush syndrome** *Rhabdomyolysis occurring as a result of muscle injury from mechanical stress.*
síndrome de Fanconi	**Fanconi's syndrome** *An idiopathic refractory anemia exhibited by pancytopenia, bone marrow hypoplasia and congenital anomalies.*
síndrome de Felty	**Felty syndrome** *Rheumatoid arthritis with leukopenia and splenomegaly.*
síndrome de Foville	**Foville's syndrome** *Caused by a lesion within the pons, there is ipsilateral facial and abducens nerve paralysis and contralateral hemiplegia.*
síndrome de fralda azul	**blue diaper syndrome** *A disorder of tryptophan absorption. Excess tryptophan is metabolized to indicans in the bowel, excreted in the urine and oxidized in the diaper to indigo, thus the blue diaper.*
síndrome de Gerstmann	**Gerstmann syndrome** *Finger agnosia, agraphia and acalculia caused by a lesion between the occipital region and angular gyrus.*
síndrome de Goodpasture	**Goodpasture' syndrome** *Glomerulonephritis, preceded by hemoptysis. The nephritis can quickly progress to death from renal failure.*
síndrome de Guillain-Barré	**Guillain-Barré syndrome** *An acute autoimmune disorder that causes nerve inflammation subsequently muscle weakness.*
síndrome de Hamman-Rich	**Hamman-Rich syndrome** *Idiopathic pulmonary fibrosis.*
síndrome de Hanhart	**Hanhart's syndrome** *Also referred to as micrognathia with peromelia. There is hypoplasia of the mandible, malformed or missing teeth, birdlike face and severe upper extremity deformities.*
síndrome de Henri	**Henri, syndrome of** *Congenital anomaly exhibited by different sized external orifices of the nostrils.*
síndrome de Horner; ptose simpática	**Horner syndrome** *A lesion of the cervical sympathetic chain causes ipsilateral myosis, ptosis and facial anhidrosis.*

Portuguese	English
síndrome de Job	**Job syndrome** *Also known as hyperimmunoglobulin E syndrome, there are high levels if IgE, a leukocyte chemotactic defect, recurrent staph infections and cold abscess formation in the skin.*
síndrome de Klinefelter	**Klinefelter's syndrome** *Presence of an extra X chromosome, it is exhibited by longer legs, narrow shoulders, small testicles and gynecomastia.*
síndrome de Libman-Sachs	**Libman-Sachs syndrome** *A verrucous endocarditis associated with disseminated lupus erythematosus; also called nonbacterial verrucous endocarditis.*
síndrome de Lyell	**Lyell's syndrome** *Also called toxic epidermal necrolysis, there are large portions of the skin that become erythematous with epidermal necrosis as seen with 2nd degree burns. This reaction can be seen with use of nevirapine or Bactrim.*
síndrome de Mallory-Weiss	**Mallory-Weiss syndrome** *Upper GI bleeding related to a laceration at the gastroesophageal junction caused by vigorous vomiting.*
síndrome de Marfan	**Marfan syndrome** *A connective tissue disease exhibited by long limbs, joint laxity and cardiovascular defects.*
síndrome de Menkes; doença do cabelo enroscado	**kinky-hair syndrome** *Inborn error of copper metabolism, noted in the first few weeks of life. Exhibited by sparse kinky hair, failure to thrive and seizures. Also called Menke's syndrome or trichopoliodystrophy.*
síndrome de mento entorpecimento	**numb chin syndrome.** *Generally associated with metastatic breast or prostate cancer, it is characterized by unilateral sensory loss of the chin and lower lip.*
síndrome de Milkmann	**Milkman syndrome** *Osteomalacia with multiple pseudofractures.*
síndrome de Morgagni	**Morgagni's syndrome** *Also called metabolic craniopathy and Stewart-Morel syndrome, it is exhibited by hyperostosis frontalis interna, obesity and neuropsychiatric disorders.*
síndrome de Mucune-Albright	**Mucune-Albright syndrome** *Polyostotic fibrous dysplasia with cutaneous brown patches, endocrine dysfunction that exhibits in females as precocious puberty.*
síndrome de patelofemoral	**patellofemoral stress syndrome** *Overuse syndrome causing anterior knee pain from excessive lateral motion.*
síndrome de Plummer-Vinson; disfagia sideropênica	**Plummer-Vinson syndrome** *Also called sideropenic dysphagia. Exhibited by iron deficiency anemia, dysphagia, esophageal stenosis and atrophic glossitis. The cause is not known.*
síndrome de Potter	**Potter's syndrome** *A group of findings associated with oligohydramnios. Renal failure is the primary problem but the infant has abnormal limbs, broad nasal bridge, low set ears and receding chin. Death usually ensues due to renal and respiratory failure.*
síndrome de Rett	**Rett syndrome.** *A rare inherited disorder causing developmental delays and is seen mostly in girls.*
síndrome de Sézary	**Sézary syndrome** *Symptoms are exfoliative dermatitis with intense itching caused by cutaneous infiltration by mononuclear cells,*
síndrome de Sjogren	**Sjogren's syndrome.** *Characterized by dryness of the mouth and eyes, it is sometimes linked to rheumatoid arthritis.*
síndrome do esvaziamento rápido	**dumping syndrome** *Characterized by rapid bowel evacuation after eating in patients with prior gastric surgery.*
síndrome do intestino irritável	**irritable bowel syndrome** *A condition exhibited by chronic diarrhea or constipation and abdominal pain; it is sometimes associated with a labile emotional state.*

Portuguese	English
síndrome do linfonodo cutaneomucoso; doença de Kawasaki	**Kawasaki syndrome** *Begins with fever for 5 days, skin rashes, strawberry tongue, lymphadenopathy and swollen hands and feet. It is known to cause coronary artery aneurysms. Also called mucocutaneous lymph node syndrome.*
síndrome do miado do gato; cri-du-chat síndrome	**cat cry syndrome** *A hereditary congenital disorder exhibited by microcephaly, hypertelorism, and cognitive deficits.*
síndrome do roubo subclávio	**subclavian steal syndrome** *Retrograde vertebral artery flow due to ipsilateral subclavian artery stenosis.*
síndrome do túnel do carpo	**carpal tunnel syndrome** *Paresthesia that results from compression of the median nerve.*
síndrome do túnel do tarso	**tarsal tunnel syndrome** *Characterized by impingement of various nerves of the ankle.*
síndrome maligna meuroléptica	**neuroleptic malignant syndrome** *A severe reaction to neuroleptic medications characterized by hyperthermia with autonomic and extrapyramidal symptoms.*
síndrome pré-menstrual	**premenstrual syndrome** *A cluster of emotional, behavioral, and physical symptoms that occur in the premenstrual phase of the menstrual cycle and resolve with the onset of menstruation.*
síndrome pseudocoma	**locked-in syndrome** *A neurologic condition characterized by a person being conscious of their surroundings but being unable to verbally communicate that understanding.*
síndrome sela vazia	**empty sella syndrome** *Compressed or flattened pituitary related to herniating arachnoid, surgery or radiotherapy.*
síndrome talâmica	**thalamic syndrome** *Caused by an infarct of the posteroinferior thalamus, there is transient hemiparesis, severe sensory loss with preserved crude pain in the hypalgic limbs.*
sístole	**systole** *The phase of the cardiac cycle in which the ventricles contract.*
sítio	**site** *Location.*
sobrancelha	**eyebrow** *Supercilium.*
sobrenome	**surname** *One's given "last" name that generally changes for women upon marriage to that of the man's surname.*
sobrevivência	**stamina** *Ability to maintain physical or mental exertion for a long period.*
sofrer	**suffer, to** *To be affected by an illness or sickness.*
sofrer de estrabismo	**squint, to** *To look at something with the eyes partially closed.*
sola de pé	**sole of foot** *Common term for plantar aspect of the foot.*
solitário	**single** *Only one.*
solteiro	**single** *Not married.*
soluçar	**sob, to** *To cry uncontrollably.*
solução salina fisiológica	**physiological saline** *0.9% normal saline.*
soluço	**hiccup** *Involuntary spasm of the diaphragm with sudden closure of the glottis; this causes a characteristic cough.*
solvente	**solvent** *Able to dissolve with other chemicals.*
som	**sound** *Vibrations that travel through air and are heard when reaching the ears.*
soma	**amount** *The total or the aggregate.*
somático	**somatic** *Referring to the body.*
sonambulismo	**somnambulism** *Sleepwalking.*
sonda	**probe** *A device used for exploration.*
sonda de canal triplo	**three way foley** *A urinary tube used for irrigation of the bladder.*
sonda de drenagem	**drainage tube** *A cannula used to allow outflow of fluids.*
sonda de Foley	**Foley catheter** *A drainage tube placed in the urinary bladder via the urethra.*

Portuguese	English
sonda de gavagem	**gavage tube** *A tube used for instillation of liquids into the stomach.*
soneca	**nap** *A brief sleep or catnap.*
sonho	**dream** *The thoughts or images occurring during sleep.*
sono	**sleep** *A nap or a snooze.*
sonolência	**drowsiness** *Sleepiness.*
sonolência	**somnolence** *Drowsiness.*
sons respiratórios	**breath sounds** *The noise heard upon auscultation with a stethoscope.*
soporífico	**soporific** *Promoting drowsiness or sleep.*
sopro	**murmur** *An abnormal heart sound heard with a stethoscope.*
sopro cardíaco	**heart murmur** *An abnormal heart sound usually related to valvular disease.*
soro	**serum** *The fluid that isolates out when blood coagulates.*
sovaco	**armpit** *A common term for axilla.*
status marital	**marital status** *Single versus married status.*
suar	**sweat, to** *The action of releasing moisture through pores of the skin.*
suave	**mild** *Slight, nominal.*
subagudo	**subacute** *A stage between acute and chronic.*
subaracnóide	**subarachnoid** *The layer of the brain covering between the arachnoid and pia mater.*
subclávio	**subclavian** *Refers to the area under the clavicle; the subclavian vein runs below the clavicle.*
subdural	**subdural** *The area between the dura mater and the arachnoid membrane.*
suberose	**suberosis** *A type of hypersensitivity pneumonitis related to inhalation of moldy cork dust.*
subfrênico	**subphrenic** *Referring to below the diaphragm.*
subjacente	**underlying** *Causative, unexposed, or fundamental.*
sublingual	**sublingual** *Situated under the tongue.*
submaxilar	**submaxillary** *Situated below the maxilla.*
substância branca	**white matter** *The brain tissue consisting of myelin sheaths and nerve fibers.*
substância cinzenta do sistema nervoso	**gray matter** *The section of the brain and spinal cord composed of branching dendrites and nerve cell bodies.*
substância cinzenta periaqueduto do cérebro	**periaqueductal gray matter** *Refers to the brain gray matter adjacent to the periaqueductal.*
substância lipotrófico	**lipotrophic substance** *A compound which causes an increase in body fat.*
sucussão	**succussion** *The presence of a splashing sound when a body cavity is moved indicating presence of both air and fluid.*
sudames	**sudamina** *White vesicles noted because of retained sweat in the layers of the epidermis.*
sufocação	**suffocation** *To die from a lack of air or inability to breathe.*
sufocar-se; asfixiar	**choke, to** *To retch, cough or fight for breath.*
sugar	**suck, to** *As in, to suction fluid.*
suicídio	**suicide** *To kill oneself intentionally.*
sujo	**dirty** *Unclean.*
sulco	**sulcus** *A groove, like in the brain.*
sulfonamidas	**sulfonamide** *A class of drugs derived from sulfanilamide that are antibacterial.*
suor	**sweat** *Moisture exuded through the pores of the skin.*

Portuguese	English
suores noturnos	**night sweats** *Profuse sweating at night occurring with tuberculosis among other conditions.*
superfecundação	**superfecundation** *The fertilization of two different ova by spermatozoa of two different males.*
superficial	**superior** *In a position above something else.*
supinação	**supination** *Turning the sole of the foot or the palm of the hand upward..*
supino	**supine** *Flat on one's back.*
suportar	**bear, to** *To endure or resist.*
suporte calcâneo	**ankle support** *A mechanical device or banding to support the ankle.*
suporte por túnel do carpo	**cock-up splint** *A splint used to maintain the wrist in dorsiflexion; used for carpal tunnel syndrome.*
suporte; órtose	**brace** *A splint.*
supositório	**suppository** *A delivery system for medication placed in an orifice.*
supra-normal	**greater than normal** *Above normal.*
supra-orbitário	**supraorbital** *Situated above the orbit.*
suprapúbico	**suprapubic** *Situated above the pubis.*
supressão	**withdrawal** *The action of being without drugs or alcohol.*
suprimento	**supplies** *Stock or reserves.*
supuração	**suppuration** *Formation of purulent material.*
sural	**sural** *Referring to the calf of the leg.*
surdez	**deafness** *Having impaired hearing.*
surdo	**deaf** *Absence of the sense of hearing.*
surdo-mudo	**deaf-mute** *Inability to hear or speak.*
surfactante	**surfactant** *A substance that reduces surface tension in the lungs.*
suspiro	**sigh** *A long deep exhalation that expresses an emotion, as in relief.*
sussurrar	**whisper, to** *To speak in a volume that is barely discernible.*
sussurro	**whisper** *Speech in a volume that is barely discernible.*
sustentar	**sustain, to** *To keep or maintain.*
sutura	**suture** *Thread used for sewing together a wound.*
sutura absorvível	**resorbable suture (chromic)** *Suture that is not intended to be permanent as it is dissolved by normal body processes.*
sutura cirúrgica inabsorvível	**non-resorbable suture (nylon)** *Suture used to be permanent as it is not removed by normal body processes.*
sutura contínua	**running suture** *A method of sewing a wound in which there is a knot at each end and continuous otherwise.*
sutura coronal	**coronal suture** *The line of intersection of the frontal bone and the two parietal bones.*
sutura de colchoeiro	**mattress suture** *A double stitch that forms a loop and there is eversion of the edges when tied.*
sutura sagital	**sagittal suture** *The line where the two parietal bones meet.*
tabaqueira anatômico	**anatomical snuff-box** *The area on the back of the hand near the base of the thumb that is between the extensor pollicus longus and extensor pollicus brevis.*
talassemia	**thalassemia** *A hereditary hemolytic anemia first observed in people from the Mediterranean area.*
talidomida	**thalidomide** *A drug used originally as a sedative, after it was found to cause congenital anomalies, its use was restricted. Now it is used for a few conditions such as multiple myeloma.*

Portuguese	English
talipe calcaneus	**talipes calcaneus** *A foot deformity exhibited by abnormal dorsiflexion.*
talipe eqüino	**talipes equinus** *A foot deformity exhibited by abnormal plantar flexion.*
talipe eqüinovaro	**talipes equinovaro** *Medical term for what is commonly known as club foot.*
talo	**talus** *The most superior tarsal bone that articulates with the tibia.*
tamanho	**size** *The dimensions of something.*
tampão	**feminine pad** *Gauze specially designed to absorb menstrual flow.*
tampão	**sanitary napkin** *Cloth or synthetic material used to absorb menstrual blood.*
tampão	**tampon** *Disposable intravaginal product used to collect blood from menstruation.*
tamponamento	**tamponade** *1. Stopping bleeding during surgery with a cotton pledget. 2. When referring to cardiac tamponade, it is the limitation of cardiac contraction because of blood or fluid accumulation in the pericardial sac.*
taquicardia	**tachycardia** *Heart rate higher than physiologic normal.*
taquipnéia	**tachypnea** *Breathing faster than normal.*
taracoscopia	**thoracoscopy** *Visualization of the thoracic cavity with a scope.*
taracotomia	**thoracotomy** *Surgical incision of the thorax.*
tarântula	**tarantula** *A large hairy spider found mainly in the tropics.*
tardio	**late** *A time later than expected.*
tarsalgia	**tarsalgia** *Pain in any of the tarsal bones.*
tarsectomia	**tarsectomy** *Surgical excision of all or part of the tarsus.*
tarso	**tarsus** *The group of seven bones of the ankle or foot (three cuneiform bones, talus, calcaneus, navicular, cuboid bones).*
tarsorrafia	**tarsorrhaphy** *Suturing the eyelids in order to tighten the palpebral fissure.*
tartamudez	**stuttering** *Involuntary repetition of the first consonant.*
tatuagem	**tattoo** *A design made by inserting indelible ink into the skin.*
tálamo	**thalamus** *A paired structure located adjacent to the third ventricle.*
tálon	**talon** *The ball of the ankle joint.*
társico	**tarsal** *Referring to any bone in the tarsus.*
tátil	**tactile** *Able to be felt.*
TC tomografia computadorizada	**CT scan** *Computerized axial tomography.*
teca	**theca** *A tendon or ovarian follicle sheath.*
tecido	**tissue** *Any of the distinct materials people are made of.*
tecido de granulação	**granulation tissue** *Vascular connective tissue forming granular protrusions on the surface of a healing wound.*
tecoma	**thecoma** *A tumor composed of theca cells.*
telangiectasia	**telangiectasis** *A condition exhibited by red, dilated capillaries on the skin.*
telemetria	**telemetry** *Use of radio signals to transmit patient data. The most common form is for electrocardiography in a patient who is ambulatory.*
temperatura	**temperature** *The degree of internal heat in a person's body.*
tempo de sangramento	**bleeding time** *The time of bleeding after a controlled standardized puncture of the earlobe.*
tenazes	**tongs** *A medical device used for holding or grasping.*

Portuguese	English
tenda de oxigênio	**oxygen tent** *A manner of giving supplement oxygen to a neonate.*
tendão	**tendon** *Fibrous tissue that connects muscle to bone.*
tendência a roer as unhas; onicotilomania	**nail biting** *A habit of chewing on one's fingernails.*
tendinite	**tendinitis** *Inflammation of a tendon.*
tenesmo	**tenesmus** *The attempt to defecate but attempts elicit pain and are ineffective.*
tenoplastia	**tenoplasty** *Surgical repair of a tendon.*
tenorrafia	**tenorrhaphy** *The surgical repair with suture of a separated tendon.*
tenossinovite	**tenosynovitis** *Inflammation and swelling of an articulation.*
tenotomia	**tenotomy** *Incision of a tendon as is done for strabismus.*
tensão	**stress** *Strain or pressure.*
terapeuta de fala	**speech therapist** *A person trained to assist people with speech and language disorders.*
terapia de manutenção	**maintenance therapy** *Continuing a form of treatment long-term.*
terapia eletroconvulsiva	**electroconvulsive therapy (ECT)** *The electrical stimulation of the brain to treat mental disorders.*
terapia físico	**physical therapy** *Treatment of disease by heat, massage and exercise as opposed to medications.*
terapia ocupacional	**occupational therapy** *Rehabilitation focusing on activities of daily living.*
teratoma	**teratoma** *A tumor made up of tissue not usually at the location (a mass of hair, teeth and gingival tissue in a leg tumor for instance).*
teratógeno	**teratogen** *A substance that induces fetal anomalies.*
terciário	**tertiary** *Third in order or designating medical care at a specialized hospital.*
terçol	**sty** *Also called hordeolum externum, it is inflammation of the sebaceous gland of an eyelash.*
terebrante	**terebrant** *Having a piercing quality.*
termômetro	**thermometer** *A device used to measure temperature.*
terrores noturnos	**night terror** *Sensation of profound fear upon wakening.*
tesoura	**scissors** *A cutting instrument with two blades, joined at the middle.*
teste de Casoni	**Casoni's test** *Hydatid fluid is injected intradermally; subsequent formation of a larger papule indicates hydatid disease.*
teste de emplastro	**patch test** *A test used to determine which substances provoke an allergic response in a patient.*
testículo	**testicle** *One of a pair of organs in the male scrotum that produces sperm.*
testo de absorção de anticorpo treponêmico fluorescente	**FTA test** *Fluorescent treponemal antibody test for syphilis.*
testo de anticorpos fluorescentes	**fluorescent antibody test (FTA test)**
testo de calcanhar-canela	**heel-shin test (heel to knee to toe test)** *A test of position sense and coordination; one moves the heel of one foot from the knee on the other foot down to the foot.*
testo de dedo-nariz	**finger nose test** *A test for dysmetria in which a person reaches out to touch their own nose with an extended finger with their eyes closed.*
testo de Finkelstein	**Finkelstein test** *Pain elicited with thumb flexion and wrist flexion is indicative of De Quervain tenosynovitis.*

Portuguese	English
testo de sussurro	**whisper test** *The examiner whispers into one ear while blocking the other ear to see if the patient can hear in the ear whispered into.*
testosterona	**testosterone** *This steroid hormone produces secondary male sexual characteristics.*
tetania	**tetany** *A condition caused by the hypocalcemic effect of hypoparathyroidism, exhibited by periodic muscle spasms, convulsions, and peri-oral numbness.*
teto	**tectum** *A roof-like body.*
teto do mesencéfalo	**tectum mesencephali** *The posterior portion of the mesencephalon including the sup. and inf. colliculi and tectal lamina.*
tetraciclina	**tetracycline** *An antibiotic used for gram positive and gram negative infections.*
tetradáctilo	**tetradactylous** *Referring to a condition of having only four digits on a hand or foot.*
tépido	**tepid** *Lukewarm.*
tétano	**tetanus** *A condition caused by Clostridium tetani which produces spasm and rigidity of voluntary muscles.*
tétrade de Fallot	**Fallot, tetrology of** *Congenital cardiac defects including ventricular septal defect, pulmonic valve stenosis or infundibular stenosis, and dextroposition of the aorta.*
tênia	**tapeworm** *A parasitic, intestinal flatworm.*
tiamina	**thiamine** *Also called vitamin B1; a deficiency causes beriberi.*
timectomia	**thymectomy** *Surgical excision of the thymus.*
timina	**thymine** *A chemical with a pyrimidine base found in DNA.*
timo	**thymus** *A body organ located in the neck and it produces T cells to improve immune function.*
timoma	**thymoma** *A tumor composed of thymic tissue and is sometimes associated with myasthenia gravis.*
timócito	**thymocyte** *A lymphocyte located in the thymus.*
timpanoplastia	**tympanoplasty** *Restoration of the tympanic membrane's continuity.*
timpânico	**tympanic** *Referring to the tympanic membrane or having a resonant quality to percussion.*
tinha	**tinea** *Medical term for ringworm.*
tinha ; tinea	**ringworm** *A fungal skin infection exhibited by pruritic well circumscribed patches on the scalp or feet.*
tinha crural	**dhobie itch** *So called because the contact dermatitis is caused by the soap used by laundry workers in India who are called "dhobie".*
tinha crural	**jock itch** *Pruritus caused by tinea cruris.*
tinha crural	**tinea cruris** *Ringworm in the inguinal region, a fungal infection.*
tinha da barba	**tinea barbae** *Ringworm on the face in the region a man shaves.*
tinha da cabeça	**tinea capitis** *Ringworm of the scalp, a fungal infection.*
tinha do corpo	**tinea corporis** *Ringworm of the body, a fungal infection.*
tinha do pé	**tinea pedis** *Ringworm of the feet, a fungal infection.*
tinha imbricada	**Malabar itch.** *Pruritus associated with tinea imbricata which is characterized by overlapping rings of papulosquamous patches. It is also known as oriental ringworm.*
tinido	**tinnitus** *Medical term for ringing in the ears. It is associated with Meniere's syndrome among other conditions.*
tintura	**tincture** *1. A very small amount of something. 2. A medicine dissolved in alcohol.*

Portuguese	English
tipagem sangüínea	**blood grouping** *Testing blood to determine which type should be used for transfusion.*
tipo sangüíneo	**blood type** *Determined and listed in the ABO system.*
tipóia	**sling** *A device used to give support to an injured extremity.*
tique	**tic** *Periodic spasmodic facial muscle contractions.*
tique doloroso	**tic douloureux** *Also referred to as trigeminal neuralgia.*
tireoidectomia	**thyroidectomy** *Surgical resection of all or part of the thyroid.*
tireotoxicose	**thyrotoxicosis** *Abnormal increase in thyroid activity exhibited by thinning hair, hypertension, tachycardia and at times atrial fibrillation.*
tireoxina	**thyroxine** *An iodine containing hormone, referred to T4.*
tireóide	**thyroid** *A gland in the neck that secretes hormones regulating metabolism.*
tirosina	**tyrosine** *An amino acid important in the synthesis of hormones.*
tíbia	**tibia** *The larger of two long bones in the lower leg.*
tímpano	**ear-drum** *Common term for tympanic membrane.*
tocoferol	**tocopherol** *Vitamin E.*
tomografia com emissão de pósitrons (PET)	**PET scan Positron emission tomography.** *Production of tomographic images revealing biochemical tissue properties by analyzing positrons emitted when radioactively tagged substances are taken in tissues.*
tonossinovite de De Quervain	**De Quervain tenosynovitis** *Inflammation of the tendons of the wrist including the abductor pollicis longus and extensor pollicis brevis.*
tonômetro	**tonometer** *A device used to measure ocular pressure in glaucoma.*
tons cardíacos fetal	**fetal heart tone** *Refers to the cardiac rate and pattern of the fetus.*
tonsila	**tonsil** *A rounded mass of lymphoid tissue, most commonly referring to the pharyngeal tonsil.*
tonsilectomia	**tonsillectomy** *Excision of the tonsils.*
tonsilite	**tonsillitis** *Inflammation of the tonsils.*
tontura epidêmica	**kubisagari** *Vestibular neuronitis.*
toque	**touch** *Tactile stimulation.*
toracocentese	**thoracentesis** *Insertion of a needle into the pleural space to drain and or obtain a specimen for analysis.*
toracoplastia	**thoracoplasty** *Surgical removal of ribs.*
torácico	**thoracic** *Referring to the thorax.*
torcicolo	**torticollis** *A condition exhibited by the head being turned to one side continuously.*
torção	**torsion** *Refers to twisting. Testicular torsion is the twisting of the spermatic cord that can lead to ischemia and gangrene of the testicle.*
torção do testículo	**testicular torsion** *Rotation of the spermatic cord resulting in testicular ischemia.*
tornozelo, maléolo	**ankle** *The area of the ankle joint.*
torpor	**torpor** *Unresponsiveness to normal stimuli.*
torso	**torso** *The trunk of the body.*
tosse	**cough** *Forceful expulsion of air from the lungs.*
tosse prolongado	**coughing fit** *An episode of prolonged, forceful coughing.*
tosse seca	**dry cough** *A cough without sputum production.*
toxemia	**toxemia** *The release of toxic substances into the blood stream from a local infection. Toxemia of pregnancy is a synonym for preeclampsia.*

Portuguese	English
toxicologia	**toxicology** *The study of the nature, effects and detection of poisons.*
toxina	**toxin** *A poison of plant or animal origin.*
toxoplasmose	**toxoplasmosis** *A disease caused by an organism from the genus Toxoplasma. One can have simple malaise to central nervous system involvement.*
toxóide	**toxoid** *A chemically modified toxin that can be used as a vaccine.*
tórax	**chest** *Thorax.*
tórax	**thorax** *The part of the body between the neck and abdomen.*
tórax em funil	**funnel chest** *Anterior thorax funnel shaped depression, also called pectus excavatum.*
tórax móvel	**flail chest** *The term used when one has multiple rib fractures causing a segment of the chest wall to move incongruently with the rest of the chest wall.*
tóxico	**toxic** *Relating to or caused by poison.*
trabalho à noite; serviço noturno	**night shift** *The late shift, typically beginning at 19:00 or 23:00 hours.*
trabalho monótono	**treadmill** *An exercise machine on a continuous belt used for walking.*
trabeculectomia	**trabeculotomy** *A surgery for open angle glaucoma.*
trabécula	**trabecule** *A connective tissue strand that goes from a capsule to the enclosed organ.*
tracoma	**trachoma** *An infection of the cornea and conjunctiva caused by Chlamydia.*
tracti; tracto	**tract** *A large bundle of fibers or a major passage in the body.*
tração	**traction** *Sustained pull on a muscle or bone to correct alignment.*
tração óssea	**skeletal traction** *Use of a pulley system to reduce a fracture.*
trago	**tragus** *The fleshy prominence anterior to the opening of the ear.*
tranfusão de troca	**exchange transfusion** *Treatment of hyperbilirubinemia in neonates.*
tranqüilizante	**tranquilizer** *A medication used to diminish anxiety.*
transabdominal	**transabdominal** *Through the abdominal wall.*
transaminases	**transaminase** *An enzyme that facilitates the transfer of an amino group to an amino acid.*
transdermico	**transdermal** *Through the skin.*
transfusão	**transfusion** *Administration of blood products intravenously.*
transpirar	**transpire, to** *To release vapor from the skin or respiratory mucosa.*
transplante	**transplant,to** *To move a body part from one location to another.*
transplante	**transplantation** *The grafting of tissues.*
transplante corneal	**corneal transplant** *Surgical replacement of a cornea with a donor cornea.*
transudação	**transudation** *The movement of body tissue through a membrane that is usually the result of inflammation.*
trapézio	**trapezium** *The lateral bone in the distal row of carpal bones.*
traqueíte	**tracheitis** *Inflammation of the trachea.*
traquelorrafia	**trachelorrhaphy** *Surgical repair of a lacerated cervix.*
traqueobronquite	**tracheobronchitis** *Inflammation of the trachea and bronchi.*
traqueostomia	**tracheostomy** *Creation of a surgical opening in the trachea so a tube could be placed in the trachea.*

Portuguese	English
traqueotomia	**tracheotomy** *Surgical incision of the trachea.*
traquéia	**trachea** *The ringed canal between the pharynx and bronchi.*
traseiro	**pillow** *An encased fabric covering soft material used for a cushion.*
tratamento (P)	**treatment** *Medical care one receives for illness or injury.*
tratamento nebulizador	**nebulizer treatment** *Administration of medication such as albuterol via a fine mist using a nebulizer.*
tratamento por ferida	**wound care** *The treatment applied to a tissue injury.*
trato extrapiramidal	**extrapyramidal tract** *Motor nerves that are not part of the pyramidal tract.*
trato gastrointestinal	**gastrointestinal tract** *The alimentary canal from the distal esophagus to the cecum.*
trato respiratório superior	**upper respiratory tract** *Generally considered the part of the respiratory tract superior to the vocal cords.*
trato urinário	**urinary tract** *The organs and canals associated with urine secretion including the kidneys, ureters, bladder and urethra.*
trauma; traumatismo	**trauma** *A physical injury or emotional shock.*
trazer	**bring, to** *To carry or transport something.*
trematódeo	**fluke** *Parasitic nematode worm; an example is Schistosoma.*
trematódeo	**trematoda** *A parasitic fluke such as Schistosoma.*
tremor	**tremor** *Involuntary contraction and relaxation of small muscle groups.*
tremor de intenção	**intention tremor** *The tremulous movement noted when a person is beginning to perform a task but not seen at rest.*
tremor; calafrio	**shiver** *A trembling.*
treonina	**threonine** *An amino acid needed for the growth in infants.*
trepanação	**trephination** *Cutting away a circular disc of bone or the cornea.*
trépano	**burr or bur** *A rotary cutting instrument.*
triagem	**screening** *An evaluation as part of a methodical study.*
triângulo femoral	**femoral triangle** *An area that is bordered by the sartorius muscle, the adductor longus muscle and the inguinal ligament.*
trichuris trichiura; tricuro	**whipworm** *A parasitic, intestinal nematode worm of the genus Trichuris.*
tricofitose	**trichophytosis** *A skin or nail fungal infection caused by Trichophyton.*
trifosfato de adenosina	**adenosine triphosphate (ATP)** *A chemical that represents the energy reserve of the muscle.*
trigeminal	**trigeminal** *Generally refers to the fifth cranial nerve.*
tripanossomíase	**trypanosomiasis** *A disease caused by a protozoa of the genus Trypanosoma that can cause sleeping sickness and Chagas' disease.*
triplegia	**triplegia** *Paralysis of three extremities.*
tripleto	**triplets** *Three infants born during one birth.*
triplóide	**triploid** *Referring to a cell with three homologous sets of chromosomes.*
tripsina	**trypsin** *An enzyme whose precursor is secreted by the pancreas that breaks down proteins in the intestine.*
tripsinogênio	**trypsinogen** *The precursor to trypsin that is secreted by the pancreas.*
triptofano	**tryptophan** *An amino acid that is a precursor of serotonin. If present in the body in appropriate levels it can prevent pellagra even if niacin levels are low.*
triquinose	**trichinosis** *A disease caused by meat infected by Trichinella spiralis causing fever and gastrointestinal effects.*

Portuguese	English
triquíase	trichiasis *Inversion of the eyelashes.*
trismo	trismus *Commonly called lockjaw, it is a spasm of the muscles supplied by the trigeminal nerve and is an early symptom of tetanus.*
trissomia	trisomy *A general category of congenital anomalies in which there is an extra set of chromosomes in the cell nucleus.*
trissomia 21	trisomy 21 *A congenital anomaly in which chromosome 21 is effected and results in Down's syndrome.*
tristeza	sadness *The state of being sad.*
tristeza	sorrow *A feeling of deep despair.*
tríceps	triceps *Referring to something having three heads like the triceps muscle.*
trígono da bexiga	trigone of bladder *Refers to the area at the base of the bladder between the openings of the ureters and the urethra.*
trocarte	trocar *A device enclosed in a catheter that is used to withdraw fluid from a body cavity.*
trocânter	trochanter *Refers to the greater or lesser trochanter; the prominences on the femoral neck.*
troclear	trochlear *Referring to a trochlea.*
trofoblasto	trophoblast *A layer of endodermal tissue that helps attach an ovum to the uterine wall.*
trombectomia	thrombectomy *Excision of a thrombus from a vein or artery.*
trombina	thrombin *An enzyme that is a catalyst for the conversion of fibrinogen to fibrin in the formation of a clot.*
trombo mural	mural thrombus *A thrombus attached to a diseased portion of endocardium.*
tromboangeíte	thromboangiitis *Inflammation and thrombosis in a blood vessel.*
tromboarterite	thromboarteritis *Thrombosis of an inflamed artery.*
trombocitopenia	thrombocytopenia *Abnormal decrease in the number of blood platelets.*
tromboflebite	thrombophlebitis *Inflammation of a venous wall associated with a thrombus.*
trombose	thrombosis *Formation of a clot in a vein or artery.*
trombose de seio cavernoso	cavernous sinus thrombosis *A blood clot in the base of the brain.*
trombose venosa profunda (TPV)	deep vein thrombosis (DVT) *A blood clot that forms within a vein, typically in the lower extremities.*
trompa de Falópio; tubo de Falópio	fallopian tubes *Either of a pair of long narrow ducts located in a female's abdominal cavity that transport the male sperm cells to the egg.*
tronco	truncal *Referring to the trunk of a body or a nerve.*
tronco cerebral	brain stem *An organ that consists of the medulla oblongata, pons and midbrain.*
tróclea	trochlea *A pulley-shaped structure such as the groove at the distal humerus.*
tubárino	tubal *Referring to a tube, as in fallopian tube.*
tuberculina	tuberculin *A solution containing M. tuberculosis or M. bovis that is used to test for tuberculosis by injecting the solution intradermally and looking for a reaction.*
tuberculoma	tuberculoma *1. A tuberculous growth in the brain. 2. A mass that is produced from enlargement of a caseous tubercle.*
tuberculose	tuberculosis *Any infectious disease caused by Mycobacterium.*
tuberculoso	tuberculous *Referring to tuberculosis.*

Portuguese	English
tuberosidade	**tuberosity** *A protuberance. For instance the iliac tuberosity is a prominence on the surface of the ilium.*
tubérculo	**tubercle** *1. A granulomatous nodule produced by Mycobacterium tuberculosis. 2. A small prominence on a bone.*
tubo de teste; tubo de ensaio	**test tube** *A glass or plastic tube used to hold a medical specimen.*
tubo endotraqueal	**cuffed endotracheal tube** *A cannula that has an balloon on the tip that can be inflated with air and placed into the trachea.*
tubo faringotimpânico	**pharyngotympanic tube** *Synonym for eustachian tube.*
tubo intravenoso	**intravenous tubing** *The tubing used to administer fluids.*
tubo nasogástrico	**nasogastric tube** *A tube that is inserted into the nose with the distal tip in the stomach; it is used for irrigation or drainage of gastric contents.*
tubovariano	**tubo-ovarian** *Referring to the fallopian tube or ovary.*
tubular	**tubular** *Referring to a hollow, round-shaped organ.*
tularemia	**tularemia** *An infectious disease caused by Francisella tularensis. The symptoms range from mild constitutional complaints to septic shock.*
tumefação	**swelling** *An abnormal enlarged from fluid collection.*
tumefação	**tumefaction** *An area of swelling.*
tumefação abdominal	**swollen (distended) abdomen**
tumefação de calcâneo	**ankle swelling** *Enlargement of the ankle region with or without pitting.*
tumor glômico	**glomus tumor** *A reddish-blue painful papule that occurs on the distal aspects of the digits.*
tumor; neoplasia	**tumor** *A benign or malignant overgrowth of tissue.*
turbinectomia	**turbinectomy** *Surgical excision of a turbinate bone.*
turgor	**turgor** *Referring to the elasticity of skin. If one pinches skin and it remains in place the patient is dehydrated.*
túbulos seminífero	**seminiferous tubules** *Used for transport of semen.*
túnica	**tunica** *Generally a covering of a body part or organ. The tunica mucosa nasi is the mucous membrane lining the nasal cavity.*
túrgido	**turgid** *Congested and swollen.*
ulcerativo	**ulcerative** *Referring to ulceration.*
ultra-som	**ultrasound** *A sound or vibration of ultrasonic frequency.*
ultra-som transretal	**transrectal ultrasound** *Insertion of an ultrasound probe into the rectum to view adjacent structures.*
ultra-som transvaginal	**transvaginal ultrasound** *Insertion of an ultrasound probe in the vagina to view adjacent structures.*
ultra-sonografia	**ultrasonography** *Visualization of body structures with the echoes of ultrasound pulses.*
um dia sim	**every other day** *On alternate days.*
uma maca	**stretcher** *A device used to carry a patient in the supine position.*
umbigo	**navel** *Umbilicus.*
umbigo; ônfalo	**umbilicus** *The scar that denotes the end of the umbilical cord.*
umbilicado	**umbilicated** *Referring to depressed areas that resemble the umbilicus.*
umidade	**wet** *Covered in moisture.*
unciforme; osso hamato	**unciform** *Another term for hamate bone in the wrist.*
uncinaríase	**uncinariasis** *Hookworm infestation of genus Uncinaria.*
ungüento; pomada	**ointment** *A petroleum jelly based topical medication.*
unha	**fingernail** *Thin horny plate over the dorsal aspect of the end of finger.*

Portuguese	English
unha	**nail** *The hard surface on the dorsal surface of the toes or fingers.*
unha do dedo do pé	**toenail** *The nail at the tip/dorsal aspect of each toe.*
unha em bico de papagaio	**parrot-beak nail** *A curved fingernail.*
unha em colher	**spoon nail** *Also referred to as koilonychia, the nail is concave and is generally associated with anemia.*
unheiro	**hangnail** *A loose piece of skin attached near the medial or lateral nail fold.*
unicelular	**unicellular** *A term describing organisms like protozoans that only have cell.*
unidade motora	**motor unit** *The complex of one motor cell and its attached muscle fibers.*
unilateral	**unilateral** *One side only.*
uniovular; unioval	**uniovolar** *Referring to one fertilized ovum.*
urato	**urate** *The salt of uric acid.*
uremia	**uremia** *An excess of urea and creatinine in the blood.*
ureter	**ureter** *The conduit between each kidney and the urinary bladder.*
ureteral; uretérico	**ureteral** *Referring to one of two tubes from the kidneys to the bladder that carry urine.*
ureterectomia	**ureterectomy** *Surgical resection of one or both ureters.*
ureterite	**ureteritis** *Inflammation of the ureter.*
ureterocele	**ureterocele** *Protrusion of the distal portion of the ureter into the bladder.*
ureterolitotomia	**ureterolithotomy** *Removal of a ureteral stone.*
ureterovaginal	**ureterovaginal** *Referring to the ureter and vagina.*
ureterovesical	**ureterovesical** *Referring to the ureter and urinary bladder.*
ureterólito	**ureterolith** *Presence of a stone in the ureter.*
uretra	**urethra** *The canal connecting the urinary bladder with the outside of the body.*
uretral	**urethral** *Referring to the urethra.*
uretrite	**urethritis** *Inflammation of the urethra.*
uretrocele	**urethrocele** *A prolapse of the urethra through the meatus.*
uretrografia	**urethrography** *Imaging of the urethra after instillation of contrast media.*
uretroplastia	**urethroplasty** *Surgical repair of the urethra.*
uretroscópio	**urethroscope** *A scope used to visualize the inside of the urethra.*
uretrotomia	**urethrotomy** *A surgical opening of the urethra.*
uréia	**urea** *A nitrogenous product of protein metabolism; excreted in urine.*
urgência	**urgency** *Emergency or priority.*
urina	**urine** *The fluid concentrated by the kidneys and expelled via the urethra.*
urina residual	**residual urine** *The amount of urine remaining in the bladder after a person voids.*
urinálise	**urinalysis** *Chemical and microscopic examination of the urine.*
urinário	**urinary** *Referring to the urine.*
urine meio do fluxo	**midstream urine** *A specimen of urine that is collected after the initial stream of urine is initiated and before one finishes urinating.*
urinol	**urinal** *Device used by men to void while in bed or sitting.*
urinômetro	**urinometer** *A device for measuring urine specific gravity.*

Portuguese	English
urobilina	**urobilin** *A brownish pigment that is an oxidized form of urobilinogen.*
urobilinogênio	**urobilinogen** *A colorless substance produced in the intestines when bilirubin is reduced.*
urocromo	**urochrome** *A yellow pigment in the urine that gives urine its color.*
urodinâmica	**urodynamics** *A study done to determine whether a person has the contractile capacity in the bladder to void spontaneously.*
urogenital	**urogenital** *Referring to the urinary and genital systems.*
urografia	**urography** *Roentgenography of the urinary tract after administration of contrast media.*
urologia	**urology** *Surgical specialty involving medical and surgical treatment of the urogenital system.*
urólito	**urolith** *Urinary calculi.*
urticária	**urticaria** *A diffuse pruritic macular rash, caused by an allergy.*
usual	**usual** *Typical or normal.*
uterino	**uterine** *Referring to the uterus.*
uterovesical; vesicouterino	**uterovesical** *Referring to the uterus and urinary bladder.*
utrículo	**utricle** *A small sac. It can refer to a division of the membranous labyrinth.*
uveíte	**uveitis** *Inflammation of the uvea.*
uvulectomia	**uvulectomy** *Excision of the uvula.*
uvulite	**uvulitis** *Inflammation of the uvula.*
úlcera	**ulcer** *A concave wound caused by a break in the integrity of skin or mucous membrane. (duodenal ulcer)*
úlcera compressivo	**pressure ulcer** *Loss in skin integrity due to a portion of the body being in the same position for too long and possibly other factors.*
úlcera de decúbito	**decubitus ulcer** *A wound caused by laying in one position for too long; also referred to as a pressure ulcer.*
úlcera duodenal	**duodenal ulcer** *A defect in the lining of the first portion of the small bowel, typically caused by H. pylori.*
úlcera gastroduodenal	**gastroduodenal ulcer** *A lesion in the mucosal lining of the stomach or duodenum.*
úlcera oriental	**oriental sore** *A stigmata of cutaneous leishmaniasis caused by a bite from a sand fly.*
último prazo	**deadline** *Cutoff date.*
úmero	**humerus** *The long bone in the upper arm.*
úraco	**urachus** *A connection between the bladder and the allantois in the fetus.*
útero	**uterus** *The hollow organ in the female pelvis where a fertilized ovum embeds and grows.*
útero retroflexão	**retroflexed uterus** *Bending back of the uterus so that the top portion pushes against the rectum.*
úvula	**uvula** *A fleshy pendent at the back of the soft palate.*
vacina	**vaccine** *A solution of attenuated microorganisms given to prevent or treat a disease.*
vacinação	**vaccination** *The act of receiving a vaccine.*
vacúolo	**vacuole** *A cavity that develops in a cell.*
vagal	**vagal** *Referring to the vagus nerve.*
vagido	**vagitus** *An infant cry that can be further defined as vagitus vaginalis in which the infant cries while its head is in the vaginal canal.*
vagina	**vagina** *The canal in a female that extends from the vulva to the cervix.*

Portuguese	English
vaginal	**vaginal** *Referring to the vagina.*
vaginismo	**vaginismus** *Involuntary contraction of the vagina muscles that causes a painful spasm.*
vaginite tricomoníase	**trichomoniasis vaginitis** *Infection related to a species of Trichomonas.*
vagotomia	**vagotomy** *Incision of the vagus nerve.*
valgo	**valgus** *Refers to a joint being abnormally angulated away from the midline of the body.*
valina	**valine** *An essential amino acid that assists with nitrogen equilibrium.*
valva mitral	**mitral valve** *The valve with two cusps between the left atrium and ventricle.*
valva tricúspide	**tricuspid valve** *The cardiac valve located between the right atrium and right ventricle.*
valvotomia	**valvulotomy** *Surgical incision of a valve.*
variação terapêutica	**therapeutic range** *The highest to lowest value that will produce a desired effect.*
varicela	**varicella** *A virus that causes chickenpox and shingles. Also called herpes zoster.*
varicela; catapora	**chicken pox, varicella** *A viral disease characterized by extremely pruritus blisters over the entire body.*
varicocele	**varicocele** *A cluster of varicose veins in the scrotum.*
varicoso	**varicose** *Referring to an abnormally distended, irregular vein.*
variz	**varix** *A twisted, distended vein, artery or lymph vessel.*
varíola	**smallpox** *Variola.*
varíola bovina	**cowpox; vaccinia** *A viral disease of cows that was used for an original smallpox vaccine.*
vascular	**vascular** *Referring to a blood vessel.*
vasculite	**vasculitis** *Inflammation of a blood vessel.*
vasectomia	**vasectomy** *The surgical separation of each vas deferens with the intent of producing a sterile person.*
vaso cororário	**coronary vessel** *Referring to a coronary artery.*
vasoconstrição	**vasoconstriction** *The process of making the blood vessels smaller which increases blood pressure.*
vasodilitação	**vasodilatation** *The process of making the blood vessels larger which decreases blood pressure.*
vasoespasmo	**vasospasm** *The abrupt constriction of a blood vessel.*
vasomotor; angiocinético	**vasomotor** *Referring to the constriction or dilation of vessels.*
vasopressina	**vasopressin** *A hormone secreted by the pituitary that facilitates the retention of sodium and water and also increases blood pressure.*
vasovagal	**vasovagal** *Referring to overstimulation of the vagus nerve, exhibited by hypotension, pallor, nausea and diaphoresis.*
vazamento	**leakage** *Unintentional escape of gas or fluid.*
vazio	**empty** *Containing nothing.*
válvula aórtica	**aortic valve** *The valve situated between the left ventricle and the aorta.*
válvula ileocecal	**ileocecal valve** *The membranous folds between the ileum and cecum.*
vegetação	**vegetation** *Abnormal growth, such as cardiac valve vegetations as found in endocarditis.*
veia	**vein** *A vessel carrying blood back toward the heart.*
veia basílica	**basilic vein** *A vein in the hand that joins the brachial veins to form the axillary vein.*

Portuguese	English
veia cava	**vena cava** *The large vein that carries deoxygenated blood to the right atrium.*
vela	**candle** *A cylindrical piece of wax with a central wick.*
velhice	**old age** *A relative term for the period of advanced years.*
velocidade de sedimentação de hemácias	**blood sedimentation rate (ESR)** *The settling time of erythrocytes in a prepared sample. This is a measure of the abnormal concentration of substances that are associated with pathological states.*
veloz	**quiet** *Making little or no noise.*
veneno	**poison** *A substance that causes illness or death.*
veneno	**venom** *A term used to describe the toxin injected via a bite or sting.*
veno jugular	**jugular vein (s)** *Includes the internal, external and anterior jugular veins.*
venografia	**venography** *Roentgenography of a vein after administration of contrast media.*
venoso	**venous** *Referring to the veins.*
ventilação	**ventilation** *The movement of air into the lungs; generally meant to suggest by an artificial process.*
ventral	**ventral** *Referring to the underside but in humans, a ventral hernia, for example, refers to an abdominal hernia.*
ventriculografia	**ventriculography** *Roentgenography of the ventricles after administration of contrast media.*
ventriculostomia do terceiro ventrículo	**ventriculostomy** *A tube placed into the third ventricle to relieve increased intracranial pressure.*
ventrículo	**ventricle** *1. One of two chambers of the heart. 2. The four interconnected cavities in the center of the brain.*
verme	**worm** *Any of long, slender, legless, soft-bodied invertebrates.*
verme da Guiné	**guinea worm** *A parasitic nematode worm that, in cases of infection, lives under the skin, formally called Dracunculus medinensis.*
verme plano	**flatworm** *A class of worms that includes parasitic flukes and tapeworms.*
verminoso	**verminous** *Referring to presence of worms.*
verruga	**verruca** *A hyperplastic epidermal lesion, sometimes referred to as plantar wart.*
verruga	**wart** *A flesh colored growth that is also called verruca.*
verruga genital	**genital wart** *The common term for Condylomata acuminata.*
verruga plantar	**plantar wart** *A viral epidermal growth on the bottom of the foot.*
verruga venérea	**venereal wart** *Common term for condyloma acuminatum.*
vertical; em pé	**upright** *Vertical or standing.*
vertigem	**dizziness** *Sensation of losing one's balance.*
vertigem	**giddiness** *A tendency to fall or dizziness.*
vertigem	**vertigo** *A sensation of imbalance with many possible causes.*
vesical	**vesical** *Referring to the urinary bladder.*
vesicovaginal	**vesicovaginal** *Referring to the urinary bladder and vagina.*
vesiculite	**vesiculitis** *Inflammation of the urinary bladder.*
vesícula biliar	**gallbladder** *The organ adjacent to the liver that stores bile and secretes it into the duodenum.*
vesícula urinária	**bladder, urinary** *Vestibule for urine prior to being expelled via the urethra.*
vesícula urinária	**urinary bladder** *The organ collecting urine from the ureters prior to discharge via the urethra.*

Portuguese	English
vesícula; empola	**blister** *Common term for bulla.*
vespa	**wasp** *Any one of a winged hymenopterous insects.*
vestibular	**vestibular** *Referring to a vestibule.*
vestido estéril	**gown** *A sterile gown used during surgical procedures.*
vestigial	**vestigial** *Rudimentary.*
vetor	**vector** *An organism that transmits disease.*
vértebra	**vertebra** *A term for each bone surrounding the spine.*
vértice	**vertex** *The crown of the head.*
véu	**velum** *A veil-like part or covering of the palate; soft palate; Velum palatinum.*
vênula	**venula** *The vessels that connect the capillary plexuses to veins.*
vibração	**vibration** *An instance of oscillation of parts.*
vilo; vilosidade	**villus** *A small vascular prominence from a membrane surface.*
vilosidades coriônicas	**chorionic villus** *Cord-like projections of a fertilized ovum.*
viloso	**villous** *Covered with many villi.*
violeta de genciana	**gentian violet** *An antiseptic derived from rosaniline.*
virilha	**groin** *The genital region.*
virilização	**virilization** *The result of androgen; a process of development of masculine characteristics.*
virologia	**virology** *The study of viruses.*
virulência	**virulence** *The potential severity of a disease or poison.*
visão	**vision** *State of being able to see.*
visão em túnel	**tunnel vision** *Constriction in the visual field as though looking through a tube or hollow cylinder. Also called tubular vision.*
visão embaçado	**vision, blurred** *Haziness of the visual field.*
visão turva	**blurred vision** *Low visual acuity.*
visão; capacidade de ver	**eyesight** *A person's ability to see.*
visceral	**visceral** *Referring to the organs in the abdominal or thoracic cavity.*
viscosímetro	**viscometer** *A device used to measure viscosity.*
viscoso	**viscous** *Having a thick, sticky consistency.*
visível	**overt** *Not hidden.*
vitelino	**vitelline** *Referring to the yolk of an egg or ovum.*
vitiligo; leucodermia	**vitiligo** *The appearance of non-pigmented white patches on otherwise normal skin; hair is usually white in the affected areas.*
vivissecção	**vivisection** *Animal surgery done for purposes of research.*
vizinhança	**affinity** *To have a natural liking for.*
vírus da imunodeficiência humana	**HIV** *Abbreviation for human immunodeficiency virus.*
vírus da varíola do macaco	**monkeypox** *A viral disease that is similar to smallpox which occurs primarily in monkeys and rarely in humans.*
vírus do papiloma humano	**HPV human papillomavirus** *The virus that causes genital warts.*
vítreo	**vitreous** *Glass appearance; used to describe the vitreous body of the eye.*
viável	**viable** *Referring to a fetus that can survive childbirth.*
vocal	**vocal** *Referring to that which emanates from the vocal cords.*
volume corrente	**tidal volume** *The amount of air inspired with each breath. One can set a ventilator to deliver a preset number of milliliters of oxygenated air with each breath.*
volume de reserva expiratório	**expiratory reserve volume** *Amount of air left in the lung after a maximal exhalation, in liters.*

Portuguese	English
volume de reserva inspiratório	**inspiratory reserve volume** *The amount of air that can be inhaled after a normal inhalation.*
volume expiratório forçado (VRE)	**forced expiratory volume per second (FEV1)** *The amount of air exhaled with maximal effort, measured in liters, over one second.*
volume residual	**residual volume (RV)** *The amount of air left in the lung after a maximal exhalation.*
volume sangüíneo	**blood volume** *The amount of blood cells/plasma in the circulatory system.*
volume sistólico	**stroke volume** *The amount of blood ejected from the ventricle with each contraction.*
volumoso	**bulky** *Voluminous or substantial.*
voluntário	**volunteer** *A person who performs work without expecting compensation.*
vomitar	**vomit, to** *To expel gastric contents out the mouth.*
voz	**voice** *The sound produced through the larynx and out the mouth.*
vóvulo	**volvulus** *Twisting of the bowel leading to obstruction and sometimes perforation.*
vômito	**vomit** *The gastric contents that are expelled through the mouth.*
vômito cíclico	**cyclical vomiting** *Periods of recurrent vomiting with no apparent pathologic cause and the person has a normal state of health between the episodes.*
vômito em borra de café	**coffee-ground emesis** *Bloody vomitus with appearance of ground coffee.*
vômito seco	**retching** *Spasm of the stomach without presence of gastric material.*
vulvectomia	**vulvectomy** *Surgical resection of the vulva.*
vulvite	**vulvitis** *Inflammation of the vulva.*
vulvovaginite	**vulvovaginitis** *Inflammation of the vulva and vagina.*
xantina	**xanthine** *A purine derivative that is found in the blood and urine after the metabolism of nucleic acids to uric acid.*
xantocromia	**xanthochromia** *A yellow tone to the skin or spinal fluid.*
xantoma	**xanthoma** *A lipid deposition on the skin exhibited by an irregular yellow patch.*
xarope	**syrup** *A thick sweet liquid.*
xerodermia	**xerodermia** *A mild form of ichthyosis.*
xeroftalmia	**xerophthalmia** *A manifestation of Vitamin A deficiency exhibited by dryness of the cornea and conjunctiva.*
xerorradiografia	**xeroradiography** *A form of radiography using photoelectric cells.*
xerose	**xerosis** *Pathological dryness of the skin or mucous membranes.*
xerostomia	**xerostomia** *A dry mouth from salivary gland hypofunction.*
zero	**zero** *No quantity.*
zigoto	**zygote** *A fertilized ovum.*
zimogênio	**zymogen** *An inactive compound that is metabolized to an active state.*
zinco	**zinc** *A chemical with atomic number 30.*
zoologia	**zoology** *The study of animals.*
zoonose	**zoonosis** *An animal-born disease that can be transmitted to humans, such as rabies.*
zônula	**zonula** *A small zone or junction.*
zumbido; tinido	**ringing in the ears** *Common term for tinnitus.*

Other books by A.H. Zemback

English-Kinyarwanda-French Dictionary
English-Kinyarwanda Dictionary
English-Kirundi-French Dictionary
English-Kirundi Dictionary
English-Swahili-French Dictionary
English-Swahili Dictionary

English-French Medical Dictionary and Phrasebook
English-Spanish Medical Dictionary and Phrasebook
English-German Medical Dictionary and Phrasebook

Printed in Poland
by Amazon Fulfillment
Poland Sp. z o.o., Wrocław